Patrick Holford, BSc, DipION, FBANT, [...] spokesman on nutrition in the media, sp[...] mental health. He is the author of over 30 books, translated into over 20 languages and selling over a million copies worldwide, including *The Optimum Nutrition Bible*, *The Low-GL Diet Bible*, *Optimum Nutrition for the Mind* and *Ten Secrets of 100% Healthy People*.

Patrick started his academic career in the field of psychology. He then became a student of two of the leading pioneers in nutrition medicine and psychiatry – the late Dr Carl Pfeiffer and Dr Abram Hoffer. In 1984 he founded the Institute for Optimum Nutrition (ION), an independent educational charity, with his mentor, twice Nobel Prize-winner Dr Linus Pauling, as patron. ION has been researching and helping to define what it means to be optimally nourished for the past 25 years and is one of the most respected educational establishments for training nutritional therapists. At ION, Patrick was involved in groundbreaking research showing that multivitamins can increase children's IQ scores – the subject of a *Horizon* television documentary in the 1980s. He was one of the first promoters of the importance of zinc, antioxidants, high-dose vitamin C, essential fats, low-GL diets and homocysteine-lowering B vitamins and their importance in mental health and Alzheimer's disease prevention.

Patrick is Chief Executive Officer of the Food for the Brain Foundation and director of the Brain Bio Centre, the Foundation's treatment centre that specialises in helping those with mental issues, ranging from depression to schizophrenia. He is an honorary fellow of the British Association of Nutritional Therapy, as well as a member of the Complementary and Natural Healthcare Council. He is also Patron of the South African Association of Nutritional Therapy.

Other books by Patrick Holford

Balance Your Hormones

Beat Stress and Fatigue

Boost Your Immune System (with Jennifer Meek)

Burn Fat Fast (with Kate Staples)

Food GLorious Food (with Fiona McDonald Joyce)

Food is Better Medicine than Drugs (with Jerome Burne)

Hidden Food Allergies (with Dr James Braly)

How to Quit Without Feeling S**t (with David Miller and Dr James Braly)

Improve Your Digestion

Natural Highs (with Dr Hyla Cass)

Optimum Nutrition Before, During and After Pregnancy (with Susannah Lawson)

Optimum Nutrition for the Mind

Optimum Nutrition for Your Child (with Deborah Colson)

Optimum Nutrition Made Easy

Say No to Arthritis

Say No to Cancer (with Liz Efiong)

Say No to Heart Disease

Six Weeks to Superhealth

Smart Food for Smart Kids (with Fiona McDonald Joyce)

Solve Your Skin Problems (with Natalie Savona)

Ten Secrets of 100% Healthy People

Ten Secrets of Healthy Ageing (with Jerome Burne)

Ten Secrets of 100% Health Cookbook (with Fiona McDonald Joyce)

The Alzheimer's Prevention Plan (with Shane Heaton and Deborah Colson)

The Feel Good Factor

The Homocysteine Solution (with Dr James Braly)

The 9-Day Liver Detox (with Fiona McDonald Joyce)

The Low-GL Diet Cookbook (with Fiona McDonald Joyce)

The Low-GL Diet Counter

The Little Book of Optimum Nutrition

The Low-GL Diet Bible

The Optimum Nutrition Bible

The Optimum Nutrition Cookbook (with Judy Ridgway)

The Perfect Pregnancy Cookbook (with Fiona McDonald Joyce and Susannah Lawson)

500 Health and Nutrition Questions Answered

Foreign editions are listed at www.patrickholford.com/foreigneditions

patrick HOLFORD

GOOD Medicine

SAFE, NATURAL WAYS TO SOLVE OVER 75 COMMON HEALTH PROBLEMS

piatkus

PIATKUS

First published in Great Britain in 2014 by Piatkus

A CIP catalogue record for this book
is available from the British Library.

ISBN 978-0-7499-5919-7

Typeset in Calluna and The Sans by M Rules
Printed and bound by CPI Group (UK) Ltd, Croydon, CR0 4YY

Papers used by Piatkus are from well-managed forests
and other responsible sources.

MIX
Paper from
responsible sources
FSC® C104740

Piatkus
An imprint of
Little, Brown Book Group
100 Victoria Embankment
London EC4Y 0DY

An Hachette UK Company
www.hachette.co.uk

www.piatkus.co.uk

Acknowledgements

Producing a book like this is a marathon – writing about a disease a day for 75 days. I am deeply grateful to my wife, Gaby, for her support and encouragement, and to Tommy and Abdullah for taking such good care of me. Also, to Jo Muncaster, my super-efficient assistant, and to Emma Jamieson, Nina Omotoso and Stephanie Fox for their help in researching and writing.

I would also like to thank Jillian Stewart and Jan Cutler for their help with editing, and Tim Whiting at Piatkus for his support and encouragement to publish this book and to make it available to as many people as possible.

Contents

Guide to Abbreviations, Measures and References

Vitamins

1 gram (g) = 1,000 milligrams (mg) =
1,000,000 micrograms (mcg, also written as μg)

Most vitamins are measured in milligrams or micrograms. Vitamins A, D and E used to be measured in International Units (iu), a measurement designed to standardise the various forms of these vitamins, which have different potencies.

6mcg of beta-carotene, the vegetable precursor of vitamin A is, on average, converted into 1mcg of retinol, the animal form of vitamin A. So, 6mcg of beta-carotene is called 1mcgRE (RE stands for retinol equivalent). Throughout this book beta-carotene is referred to in mcgRE.

1mcg of retinol (1mcg RE) = 3.3iu of vitamin A
1mcg RE of beta-carotene = 6mcg of beta-carotene
100iu of vitamin D = 2.5mcg or 1mcg of vitamin D = 40iu
100iu of vitamin E = 67mg
1 pound (lb) = 16 ounces (oz)
2.2lb = 1 kilogram (kg)
1 pint = 0.6 litres
1.76 pints = 1 litre

In this book 'calories' means kilocalories (kcals).

Disclaimer

Although all the nutrients and dietary changes referred to in this book have been proven safe, those seeking help for specific medical conditions are advised to consult a qualified nutrition therapist, clinical nutritionist, doctor or equivalent health professional. The recommendations given in this book are solely intended as education and information, and should not be taken as medical advice. Neither the author nor the publisher accepts liability for readers who choose to self-prescribe. All supplements should be kept out of the reach of infants and children.

Introduction

Never a week goes by without someone asking me what they can do for this or that condition. Not everyone has the time or the inclination to read whole books on specific subjects, or attend workshops or see practitioners. After 30 years of clinical and research experience, and treating thousands of people, I thought it would be useful to have one resource that sets out what really works for the most common health problems we experience – not by suppressing symptoms, but by understanding why we get sick in the first place and dealing with the root causes.

This book is a guide to the most effective, safe and natural ways to help prevent and reverse many diseases. Use this book to restore your health and to help protect your body from ill health in the future. The recommendations that you will find are based on the principles of good medicine, defined as:

- It is proven to work – it prevents or helps reverse disease processes.

- It is good for your health, even if you are not sick.

- It conforms to your natural design and evolutionary principles.

- It does no harm.

The book covers over 75 of the most common health problems and gives you simple things that you can do to prevent or reverse your health condition. Each one is tried and tested and proven to work, both in clinical research and in practice with people like you. You'll also find case studies of people who applied many of these approaches and whose health improved.

Almost all the suggestions can be followed alongside other treatment approaches and I will indicate those that are not compatible or those that have contraindications.

Before we get started, it's good to have a general idea of why we get sick and why this natural approach makes so much sense.

Why do we become sick?

The vast majority of health conditions you are likely to suffer from in life, especially the chronic diseases, are primarily the result of too much 'bad stuff' and not enough 'good stuff'.

If we think of our health as a seesaw, we want to be balanced towards the good side of the seesaw: when we list to the left we have bad health; in the middle we have what I would call average–poor health; but to the right we have good health.

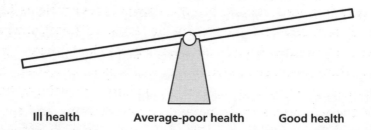

Ill health   Average-poor health   Good health

Too much of the bad stuff *and/or* not enough of the good stuff

When you repeatedly go for the 'bad stuff' – a poor diet based on refined foods, a lack of exercise, and/or taking pharmaceutical drugs to address ill health – your health 'seesaw' lists towards the bad side. Your body goes into an unhealthy 'inflammatory' state, and all kinds of body systems become out of balance.

The causes of disease

'When enough sins [against nature] have accumulated disease suddenly results.'

Hippocrates (c.460–c.377BC)

More than 2,000 years ago, the visionary and founder of medicine, Hippocrates, saw clearly that there is a cause, or a combination of causes, for every disease, and he set out to discover them. It is amazing how much of what he said still applies today, even though he had none of the diagnostic tools and insight from decades of research that we now have to draw on. In his day, the convention was that diseases were caused by 'the gods' and sacrifices had to be made. He didn't believe this. Ironically, today's equivalent excuses for diseases are that they are all in the genes and you have to take drugs to 'manage' the disease or even to prevent it occurring in the first place. I don't believe that either in most cases, although there is sometimes a role for drugs in acute situations.

Diseases are not caused by a deficiency of drugs

Your pain, your cancer, your indigestion, acid reflux, low mood, anxiety, insomnia, asthma, eczema, angina, sinus problems, high blood pressure, high cholesterol (which is not a disease), or whatever it is you suffer from, is not caused by a lack of drugs.

In truth, so-called modern medicine has been hijacked by the pharmaceutical industry and many doctors, unwittingly, have lost the real art of medicine and communication, and spend much of their time simply dispensing drugs. Some spend more time looking at their computer than looking at you! We have now reached the crazy position where people who are not sick are being prescribed drugs at vast expense to the taxpayer, only to suffer significant side effects as a result.

What is more, in the US, medical intervention has become the fourth leading cause of death. If we had accurate figures for all countries, the same may be true where you live. Thousands of people die from medical drugs, and hundreds of thousands, if not millions, experience adverse side effects. Here is just one example: taking statins to lower your cholesterol increases your risk of diabetes by up to 25 per cent, and creates memory problems and muscle aches, but it does very little to reduce your risk of heart disease if you didn't have it in the first place. The vast majority of drugs intended for long-term use and 'management' of chronic conditions don't pass the first law of good medicine, which is: first do no harm.

First do no harm

This law was another of Hippocrates' fundamental principles. At one time, when a doctor became qualified he or she would swear this oath, but that's no longer required in most medical schools in the UK. Meanwhile, 86 per cent of deaths in the EU are from chronic diseases. Seventy to eighty per cent of so-called 'healthcare' costs (which are mainly drugs) are spent on chronic diseases – no less than €700 billion in the EU. But the problem with drug-based medicine is that it can, and does, do harm.

Today, assessments of drugs report the 'numbers needed to treat for benefit' (NNTB) and also the 'numbers needed to treat for harm' (NNTH), referring to the number of people who will have adverse reactions when taking the drugs. To explain this, if the NNTB is four this means that if four people take the treatment one person will benefit. If the NNTH is eight this means that one out of eight people will be harmed. In this example, for every two people that are helped by taking the drug, one person will be harmed. Those aren't good odds, so these are the odds you ought to know from your doctor when he or she prescribes you a drug.

The vast majority of the recommendations in this book have no NNTH that I'm aware of – no risk of harm or adverse reaction in the doses recommended. In the few where I know of one, I will let you know. I will also indicate if you need to lower the dose of some nutrients as you get better, because you won't be needing so much. That's another sign of good medicine: it actually reverses the disease so that you no longer need to take the medicine. If you've been told you will be on a drug 'for life', that means the process of taking the treatment does not 'cure' the disease, it just suppresses it.

Prevention is much better than cure

Less than 3 per cent of healthcare costs are spent on real prevention, on tackling the actual contributors, the 'sins against our natural design', that lie behind disease.

These include poor diet, a lack of exercise, stress, poor posture, smoking and drinking, pollution, lack of sunlight, insufficient sleep, and a lack of love and fun. Once your seesaw of health is tilted towards disease, however, simply addressing those problems – and that's no mean feat – would be unlikely to eradicate all your health issues. It would almost certainly help, but you would need a great deal more of the good stuff and virtually none of the bad stuff to rebalance your health and to undo the damage. Once you have regained your health you no longer need to be so extreme – you will find that a healthy diet and lifestyle and just a few supplements will maintain your good health.

When enough blessings from nature have accumulated, health returns

This is a simple principle that most dieticians and doctors don't seem to grasp. When your system is sick, you need much more nutrients to restore health. To give you an example, I supplement 2,000mg of vitamin C a day – that's equivalent to about 40 supermarket oranges. It sounds like a lot, but it's what gorillas are given in London Zoo. Why? Because that's what we, and they, would achieve in the way of vitamin C when living in a tropical jungle and eating fresh foods – that's what keeps you healthy. It's consistent with our evolutionary design. If I have the first sign of a cold, I take 1,000mg of vitamin C an hour until I am well.

That's because having a very high blood vitamin C level knocks just about any virus on the head.

I aim to eat a red onion every day, I often eat olives and I use turmeric liberally on my food. This is all good for health, and I'll be discussing why later in the book. If I had arthritis, however, I would supplement a concentrate of curcumin (at least 500mg), which is the active ingredient in turmeric, plus quercetin, the active ingredient in red onions, and oleocanthal, the active ingredient in olives. I'd be taking, for example, 500mg of quercetin a day, because it works as a natural painkiller. An onion contains 20mg of quercetin, so that supplement is equivalent to 25 onions! (I'll show you exactly what to do in the Arthritis section.)

I also supplement 30mcg a day of the essential mineral chromium and avoid refined foods, which have up to 98 per cent of their chromium content removed. My whole-food diet guarantees me a further 30mcg, making 60mcg in total. That helps to keep me healthy. If I had diabetes, however, I would supplement 600mcg of chromium – ten times this amount – because it helps. (I'll show you exactly what to do in the Diabetes section.) Chromium restores insulin sensitivity and stabilises blood sugar levels, and this is assisted by eating a diet that has a low glycemic load (a low-GL diet) designed to keep your blood sugar level even. The diet also helps to remove sugar cravings, which, together with stabilising blood sugar, is essential for treating diabetes.

Nature has provided us with nutrients that, in concentrated amounts, restore function when you are dysfunctional. In other words, you can use concentrated amounts of nature's nutrients to push your health towards the right-hand (good) side of the seesaw if you become sick.

As well as having more of the nutrients, you need fewer of the anti-nutrients (which are, for example, a poor diet, a lack of exercise or too much stress). I prefer to call these 'adaptogens' and 'anti-adaptogens', however, because some of the approaches you will find in this book that help you adapt back to health are not truly nutrients. A nutrient is defined as something you can't live without. You can live without turmeric, for example, so it's not an essential nutrient, but it does help you to stay healthy. If the C2/C3 vertebrae in your neck are out of alignment, an osteopath or chiropractor can get them back into alignment and this might stop your headaches. That treatment is an 'adaptogen', but it's not a nutrient. Staying up until three o'clock in the morning, never getting outdoors for your daily sun exposure (which makes essential vitamin D in your body) and drinking endless cups of coffee are 'anti-adaptogens', because they work against your natural design and they eventually rob you of your health.

The causes of most diseases are many

We all know the saying that it's the last straw that breaks the camel's back. We recognise the last straw as something we feel we can definitely pinpoint as the cause of illness: stress or eating badly, or drinking too much, or an accident we had or the bust-up with our partner that caused the headaches/arthritis/asthma or whatever. The truth is that most diseases happen only when you've lost your resilience – you've pushed that seesaw too far to the left – as a result of many years of accumulated bad health habits. The trick to restoring health is to push the seesaw the other way, giving it larger quantities of the positive adaptogens to compensate for the anti-adaptogens that affected our health in the past.

For each disease I'll show you the main factors that increase your risk, as well as the main factors that decrease your risk, so that you know what to focus on changing.

The good medicine solutions I give in the book restore function where there was dysfunction. Some people have called this science of restoring function 'functional medicine'; others call it 'orthomolecular medicine', but in the 1980s I called it 'optimum nutrition', although we are all talking about the same thing. When you increase your health reserve through good medicine, your body will have resilience, so that the slightest 'insult' or period of unavoidable stress will not tip you into ill health once again.

Trust evolution and your natural design

The design of your body is utterly remarkable; it has been shaped by millions of years of evolution. Our fastest computers are nowhere near as complex as the brain, for example.

Would you rather restore your health by conforming to your body's natural design or gamble on taking a hi-tech drug that has been designed to block some part of your body's natural chemistry – for example, stopping you from making cholesterol or stomach acid? If the former, you are reading the right book. If the latter, good luck! But why not hedge your bets and follow the advice in this book as well?

Some doctors say that you don't need your appendix, or your tonsils or adenoids; they just become inflamed and infected, so why not take them out? If a person is getting, for example, repeated tonsillitis, however, that means they are reacting to something, which is often an unidentified food allergy, with dairy products being a common candidate. People are also removing their breasts or prostate to prevent cancer, when the biggest driver of cancer is what you eat and how you live, not the genes you inherit.

The reason people suffer with problems such as tonsillitis is because they are not living in a way that is consistent with how the body is designed. You are not designed to drink lots of milk as an adult, but an allergy to milk is a major cause of tonsillitis and it also increases the risk of breast and prostate cancer. (No wild animal, for example, consumes milk as an adult.) You are not meant to be eating refined, fibreless foods, and this is a major cause of appendicitis. You have to enquire into the fundamental causes of your diseases if you want to solve them. Real freedom, health and happiness come from conforming to your natural design, not trying to cheat it.

Drugs are not, by their very nature, part of the body's natural design. Of course, there is a role for short-term medication such as antibiotics, and life-saving operations, but this should be a small part of medicine, not the mainstay. If you've been told you need to be on long-term medication, that means there is something you are doing that is against your body's natural design.

Good medicine is based on scientific evidence

I believe in good science, and you'll find that every remedy and recommendation made in this book is based on good science. It is proven and works. Every recommendation has been tried and tested by the clients of thousands of nutritional therapists who have trained with me at the Institute for Optimum Nutrition. If you would like to work with a registered nutritional therapist to solve your health issue I'll show you how to find one in your area (see Resources).

The goal now is to get you started doing the right things – and not doing the wrong things – that will help to tilt that seesaw of health to the right, towards good health.

It will mean some changes, and change is always difficult at the beginning. Even a simple action that you always do in one way will take time to change to another way; for example, if I ask you to cross your arms, and then to try crossing your arms the other way round, you'll probably find that it feels quite strange. If you did this every day, however, it would soon feel normal. It takes three weeks to break a habit, six weeks to make a new habit, and 36 weeks to hard-wire a habit, but if you carry on as you were you can't expect to see improvement. With this book, you will find that creating good habits will bring you the kind of results that will make lifestyle changes something that you welcome, as you will be able to reap positive rewards.

How to use this book

Part 1 of the book is arranged in alphabetical order by condition. Find the main condition you want to resolve. You will see that each condition has the following sections:

- **Good medicine solutions** Each one explains how the suggestion works and what you need to do.

- **Best foods/worst foods** shows you which foods to increase in your diet and which ones to minimise or avoid completely.

- **Best supplements** An example supplement programme.

Some conditions also include the following:

- **I used to have . . .** This gives you a real-life case story to inspire you.

- **Cautions** If there's a drug that interferes with a recommended remedy, or anything else you need to be cautious about, such as lowering the dose of a nutrient once you get better, I will let you know here.

- **Dig deeper** The title of a book or a website to visit if you want to find out more. (Key study sources are also given in the References at the back of the book for those who want to examine the evidence for themselves.)

Read each of the good medicine solutions. Then ask yourself which of these you would find easiest to do, and which of these you would find hardest. Often, the hardest ones make the most difference, especially if they are a big part of the reason you developed the health problem in the first place. You have to be honest with yourself about this.

Now pick at least three that you will commit to doing for six weeks. Check that these are really doable. What are your odds of success? You want to be close to 100 per cent. Organise yourself so that you have everything you need to get started. Make an agreement with yourself to start on a particular day. Stick your action plan on your fridge. Share this with at least two other people and ask them to ask you how you are doing in six weeks' time.

Part 2 also gives you concrete advice to support some of the solutions; for example, if the solution is to follow a low-GL diet, or increase your antioxidants, or check and lower your homocysteine level with B vitamins, how do you do this? The relevant chapter in Part 2 shows you how.

On my website (see Resources) there are a number of support services to help keep you on track, motivated and informed. You can: ask questions on my blogs about your health issues; read articles about your specific health issues; keep informed on new research findings; discover what has or hasn't worked for others; share your own successes; receive your own personal 100% Health Programme, based on my online 100% Health Questionnaire; and find a nutritional therapist to guide you back to health.

You are designed to be healthy, and if you start applying the principles of good medicine, you will soon be on the road to good health. This does require some discipline to start with, to make new behaviours, but in six weeks those new ways of living will become your new habits.

There are lots of commercial interests enticing you to eat bad foods, drink too much of the wrong things and take prescription drugs. Your mind often tricks you into being lazy, to take the route of immediate gratification, and to keep doing the things that made you sick in the first place, but you have to take control of your own life. Only you – not your doctor nor I – have the power to transform your health. You have the power to get yourself back to good health.

I wish you the courage and perseverance to change, and the best of health and happiness as a consequence.

Patrick Holford

PART 1

The A–Z of Common Diseases

What should you do to support your recovery when you have any of the 76 most common diseases? In this part of the book I give you up to six actions that you can take both to help you address the underlying cause of a health problem and to enhance your body's ability to fight off disease and return to a state of health.

In many cases this involves cleaning up your diet, making simple lifestyle changes and taking high potencies of nutrients or herbs. It takes much larger amounts of nutrients to reverse a disease process than it does to maintain a healthy equilibrium, so these added extras will become unnecessary once you are well.

ACNE

Good medicine solutions

1. Avoid dairy products for a trial period

A number of trials have shown a clear link between dairy product intake and acne.[1] Some people are unknowingly allergic or intolerant to milk, but nevertheless milk promotes a hormone called insulin-like growth factor (IGF-1) in all of us and possibly also oestrogens. IGF-1 levels peak in teenage years, doubly so if you consume a lot of dairy products, and may be a factor in acne if they become too high.

Oestrogen dominance is also a common cause of acne in adult females. A diet high in meat and milk can contribute to oestrogen dominance in both men and women. Being overweight has the same effect, because fat cells, whether in meat, or you because of excess weight, make oestrogenic hormones. I recommend a trial period when you avoid dairy products for up to two weeks, as well as reducing meat in favour of fish and vegetarian sources of protein, to help identify if milk and meat are contributory factors for you. Only total avoidance can produce a result if you are allergic.

A high-fat diet, especially if you eat damaged fats in processed and fried foods, may also contribute to acne, so reducing meat and dairy products also tends to lessen fats.

Eat more beans and greens. Greens, especially broccoli, contain compounds called indole-3-carbinol (I3C) and di-indolylmethane (DIM), which help the liver to break down excess circulating oestrogens. I3C or DIM can also be supplemented if dietary changes don't do the trick. These are more relevant to women than men, because women have higher oestrogen levels. Also, beans and lentils contain phytoestrogens that lock onto oestrogen hormone receptors but don't send a 'growth' signal. In this way they lessen the oestrogen load, which might help if oestrogen dominance is contributing to your skin condition.

Oestrogen is counteracted by progesterone. Progesterone is produced only during a cycle in which ovulation (the release of an egg) occurs. Some women have anovulatory cycles, which lead to relative oestrogen dominance. If your skin is worse at certain times of the month, or even every other month, this is a possibility. A nutritional therapist can arrange a salivary hormone test to see if your hormones are in balance, and advise you what to do if not.

2. Cut right back on sugar

High-sugar and high-glycemic load (GL) diets (explained in Chapter 1, Part 2) are strongly linked to bad skin. Too much sugar or fast-releasing carbohydrates in white bread, cereals, white rice, pastries, sweets and sugared drinks, as well as too much fruit juice, creates spikes in your blood sugar level. This, in turn, causes the release of the hormone insulin, which promotes sebum production. The increased circulating sugar can also feed infections in the skin.

Cut right back on sugar and always choose low-GL foods, such as wholegrain pasta or brown rice instead of white. This, plus eating protein with carbohydrates, are immediate ways to lower the GL of your diet. Eating fish with brown rice, or an apple with some almonds, will help to keep your blood sugar level even. This not only helps your skin in the short term but it also helps weight loss, reducing the fat cells that increase oestrogen load.

See Chapter 1, Part 2 for details on how to follow a low-GL diet. Meanwhile, avoid all sugar, and foods or drinks containing added sugar.

3. Increase your intake of zinc

The need for zinc is especially high during the teenage years, because it is involved in growth and sexual maturation, but most people consume only about half the basic amount needed of 15mg a day.

A number of topical treatments including zinc have proven effective against acne. It is certainly worth making sure you are taking in at least 15mg, and preferably 20mg, a day, especially if you are a teenager. A good-quality multivitamin–mineral should provide 10mg, which is enough if your diet is rich in fish, eggs, lean meat, nuts, seeds, beans and lentils. (Any seed that you can plant in the ground has to be quite rich in zinc, because plants cannot grow without it, which is why seeds, beans and lentils are good choices.)

Zinc, especially combined with vitamin C, is an antimicrobial agent that helps to kill infections in the skin. A good supplement programme should include both zinc and at least 1,000mg of vitamin C. Some skin creams also contain zinc, which can act locally. The use of zinc ascorbate, which combines both zinc and vitamin C (ascorbate), would be particularly effective.

The conventional approach to clear acne includes using anti-microbial skin cleansers and antibiotics. Although effective, the latter is quite a drastic approach and it fails to address the key question as to why a person is getting spots. Acne spots are usually caused by excessive sebum (oil) production in the skin, which oxidises, creating a sealed pore in which infection can develop. Although the antibiotics may work in the short term, they wipe out healthy bacteria in the gut, which is a primary means by which the gut is protected. Their use should therefore be a last resort.

Localised cleansing with an antimicrobial cleanser helps to break down the obstructions stopping normal sebum drainage and reduces skin infections.

4. Use vitamin A- and C-based skin creams

Among the most commonly prescribed treatments for acne are retinoids, which are vitamin A-like drugs, sufficiently differ-ent from natural retinol, and hence patentable. Many of these retinoids are also considerably more toxic than natural vitamin A and hence there is a need for real caution regarding their use, especially in pregnancy. Retinoids are often given in capsule form, one of the most commonly prescribed being isotretinoin, but increasingly common is the use of skin gels and creams containing retinoids. The reason they are thought to work is by decreasing the production of sebum.

The natural alternative is to use creams or gels that contain natural retinol, which comes in various forms, such as retinyl palmitate and retinyl acetate, that can penetrate the skin. These are also highly effective. Some skin-care products also contain vitamin C as ascorbyl palmitate, although ascorbyl tetraiso-palmitate is more absorbent. These are extremely effective. Vitamin A creams also help to prevent flaky skin blocking the drainage of sebum.

The issue with vitamin A creams is that if they are too concentrated they can irritate the skin. By increasing the amount of vitamin A gradually, the skin produces more receptors for vitamin A. For this reason, it is best to find skin creams, such as Environ, that contain graded amounts of vitamin A and, ideally, be guided by a skin-care therapist or dermatologist.

Vitamin A can also be supplemented internally. It is far less toxic than the synthetic retinoids, and although the general advice is not to exceed 3,000mcg (10,000iu) in pregnancy, I have seen no convincing evidence that this is necessary. However, for the sake of caution, do not exceed 3,000mcg (10,000iu) if you are a woman of child-bearing age. If you are male or extremely unlikely to get pregnant, I recommend 3,000mcg twice a day for at least a month to help reduce sebum production. A good multivitamin should provide at least 1,500mcg (5,000iu) so you'll need to supplement extra vitamin A, which is available in small capsules.

Vitamin C, at an intake of at least 1,000mg, taking either 500mg or 1,000mg twice a day, often helps reduce acne for reasons that are not completely clear. It may prevent the oxidation of sebum and oils in the skin, or act as a natural antibiotic.

Best foods

- Vegetables – raw or steamed
- Fruit – berries, cherries, plums, apples, pears
- Fish
- Raw nuts and seeds
- Beans and lentils (pulses)
- Water – drink the equivalent of eight glasses a day, including hot drinks

Worst foods

- Sugar
- Refined 'white' foods
- High-fat foods, such as meat and cheese, especially processed or fried food
- Milk, cheese, cream and other dairy products
- Meat

Best supplements

- 2 × high-potency multivitamin–minerals providing 10mg of zinc, 1,500mcg (3,000iu) of retinol vitamin A, plus B vitamins, vitamin C, selenium

- 2 × vitamin C 1,000mg

- 1 × zinc 10mg (making 20mg in total, including the zinc in the multivitamin)

- 2 × vitamin A (retinol) 5,000iu. If you are pregnant and taking a multivitamin–mineral with 5,000iu, then take only 1 extra vitamin A 5,000iu. Otherwise 5,000iu (1, 500mcg) × 3 is fine, giving 15,000iu in total.

CAUTIONS

- Limit your intake of vitamin A to 3,000mcg (10,000iu) if pregnant.
- Increase the dose of vitamin A in skin creams gradually to avoid irritation, as advised by a skin-care therapist.
- If you have had a course of antibiotics, always follow with two weeks of probiotics, which are beneficial bacteria (*Lactobacillus acidophilus* and bifidobacteria) in order to recolonise the gut.

DIG DEEPER

To find out more on this subject, read *Solve Your Skin Problems* (Patrick Holford and Natalie Savona), which includes key referenced studies.

ADHD AND HYPERACTIVITY

General information

It is common for children with attention deficit hyperactivity disorder (ADHD) to have three basic problems: they can't pay attention, they are hyperactive, and they act on impulse. It can, however, be difficult to draw the line between the behaviour of a child that is within the normal limits of high energy and abnormally active behaviour. You can use a free online hyperactivity/ADHD check at Food for the Brain (see Resources) to help you decide whether your child is hyperactive.

Good medicine solutions

1. Avoid sugar and refined carbohydrates

Dietary studies consistently reveal that hyperactive children eat more sugar than other children, and reducing sugar has been found to halve disciplinary actions in young offenders. Other research has confirmed that the problem is not sugar itself but the forms it comes in, the absence of a well-balanced diet overall and abnormal glucose metabolism. A study of 265 hyperactive children found that more than three-quarters of them displayed abnormal glucose tolerance; that is, their bodies were less able to handle sugar intake and maintain balanced blood sugar levels.

In any case, when a child is regularly snacking on refined carbohydrates, sweets, chocolate, fizzy drinks, juices and little or no fibre to slow the glucose absorption, the levels of glucose in their blood will seesaw continually and trigger wild fluctuations in their levels of activity, concentration, focus and behaviour. These, of course, are also the symptoms of ADHD.

The advice is, therefore, to remove from the diet all forms of refined sugar and any foods that contain it, replacing them with frequent consumption of whole foods and complex carbohydrates (brown rice and other whole grains, oats, lentils, beans, quinoa and vegetables) throughout the day. The fibre in these foods helps to slow-release sugars. Carbohydrates should always be balanced with protein to improve glucose balance; for example, eat nuts with fruit or fish with rice. Also, avoid stimulants, such as caffeinated drinks, and even apparently 'natural' ones, such as guarana, which is a stimulant similar to caffeine. In essence, this means following a low-GL diet, as explained in Chapter 1, Part 2.

Supplementing 200mcg of chromium also helps to stabilise blood sugar, this dose is appropriate for children aged over 10, with half this dose for younger children.

2. Increase your omega-3 intake

The omega-3 essential fats have a calming effect on many children with hyperactivity and ADHD. Many children with ADHD/hyperactivity have visible symptoms of essential-fat deficiency, such as excessive thirst, dry skin, eczema and asthma.

It is also interesting that boys, whose requirement for essential fats is much higher than girls', are also much more likely to have ADHD. Researchers have theorised that ADHD children may be deficient in essential fats for two reasons: their dietary intake from foods such as fish, seeds and nuts is inadequate (although this is not uncommon); and their need is higher, their absorption is poor, or they are less efficient at converting these fats from nuts and seeds, for example, into the more biologically active fats that are found in oily fish – namely docosahexaenoic acid (DHA). Also, they are less able to convert DHA into prostaglandins, which then affect brain function.

The conversion of essential fats can be inhibited by most of the foods that cause symptoms in children with ADHD, such as wheat, dairy and foods containing salicylates (discussed below). This conversion is also hindered by deficiencies of the various vitamins and minerals that help the enzymes driving those conversions: vitamins B_3 (niacin), B_6, C, biotin, zinc and magnesium. Zinc deficiency is common in children with ADHD.

Research carried out at Purdue University in the US confirmed that children with ADHD have an inadequate intake of the nutrients required for the conversion of essential fats into prostaglandins, and have lower levels of eicosapentaenoic acid (EPA), DHA and arachidonic acid (AA) – a brain-essential omega-6 fat – than children without ADHD. Supplementation with all these omega-3 essential fats, pre-converted, along with the omega-6 essential fat gamma-linolenic acid (GLA), has been shown to reduce ADHD symptoms, such as anxiety, attention difficulties and general behaviour problems. A UK trial using omega-3 and omega-6 fish oil supplements has proven the value of these essential fats in a double-blind trial involving 41 children aged 8–12 years who had ADHD symptoms and specific learning difficulties. Those children receiving extra essential fats in supplements were both behaving and learning better within 12 weeks.[1]

To ensure adequate essential fats in the diet, eat fish at least twice a week, seeds on most days and supplement omega-3 fish oils. Look for a supplement that contains EPA, DHA and GLA.

The best fish for EPA, the type of omega-3 fat that's been most thoroughly researched are, per 100g (3½oz) portion: mackerel (1,400mg), herring/kipper (1,000mg), sardines (1,000mg), fresh (not tinned) tuna (900mg), anchovies (900mg), salmon (800mg) and trout (500mg). Tuna, being high in mercury, is best eaten no more than twice a month. Although small tuna pose less of a risk – Indian Ocean yellow fin has less mercury, for example – it is hard to know where the tuna you buy is sourced.

The best seeds to eat that contain omega-6 and omega-3 fats are chia, flax and pumpkin seeds. Flax seeds are so small that they are best ground and sprinkled on cereal. Chia seeds do not need grinding, as the outer husk dissolves on contact with liquid. Alternatively, use flaxseed oil; for example, in salad dressings. Although technically providing omega-3, only about 5 per cent of the type of omega-3 (alpha linolenic acid – ALA) contained in these seeds is converted in your body into EPA, so fish sources are preferable.

3. Check for and remove potential allergens

Of all the avenues so far explored, the link between hyperactivity and food sensitivity is the most established and worthy of pursuit in any child showing signs of ADHD. Food allergies can be of two types: type 1 is the classical, severe and immediate allergy, most commonly associated with peanuts and shellfish. This allergy involves an antibody called IgE, and most people discover if they have this type of allergy early in life, since the reaction is so immediate and severe. The second type involves the IgG antibody, which works in quite a different way. Symptoms of these allergies can be many and varied, and may take many hours to appear. These allergies often go undetected for this reason. (See Allergies on page 31.)

One survey from the US found that hyperactive children are seven times more likely to have food allergies than other children. A separate investigation by the Hyperactive Children's Support Group found that 89 per cent of children with ADHD reacted to food colourings, 72 per cent to flavourings, 60 per cent to monosodium glutamate (MSG), 45 per cent to all synthetic additives, 50 per cent to cow's milk, 60 per cent to chocolate and 40 per cent to oranges.

Other substances often found to induce behavioural changes are wheat, corn, yeast, soya, peanuts and eggs. Symptoms strongly linked to allergy include nasal problems and excessive mucus, ear infections, facial swelling and discolouration around the eyes, tonsillitis, digestive problems, bad breath, eczema, asthma, headaches and bedwetting.

A considerable number of hyperactive children may benefit from eliminating foods that contain artificial colourings, flavours and preservatives; processed and manufactured foods; and 'culprit' foods identified by either an exclusion diet or blood test for allergies or intolerances. Some parents have also reported success with the Feingold diet, by removing not only all artificial additives but also foods that naturally contain compounds called salicylates.

Researchers at the University of Sydney in Australia found that three-quarters of 86 children with ADHD reacted adversely to foods containing salicylates. These include prunes, raisins, raspberries, almonds, apricots, canned cherries, blackcurrants, oranges, strawberries, grapes, tomato sauce, plums, cucumbers and apples. As the list of foods containing salicylates is very long and contains many otherwise nutritious foods, cutting them all out should be considered only as a secondary course of action, and must be carefully planned and monitored by a nutritional therapist.

Understanding how a low-salicylate diet helps hyperactive

children does offer a useful alternative to such a drastic course of action. Salicylates inhibit the conversion and utilisation of essential fats, which are often low in hyperactive children. Instead of avoiding salicylates, it may help simply to increase the supply of essential fats.

4. Increase vitamins and minerals

Although it is unlikely, on the basis of the studies to date, that ADHD is purely a deficiency disease, most children with this diagnosis are deficient in certain key nutrients, and do respond very well to taking more vitamins and minerals.

Zinc and magnesium are the most commonly deficient nutrients in people with ADHD. In fact, symptoms of deficiency in these minerals are very similar to the symptoms of ADHD. Low levels of magnesium, for example, can cause excessive fidgeting, anxious restlessness, insomnia, coordination problems and learning difficulties (if accompanied by a normal IQ).

Polish researchers studying levels of magnesium in 116 children with ADHD found that 95 per cent of them were deficient – a much higher percentage than that among healthy children. The team also noted a correlation between levels of magnesium and severity of symptoms. Supplementing 200mg of magnesium has been shown to reduce hyperactivity in children with ADHD.

Dr Neil Ward of the University of Surrey has made a discovery that could explain the link between ADHD and such deficiencies. In a study of 530 hyperactive children, Ward found that, compared to children without ADHD, a significantly higher percentage of children with the condition had had several courses of antibiotics in early childhood,[2] and further investigations revealed that these children had lower levels of various essential minerals. It is possible that antibiotics have a disruptive effect on beneficial gut flora and consequently on overall digestive health, impairing absorption.

'I used to have . . . '

Eight-year-old Richard was diagnosed with ADHD. He was 'out of control' and his parents were at their wits' end. Through bio-chemical testing at the Brain Bio Centre, near London, it was found that he was allergic to dairy products and eggs and was very deficient in magnesium. Dietary analysis revealed that he consumed excessive amounts of sugar every day. The Centre recommended cutting down his sugar intake significantly, cutting out dairy and egg products and supplementing magnesium and omega-3 essential fats. Within three months, his parents reported that Richard had calmed down considerably and had become much more manageable.

Best foods

- Whole foods, such as beans and lentils (pulses)
- Oats (helps keep blood sugar level even)
- Vegetables
- Fruit – apples, pears and berries
- Oily fish (salmon, mackerel, herring, kippers, sardines)

Worst foods

- Sugar
- Caffeinated drinks
- Refined carbohydrates (white bread, cereal, pasta, rice)
- Bananas, grapes, raisins (these are especially high in sugar)

Best supplements

- 1–2 × high-potency multivitamin–minerals, dose dependent on age of child (follow the dosage guidelines on the product) but check that it has at least 5mg zinc, 100mg of magnesium and B vitamins

- 1–2 × essential omegas with fish-oil-derived omega-3 (EPA, DHA), plus omega-6 (GLA) from borage or evening primrose oil, providing at least 500mg of EPA, DHA and GLA combined

Optional

- Extra zinc up to 15mg a day for teenagers
- Extra magnesium up to 300mg a day for teenagers
- (Halve these doses for much younger children from ages 4 to 10 years.)

DIG DEEPER

To find out more on this subject, read *Attention-Deficit Hyperactivity Disorder* (Basant Puri). Food for the Brain and the Brain Bio Centre, near London, specialise in the nutritional treatment of ADHD and related conditions – see Resources.

ALCOHOL DEPENDENCE/CRAVINGS

General information

Alcohol switches off adrenalin, making drinking an attractive way to chill out. The problem is that the more you drink the more you need for an effect. After a while, it gets hard to switch off without having a drink, and many people start to become somewhat dependent on alcohol. If you are having an alcoholic drink every day, and you have been doing this for months or years, or if you crave a drink if you haven't had one, you may have developed a level of dependency. You can break this by having a break from drinking, and taking steps to rebalance your brain and body. If, however, you're beyond this point, and would suffer considerable withdrawal effects if you stopped alcohol, or if you don't even believe you would be able to stop, you may have developed an addiction, in which case it is important to seek professional help.

Good medicine solutions

1. Follow a low-GL diet

Regular alcohol consumption disrupts your blood sugar control, so the way to help alcohol dependency or cravings is to keep your blood sugar balanced, as well as not drinking alcohol for a period to clear your system and break the cycle of cravings. When you stop drinking alcohol, which should be for at least two weeks, it is vitally important to eat a healthy low-GL diet because this is what will keep your blood sugar level even. (See Chapter 1, Part 2 for details on how to follow a low-GL diet.)

One of the key principles is eating little and often. This means always having breakfast, lunch, dinner and two snacks. A late-afternoon snack is vital for avoiding blood sugar lows in the evening. This is because a blood sugar dip often triggers a craving for alcohol or sugar. When this is accompanied by the need to switch off the stress after a hard day's work, it can hard to resist pouring yourself a drink. I'll be explaining below how specific amino acids can help you with this.

Most regular alcohol consumers, especially those who crave it, have poor blood sugar control and are strongly likely to be what is known as 'insulin resistant'. This means that the body produces more insulin because the cells have become less sensitive to its effects. Insulin helps to normalise blood sugar balance. The essential mineral chromium is required for the insulin receptor to work, so as well as following a low-GL diet, which helps to stabilise blood sugar, supplementing 200mcg of chromium two or three times a day will improve insulin sensitivity and reduces cravings for both sugar and alcohol. Chromium, then, is well worth supplementing, especially during the first week of quitting.

2. Supplement amino acids

Alcohol mimics and depletes the brain's feel-good neurotransmitters. These include:

- Serotonin, which makes you feel good and from which the body makes melatonin, necessary for a good night's sleep (see below).

- Gamma-amino-butyric acid (GABA), an amino acid (a protein building block) that switches off adrenalin. Alcohol promotes GABA in the short term, which is why it makes us feel relaxed, but it depletes GABA in the long term, making us feel more anxious and unable to relax.

All neurotransmitters are made directly from amino acids found in food protein. Generally, it is good to eat protein-rich foods such as nuts, seeds, eggs and fish; however, by supplementing specific amino acids you can enhance the brain's ability to recover.

GABA is available as an amino acid in some countries (for example, the US), but not in the UK. If you live in the US, taking 2 × 500mg helps to relax and balance brain function in the evening. GABA is made from the amino acids taurine and glutamine. Some UK-based supplements provide these instead.

Glutamine is worth supplementing, because it also helps reduce cravings for alcohol. It also heals the gut, which becomes damaged by too much alcohol. Glutamine is best taken as a powder: take 1 heaped teaspoon (5g) in a glass of cold water last thing at night or in the afternoon on an empty stomach, as it is more easily absorbed without food.

We have seen above that serotonin, from which the brain makes melatonin, is essential for sleep. It is made from the amino acid tryptophan. The most potent form of tryptophan is 5-hydroxytryptophan (5-HTP) (see below).

3. Increase fish and take fish oils

Alcohol depletes essential fats and, in excess, it disturbs the delicate gut membrane. As we have seen, glutamine helps to heal the gut. Although omega-3 fats are essential to the body and needed by everyone, it is doubly important to increase your intake of these essential fats when you are stopping alcohol. Essential fats are the key components of receptors, the 'docking ports' for the brain's neurotransmitters, and increasing omega-3 fats, in particular, appears to increase serotonin, or at least make your brain's own feel-good chemicals work better.

It is worth supplementing at least 1,500mg of fish oils (two capsules) a day. Also, eat oily fish and omega-3-rich seeds such as pumpkin, chia and flax seeds. (For more details on essential fats see Chapter 3, Part 2.)

4. Get a good night's sleep

Although it might appear that alcohol helps you to sleep, the truth is that it disturbs the normal sleep cycle. Alcohol suppresses rapid eye movement (REM) sleep, which is the dreaming phase of sleep, and decreases deep sleep;[1] drinkers wake up more frequently in the night. What most people are not aware of is that the lack of REM sleep due to alcohol can also cause sleep disturbances when the person gives up drinking. When alcohol is removed, there is a rebound of REM sleep. The body attempts to make up for the REM sleep that it has missed.

The brain needs the amino acid 5-HTP to make serotonin and melatonin for a normal sleep cycle, so supplementing 5-HTP often helps to improve the quantity and quality of undisturbed sleep. People have different sensitivities to 5-HTP, which is best taken in doses of between 50mg and 200mg, one hour before bed. Start with the lower dose and work up until you have the best effect. GABA, discussed earlier, also helps to switch off the stress hormones that can also make it difficult to get to sleep.

Another way to switch off the stress hormones is to listen to music designed to induce alpha waves in the brain, which are essential to enable the body to fall asleep. Many people have found the CD *Silence of Peace*, composed by John Levine, very effective for this purpose (see Resources).

Best foods

- Oily fish (salmon, mackerel, herring, kippers, sardines)
- Chia seeds
- Flax seeds
- Pumpkin seeds
- Raw nuts
- Free-range eggs
- Oats, oatcakes
- Fresh fruit
- Fresh vegetables
- 8 glasses of water a day
- Green tea and herbal teas

Worst foods

- Sugar and refined foods (these affect blood sugar)
- Caffeinated drinks after midday (these affect sleep)

Best supplements

- 2 × high-potency multivitamin–minerals providing B vitamins, 10mg zinc and 100mg magnesium

- 2 × vitamin C 1,000mg

- 2 × essential omegas providing at least 1,500mg of fish-oil-derived omega-3, plus omega-6 from borage or evening primrose oil

- 1 teaspoon glutamine powder taken in cold water last thing at night on an empty stomach

- 2 × GABA 500mg, taken on an empty stomach in the evening or a formula containing glutamine and taurine

- 1 × 5-HTP 100mg one hour before bed, or 2 × 5-HTP 50mg morning and evening

- 2 × chromium 200mcg

CAUTIONS

Some people feel nauseous when first taking 5-HTP. If that happens, lower the dose, but continue to take it. For most people this effect passes within two or three days. 5-HTP is not recommend for those taking antidepressant drugs unless under the guidance of a health-care practitioner.

Glutamine, in quantities beyond 5g a day, is not recommended for those with advanced liver cirrhosis or kidney disease.

DIG DEEPER

To find out more on this subject, read *How to Quit Without Feeling S**t* (Patrick Holford, James Braly, David Miller), which includes key referenced studies.

ALLERGIES

Good medicine solutions

1. Test and identify your allergies

The first step towards identifying whether you have an allergy is to get properly diagnosed. Many people believe, incorrectly, that they have an allergy – for example, if they bloat after eating a certain food – but allergy-like symptoms can be caused by an inability to digest a compound in a food. Lactose intolerance, for example, is an *inability to digest* milk, but it is not an allergy.

Allergies involve the immune system producing antibodies that target a substance. One kind of antibody, called immuno-globulinE (IgE), produces a fairly immediate reaction to an aller-gen; for example, to peanuts or shellfish. The most common method of testing for IgE allergies is with a skin-prick test. The substance (for example, milk or pollen) is put on the skin, which is then pricked. If the area goes red after ten minutes, this indi-cates an allergic reaction. The problem with this method is that you have to guess what is likely to be a culprit. Usually about ten foods are tested in this way.

Another kind of antibody, responsible for many food reac-tions, is called immunoglobulinG (IgG). The symptoms are often less severe than IgE reactions, and not so immediate. IgG-based reactions are often called food intolerances. Your reactiv-ity can be tested for multiple foods using a small blood sample in a laboratory process called ELISA. This also quantifies the scale of reaction. The advantage of this kind of testing is that it identifies likely culprits in your daily food that you can then eliminate to see if your symptoms subside. Three in four people who avoid their IgG-positive foods notice a definite improve-ment in symptoms. Testing allows for a more informed means to suspect foods that you might not have thought of poten-tially offending your immune system. This is more effective and accurate than the conventional 'elimination diet', which is based on avoiding a list of more common allergens, then rein-troducing them one at a time to identify the likely culprit. This method of testing does not require much blood to be taken, so you can buy a home test kit and then send it to a laboratory (see Resources).

Coeliac disease is caused by a strong reaction to gluten; however, recent research has identified that a specific kind of protein within gluten, called gliadin, is the cause of at least eight out of ten cases of coeliac disease. Gliadin is found in wheat, rye and barley, but not in oats, and stimulates production of a different kind of antibody called IgA anti-tissue transglutaminase (IgATT). It can be tested with a specific IgATT home test kit (see Resources).

2. Avoid or rotate your suspect foods

If you have an IgE-based allergy the only 'cure' is lifelong avoidance. Even when avoiding the allergen it is possible to accidentally be exposed to it, such as eating a food that is slightly tainted, but following the advice below may help to reduce the severity of those reactions.

If you have had a reliable IgG food intolerance test it will grade your severity of reaction. For stronger reactions, you'll be advised to avoid the food completely. For very mild reactions you may be advised to 'rotate' the food, which means eating it no more than once every four or five days. This is because sequential consumption of an allergy-provoking food 'primes' the immune system to react, but leaving a space allows the immune system to 'forget' that it wants to react.

Unlike the more severe IgE allergies, IgG reactions do not last a lifetime, because the antibody, when it dies off over a period of three to four months, leaves no 'memory' behind of the food or substance you're reacting to. If you continue to eat the food, however, your body may continue to produce IgG antibodies against it. If you can strictly avoid your food intolerances for four months, all the antibodies that were primed to react will have died off. Providing you then follow the guidelines below, you'll probably no longer react, or react as strongly, to many of your food intolerances. Those that stay reactive are more likely to be IgE based.

3. Improve your gut health

Among the main reasons for developing food allergies are gut problems causing increased intestinal permeability. The gut membrane is exceedingly thin and the cells that comprise it are replaced every four days. Alcohol, antibiotics, anti-inflammatory drugs (painkillers), gliadin in wheat, coffee and fried foods all irritate the gut. So too does anything that you are allergic to or that causes excessive bloating.

The first line of defence in the gut is the beneficial bacteria called probiotics. The two main strains are *Lactobacillus acido-philus* and bifidobacteria. By supplementing these you effectively 're-inoculate' the gut. This is well worth doing if you have taken a course of antibiotics, or if you have had a gut infection or a binge on alcohol.

You make 10 litres (17½ pints) of digestive juices a day containing a variety of digestive enzymes. A lack of certain digestive enzymes – for example those necessary for digesting beans, greens or milk – can cause bloating in some people. If food isn't properly digested, and if the gut wall does not have good integrity (which is called increased permeability), whole food protein can cross the gut wall, triggering an allergic reaction because the immune system will recognise it as an enemy. Supplementing a broad range of digestive enzymes can make a big difference.

Gut cells use an amino acid, glutamine, for energy. Taking glutamine helps to replenish gut cells and reduce permeability. If you know your gut is compromised, take 1 heaped teaspoon (5g) of glutamine powder in cold water on an empty stomach before bed to 'heal' the gut.

Some digestion-friendly supplements contain probiotics, digestive enzymes and glutamine. Supplementing these for a month is a great way to support gut health, thus reducing allergic potential.

4. Reduce inflammatory foods

Any food you are allergic to becomes an inflammatory food, because an allergic reaction is part of an inflammatory response by the body. Most of the symptoms you think of when you have flu – aching, mucus production, fatigue, raised temperature – are caused by the body going into 'red alert' mode.

Many of the body's chemicals that are produced to trigger an inflammatory response are made from a type of fat called arachidonic acid (AA) which is found in very high amounts in milk products and meat. Avoiding these foods helps to reduce inflammation.

Also helpful is avoiding coffee, which raises several inflammatory substances. Sugar has a similar effect, but primarily because big fluctuations in blood sugar levels trigger hormonal changes that can encourage inflammation.

5. Increase anti-inflammatory foods

Conversely, there are compounds in food that help to switch off inflammation. The best known are quercetin in red onions, curcumin in turmeric, oleocanthal in olives, bromelain in pineapple, vitamin C – which is an antihistamine – in berries and broccoli, sulphur in eggs, onions and garlic. You can get supplements containing combinations of these, which are much more potent than just eating the foods. A red onion, for example, contains 20mg of quercetin but supplements providing 500mg have a major anti-inflammatory and anti-allergy effect.[1] Combinations of these are particularly powerful, both for reducing allergic potential and in calming down a reaction.

The omega-3 fats in oily fish are also powerful anti-inflammatory agents (see Chapter 3, Part 2).

The body produces oxidants as part of an inflammatory reaction; therefore any food high in antioxidants is also likely to be anti-inflammatory. Foods with strong colours, such as beetroot, blueberries, strawberries, watermelon, tomatoes, carrots, mustard, turmeric, broccoli, avocado, asparagus and other greens, all help to reduce inflammation and thus allergic potential.

'I used to have . . .'

I met Sonia on a breakfast television show. She was described as one of Britain's worst hay fever sufferers. An IgG food intolerance test identified that she reacted to milk and eggs. She eliminated those foods, started taking a digestive-support supplement and an anti-allergy supplement, and began eating a diet high in anti-inflammatory foods. After ten days, almost all of Sonia's symptoms were gone.

> 'After a diet of healthy fresh fruit, vegetables and oily fish, I've noticed a huge difference in energy levels. Not only have I conquered my hay fever but it has also been a very easy diet to follow. I don't feel like I've missed out on anything, except for an occasional desire for cheese. I look at it as an eating plan, not a diet, and something that I will follow for the foreseeable future. I wish I had known all this ten years ago!'

Since then, Sonia hasn't had to take a single antihistamine. One year later, she remains symptom-free and is no longer allergic to eggs. Milk, however, is still a problem. During hay-fever season she supplements an anti-inflammatory formula.

Best foods

- Red onions and garlic
- Turmeric and mustard
- Broccoli and green vegetables
- Beetroot
- Blueberries and other berries
- Carrots, sweet potato and butternut squash
- Oily fish (salmon, mackerel, herring, kippers, sardines)

Worst foods

- Milk
- Meat
- Wheat
- Coffee
- Sugar
- Alcohol

Best supplements

- 2 × high-potency multivitamin–minerals

- 2 × vitamin C 1,000mg

- 2 × essential omegas with fish-oil-derived omega-3, plus omega-6 from borage or evening primrose oil (ten times more omega-3 than -6)

- 2 × anti-inflammatory formula, containing a combination of quercetin, vitamin C, glutamine, MSM (sulphur), bromelain

Or

- 2 × quercetin 250mg

Optional

- 1 × digestive enzymes, probiotics, glutamine with each meal for 30 days

DIG DEEPER

To find out more on this subject, read *Hidden Food Allergies* (Patrick Holford and Dr James Braly), which includes key referenced studies.

ANGINA

Good medicine solutions

1. Take CoQ_{10}, plus carnitine – the dynamic duo

Both coenzyme Q_{10} (CoQ_{10}) and carnitine are known as 'semi-essential nutrients' that are vital for heart function. This means that your body can make them, but it doesn't make enough for optimal health, especially if you have angina, with compromised circulation of nutrients. Your heart can therefore benefit from a greater intake of these two heart-friendly nutrients.

More than half of your heart's energy comes from fat, and since it's working hard every second, it needs a steady supply. Carnitine is the delivery boy that brings in fatty acids to process for energy. It also takes away the toxic by-products, including damaged fats. Carnitine helps your heart to liberate the energy it needs efficiently.

A number of studies confirm its usefulness, particularly if there's stress on the heart. One showed that 2g a day of L-carnitine helped angina sufferers recover more quickly. They exhibited sufficient improvement to be able to start exercising.[1]

There are actually three different kinds of carnitine, which all work in terms of improving heart-muscle function. If you had to pick one, propionyl l-carnitine (PLC) would probably be the best, because it specifically helps heart and peripheral-muscle function. You can purchase PLC on its own or in carnitine complexes that provide all three types. The latter are better for overall health. Take 250–500mg of carnitine two to four times a day.

Alongside 30mg of CoQ_{10} taken two to four times a day, carnitine can work wonders. CoQ_{10} is an antioxidant made by the body that helps heart and all muscle cells to become more efficient. With over a hundred published studies, there is no doubt that it helps the heart, and all other muscle cells, to become more efficient. People with angina have fewer attacks and an increased exercise tolerance when taking it. CoQ$_{10}$ also prevents nitric oxide from being disarmed by oxidation, thus promoting vasodilation in the arteries. It improves heart function within four weeks at a dose of 100mg a day.

Although these two nutrients work in different ways, they both support your heart and brain by helping to provide a consistent, high level of energy and by reducing the toxic by-products of energy production.

2. Follow a low-GL diet

Sugary and refined foods, and eating too much carbohydrate, raises blood sugar levels and, in turn, leads to raised insulin levels and insulin resistance. Both raised insulin and raised blood sugar damages blood vessels and raises blood pressure. Therefore, it is vital to follow a low-GL diet (explained in Chapter 1, Part 2). My low-GL diet is also high in soluble fibres (such as oats), and plant sterols (such as beans), which further help cardiovascular health (see High Cholesterol page 202).

3. Increase your omega-3 intake

Supplementing reasonably high doses of omega-3 fish oils has been shown to help reduce angina symptoms, as well as reducing cholesterol and triglycerides, and helping to prevent further cardiovascular problems in those at risk.

Although eating oily fish generally reduces the level of risk, the benefit for reducing angina requires a total daily intake of about 1,000mg of eicosapentaenoic acid (EPA), which means two omega-3-rich fish oil capsules a day.

There are three kinds of essential fat found in fish – EPA, docosapentaenoic acid (DPA) and docosahexaenoic acid (DHA). Both EPA and DPA have proven heart benefits. When choosing a fish oil capsule, add up the total EPA and DPA. Good supplements provide 300–400mg per capsule. Therefore, two capsules provides up to 800mg. A serving of mackerel, herring or salmon will give you about 700mg. If you eat these oily fish three times a week and supplement at least 600mg of EPA, plus DPA, and eat omega-3-rich seeds and nuts, such as chia or flax seeds and walnuts, you'll achieve 1,000mg of EPA.

Vegetarians should note that, as good as these seeds and nuts are, only about 5 per cent of the type of omega-3 fat (alpha linolenic acid – ALA) contained in them converts into EPA, so relying on seeds, nuts or their oils will not confer the benefit of concentrated fish oil supplements and eating oily fish.

4. Take homocysteine-lowering B vitamins

One of the most reliable predictors of cardiovascular death is your blood level of homocysteine, not cholesterol. Homocysteine is a toxic amino acid that can directly damage the arteries and heart, and it accumulates if you have an insufficient intake of B vitamins (B_2, B_6, B_{12}, folic acid).

If your doctor hasn't tested your homocysteine level, you can test it yourself using a home test kit (see Resources). Ideally, you want your level to be below 7mcmol/l, but certainly not above 10. Risk for cardiovascular disease is far greater in those with a level above 15.

Homocysteine is easily lowered by taking a supplement containing vitamins B_2, B_6, B_{12} and folic acid. The best supplements also contain zinc and tri-methyl-glycine (TMG), which is an amino acid that, along with zinc, helps to break down homocysteine. The doses required to lower homocysteine are much higher than the basic recommended daily allowance (RDA) levels of nutrients, especially for vitamin B_{12}, which is poorly absorbed in older people, some more than others. Therefore, most homocysteine-modulating supplements provide around 500mcg of B_{12}. (The EU RDA is 1mcg.) The amount you need depends on your homocysteine level (see the chart on page 420 in Chapter 4, Part 2).

A study in the *American Journal of Cardiology* found that cardiovascular patients with high homocysteine levels (above 15mcmol/l) who were treated with B vitamins cut their risk of death by a quarter over ten years.[2] Among those not given the B vitamins, 32 per cent had died, compared to only 4 per cent of those given high-dose vitamins. This means that those on placebo were eight times more likely to die than those on B vitamins.

5. Increase your intake of magnesium and potassium, and reduce salt

Increasing your intake of magnesium and potassium from vegetables, nuts, beans and seeds, and reducing salt from cured meats, cheese and salted foods immediately lowers your blood pressure, which means a better flow of blood and oxygen to the heart, reducing angina symptoms. See High Blood Pressure, page 195, for more details and a fuller list of foods to eat or avoid. Make sure your supplement programme includes 300mg of magnesium.

6. Reduce stress

Don't underestimate the effect of stress on both raised cholesterol and blood pressure. Stress immediately generates adrenal hormones, which raise blood pressure and cardiovascular risk as part of the 'fight–flight' reaction. If you are often in a stressed state, this raises cholesterol. (See page 195 on High Blood Pressure for more on this.)

Although there are practical steps you can take to reduce your stress levels, one of the most important skills to learn is how to master your own stress response the moment it occurs, or in preparation for a potentially stressful situation. (For more information on these stress-reducing techniques see Chapter 6, Part 2.)

7. Consider chelation therapy

If you are already pulling out all the nutritional stops but not making progress, one way to speed up the breakdown of arterial plaque is through chelation therapy. This involves the infusion of the chelating agent, EDTA, which latches onto calcium in arterial plaque and helps to break it down. It's approved by the FDA (Food and Drug Administration) in the US for treating hypercalcaemia (high calcium in the blood). High levels of coronary-artery calcium is very predictive of a worse outcome in those with cardiovascular disease.

A chelation infusion usually takes two hours, and will be carried out a number of times, usually over a two- or three-month period. Chelation therapists also give combinations of nutrients in the intravenous infusion, similar to those I recommend here. This is especially important, because EDTA also chelates (that is, removes) other beneficial minerals such as magnesium, which must be replaced through supplementation. Vitamin C is also a natural, but weaker, chelating agent that does, however, appear to enhance the effectiveness of EDTA. Supplementing at least 2g of vitamin C is associated with many cardiovascular benefits, including lowering blood pressure.

Chelation therapy is certainly something you might want to consider if other options aren't working or desirable. For experienced doctors practising chelation therapy, see Resources. If you have an open-minded cardiologist or doctor, this is an option you might want to discuss with them.

Best foods

- Oily fish (salmon, mackerel, herring, kippers, sardines)
- White fish
- Chia seeds and pumpkin seeds
- Almonds
- Oats

- Beetroot
- Beans and lentils (pulses)
- Green vegetables and peas

Worst foods

- Sugar
- Salt
- Bacon and salted meats
- Cheese
- Coffee

Best supplements

- 2 × high-potency multivitamin–minerals providing 100mg of magnesium

- 2 × vitamin C 1,000mg (there is no harm in doubling this amount)

- 2 × high-potency omega-3-rich fish oil capsules (giving around 800mg of EPA, plus DPA)

- 2 × magnesium 100mg (giving a total of 300mg with your multivitamin)

- X* × homocysteine-modulating B vitamin formula (*dose and need dependent on your homocysteine score, as explained in Chapter 4, Part 2, page 420)

CAUTIONS

If you are on blood-thinning medication, or have a history of stroke, see your doctor before taking omega-3 fish oils, as they also reduce blood clotting. Too much blood thinning may increase the risk of cerebral haemorrhage.

DIG DEEPER
To find out more on this subject, read *Say No to Heart Disease* (Patrick Holford), which includes key referenced studies.

ANXIETY AND STRESS

Good medicine solutions

1. Follow a low-GL diet and supplement chromium

The state of anxiety is associated with raised levels of the stress hormones adrenalin and cortisol. When your blood sugar dips (often a rebound from blood sugar highs) it promotes the release of adrenal hormones. Stimulants such as caffeine and nicotine cause the same reaction. The first step towards reducing anxiety, therefore, is to balance your blood sugar by eating a low-GL diet containing slow-releasing carbohydrates eaten with protein and to avoid, or at least considerably reduce, your use of stimulants and alcohol (see below). This alone has a major effect in reducing anxiety. (See Chapter 1, Part 2 for details on how to follow a low-GL diet.)

The mineral chromium helps to even out blood sugar by making you more sensitive to insulin – that's the hormone that keeps blood sugar level even. It is particularly effective in those with symptoms of depression associated with sugar cravings, and feeling tired and oversensitive. If that sounds like you, try supplementing 200mcg of chromium twice a day, with breakfast and lunch.

2. Stop taking stimulants and reduce alcohol

The reason we use stimulants is to increase adrenal hormones and with them the feelings of energy and motivation. But the more you have, the more you need until you can't function without them – feeling 'flat'. It takes only a few days to recover your natural energy through eating a low-GL diet and taking the right supplements.

If you are prone to anxiety and feeling stressed, the worst thing is to consume lots of caffeine, so step one for reducing anxiety is to become caffeine-free. The highest amounts of caffeine are found in strong coffee and high-caffeine energy drinks. There's also some in tea, but tea is more calming due to the presence of an amino acid called theanine. So it is better than coffee, but you still need to limit your intake to two weak cups a day.

Nicotine is another stimulant, and quitting smoking is essential for reducing levels of anxiety, even though you may have become addicted precisely because a cigarette helped you to calm down.

Alcohol, at least for the first hour after drinking it, is a relaxant because it switches off adrenalin by promoting gamma-aminobutyric acid (GABA) (see below). This is why it is a highly effective way to unwind. But, similar to nicotine, the effect of using alcohol on a daily basis is the opposite. You become more stressed. Also, alcohol disturbs the normal dreaming cycle and the net effect is that you wake up more tired and irritable, in need of more caffeine in the day, then alcohol again in the evening. It's a vicious cycle. To reduce anxiety, it is important to drink lightly, and even take a break from alcohol altogether for a couple of weeks.

3. Supplement GABA and taurine

GABA is the main inhibitory or calming neurotransmitter in the brain. It not only switches off stress hormones but it also helps promote serotonin, thereby affecting your mood. For these reasons, having enough GABA in your brain is associated with feeling relaxed and happy, whereas having too little is associated with anxiety, tension, depression and insomnia.

As well as being a neurotransmitter, GABA is also an amino acid. This means that it's a nutrient and, by supplementing it, you can help to promote normal healthy levels of GABA in the brain.

There is one problem, however. In the EU, GABA has been classified as a medicine, making it no longer available over the counter in the UK. You can buy GABA supplements on the internet from countries such as the US, however.

If you are able to buy it, supplement GABA 500–1,000mg once or twice a day, to act as a highly effective natural relaxant. But note that although it is not addictive, this doesn't mean that there are no side effects in large amounts. Up to 2g a day has no reported downside; however, if you go up to 10g a day, this can induce nausea or even vomiting and a rise in blood pressure. Therefore, use GABA wisely, especially if you already have high blood pressure, starting with no more than 1,000mg a day, and do not exceed 3g a day. If you take it in the evening, it also helps you get to sleep.

Taurine is another relaxing amino acid, similar in structure and effect to GABA. Many people think taurine is a stimulant because it is used in so-called energy drinks, but it is not. It helps you relax and unwind from high levels of adrenalin, much like GABA.

Taurine is highly concentrated in animal foods such as fish, eggs and meat. Vegetarians are therefore more likely to be at risk of deficiency. Try 500–1,000mg of taurine twice daily. There are no known cautions or adverse effects at reasonable doses.

3. Take relaxing herbs – valerian, hops and passion flower

Valerian (*Valeriana officinalis*) is an excellent anti-anxiety herb. As a natural relaxant it is useful for several disorders such as restlessness, nervousness, insomnia and hysteria, and it has also been used as a sedative for 'nervous' stomach. Valerian acts on the brain's GABA receptors, thereby simulating the effects of the neurotransmitter GABA, which switches off adrenalin. This enhances the GABA receptors' activity, offering a similar tranquillising action as the Valium-type drugs but without the same side effects. As a relaxant, you need to take 50–100mg twice a day, and double this amount 45 minutes before retiring for a good night's sleep.

Since valerian increases the power of sedative drugs, including muscle relaxants and antihistamines, don't take it if you are on medication without your doctor's consent. Valerian can also interact with alcohol, as well as certain psychotropic drugs and narcotics.

Hops (*Humulus lupulus*) are an ancient remedy for a good night's sleep and probably included in beer for that reason. Hops help to calm nerves by acting directly on the central nervous system, rather than affecting GABA receptors. You need about 200mg per day, but the effect is much less than valerian and most effective when taken in combination with this and other herbs, such as passion flower.

Passion flower (*Passiflora incarnata*) was a favourite of the Aztecs, who used it to make relaxing drinks. It has a mild sedative effect and promotes sleep, in a similar way to hops, with no known side effects at normal doses. Passion flower can also be helpful for hyperactive children. You need about 100–200mg a day.

Combinations of these herbs are particularly effective for relieving anxiety and can really help break the pattern of reacting stressfully to life's challenges.

4. Increase magnesium – the calming mineral

Magnesium is another important nutrient that helps you relax. It's also commonly deficient and depleted by chronic stress. Magnesium not only relaxes your mind but also your muscles, and symptoms of deficiency include muscle aches, cramps and spasms, as well as anxiety and insomnia. Low levels are commonly found in anxious people, and supplementation can often help. You need to take about 500mg of magnesium a day. Seeds and nuts are rich in magnesium, as are vegetables and fruit, but especially dark green leafy vegetables such as kale or spinach. I recommend eating these magnesium-rich foods every day, which should provide 200mg, and supplementing an additional 300mg. If you are especially anxious and can't sleep, take your magnesium in the evening, a couple of hours before bed.

5. Practise stress-reduction techniques

Some people need a little extra help to learn how to switch out of the adrenalin state. There are breathing and meditation techniques for this, as well as psychotherapeutic avenues to explore in dealing with the perceived stresses and causes of anxiety, and many of them can be extremely helpful. I have been particularly impressed by HeartMath techniques (explained in Chapter 6, Part 2) and also the effects of 'vital energy' exercises such as yoga, t'ai chi and Psychocalisthenics®.

'I used to have . . . '

Managing a chain of supermarkets had left Andrew very stressed. During the day he'd drink several cups of coffee and in the evening he'd relax with a beer or some wine, because otherwise he would experience difficulty sleeping. He was also gaining weight. He decided to go on a low-GL diet, quit drinking coffee and booze, and take some supplements. Three weeks later he said:

'My energy is through the roof, I don't feel stressed and I have no problem sleeping, and I'm waking refreshed.'

Best foods

- Dark green vegetables – kale, spinach
- Nuts and seeds, especially almonds and pumpkin seeds (rich in magnesium)
- Green tea (in moderation)
- Whole foods

Worst foods

- Caffeinated drinks
- Alcohol
- Sugar
- Refined carbohydrates

Best supplements

- 2 × high-potency multivitamin–minerals providing B vitamins, 10mg zinc and 100mg magnesium

- 2 × vitamin C 1,000mg

- 2 × essential omegas with fish-oil-derived omega-3, plus omega-6 from borage or evening primrose oil

- 2 × GABA 500mg, taken on an empty stomach in the evening

Or

- a formula containing glutamine, taurine, magnesium and herbs

- 2 × valerian 50–100mg

Optional

- 2 × chromium 200mcg

> ### CAUTIONS
>
> Don't exceed 3,000mg of GABA, and consult your doctor before taking GABA or valerian if you are on tranquillising medication or sleeping pills. Also, do not combine with alcohol.

DIG DEEPER

To find out more on this subject, read *The Feel Good Factor* (Patrick Holford), which includes key referenced studies.

ARTHRITIS

General information

Arthritis means inflammation of the joints. There are two kinds: osteoarthritis and rheumatoid arthritis. Osteoarthritis is far more common and relates to the gradual degeneration of the joints relating to what is often termed 'wear and tear'. Rheumatoid arthritis is an autoimmune disease, meaning that the immune system is in a state of systemic inflammation, which is affecting the joints. For example, it tends to affect both sides of the body, and not just joints under stress, perhaps through carrying excess weight, or through injury or bad posture.

Good medicine solutions

1. Test for, and avoid, allergies

Inflammation often happens because you are eating something you're allergic to. An allergy might not be the only cause of inflamed joints – bad posture and carrying too much weight are other possibilities – but it can certainly increase inflammation. Most painkillers damage the gut, making it more permeable, which further increases your risk of allergy. Some people benefit tremendously from allergy testing to isolate the allergens identified, then by avoiding them. (See Allergies on page 31 to find out more about the best methods for testing and treating hidden food allergies and intolerances.)

2. Increase your omega-3 intake

It's a popular misconception that fish oils lubricate your joints. What they actually do is reduce pain and inflammation by counteracting the inflammatory chemicals in the body that non-steroidal anti-inflammatory (NSAID) drugs suppress. There's plenty of research to show that fish oil supplementation can reduce the inflammation of arthritis. A recent analysis of 17 high-quality trials showed that supplementing omega-3s for three to four months substantially reduced joint pain intensity, morning stiffness and the number of painful and/or tender joints in patients with rheumatoid arthritis or joint pain. NSAID drug use was also reduced by 40 per cent. An effective amount to take is the equivalent of 1,000mg of eicosapentaenoic acid (EPA), the most potent kind of anti-inflammatory essential fat, a day. This is achieved with two high-potency omega-3 fish oil capsules a day, plus eating oily fish (salmon, mackerel, herring, kippers, sardines) three times a week and omega-3-rich seeds most days, the best being chia seeds, followed by flax seeds.

3. Eat and supplement nature's anti-inflammatories

The experience we call pain is triggered by certain chemicals called inflammatory mediators, which our bodies produce in response to some kind of damage. These cause swelling, redness and pain. Most inflammatory mediators are made from a type of fat, called arachidonic acid (AA), which is found in high quantities in meat and milk – a good reason to go light on these foods if you're in pain.

Some food extracts naturally dampen down the production of the inflammatory mediators, without the side effects associated with painkiller drugs. My favourites are:

Olive extracts Oleocanthal is a natural painkiller found in olives. It gives you that 'back of the throat' taste, not dissimilar to aspirin. Hydroxytyrosol, another extract from olives, is incredibly rich in certain polyphenols. Red grapes and red onions (both of which also contain the natural anti-inflammatory quercetin) contain polyphenols, as does green tea. But with an antioxidant content over ten times greater than vitamin C, hydroxytyrosol is the most powerful.

Turmeric This bright yellow spice contains the active compound curcumin, which has a variety of powerful anti-inflammatory actions. Studies show it works as well as anti-inflammatory drugs but without the side effects. It has been used for hundreds of years with no evidence of any downsides, even in high doses of 8g a day. You need about 500mg a day of curcumin extract, or 1 teaspoon of turmeric.

Hops An extract in hops, called iso-oxygene, is a natural painkiller. You need about 1,000mg a day of a hop extract.

Quercetin This potent anti-inflammatory, found in red onions, also helps to stabilise collagen, the material needed by the body to maintain healthy joint tissue. You need about 500mg a day. A red onion gives you 20mg.

Eating plenty of strongly coloured fruits, vegetables, herbs and spices – such as blueberries, mustard, beetroot, kale, red onions, turmeric and cayenne – as well as eating olives and lots of oily fish, increases dietary anti-inflammatories.

Although it's great to eat lots of the above to get a good

anti-inflammatory effect, you need to take much greater quantities as provided in supplements containing concentrated extracts of a combination of these natural painkillers.

4. Take glucosamine and MSM for rebuilding

When the body goes into a state of inflammation, the experience of pain serves to motivate you to immobilise a damaged joint; prolonged inflammation, by comparison, causes more and more damage to the cartilage, especially if the joint in question is a weight-bearing joint, such as the knees, hips or lower back. Glucosamine and methylsulfonylmethane (MSM), a form of sulphur, are vital for rebuilding cartilage, as is vitamin C, which makes collagen – the intracellular 'glue'.

Although the body can make glucosamine, if you have damaged joints you are unlikely to make enough – unless you are in the habit of munching on prawn shells, which is the richest dietary source. Studies show that glucosamine slows down the progression of osteoarthritis, and several studies show that glucosamine can be as effective as regular painkillers in easing arthritic pain and inflammation, but without the side effects. Most of the research has been carried out using glucosamine sulphate, but the most absorbable form is glucosamine hydrochloride.

If you think of building bone as similar to building something for the home, glucosamine is like the wood, but you also need nails to hold everything together – and that's where sulphur comes in. Some people have reported tremendous relief from arthritis by supplementing 1–3g of one of the most effective sources of sulphur, MSM. The combination of both glucosamine and MSM is particularly effective. I recommend that you supplement 1,000–3,000mg of glucosamine sulphate (or glucosamine hydrochloride) a day together with 600–2,000mg of MSM. The lower end of the range is enough if you want to support your joints and prevent their degeneration, while the higher end of the range is for those who want to maximise recovery.

5. Take bone-friendly minerals and vitamin D

Minerals are important for building bone, but the mineral calcium can only be driven into bone if there is sufficient vitamin D, which is made from sunlight. The richest dietary source of vitamin D is oily fish, but even that doesn't give you an optimal amount. A good multivitamin may supply 15mcg of vitamin D (600iu). To support healthy bones, supplement at least 400mg of calcium, 150mg of magnesium, 10mg of zinc and 50mcg of boron. These, plus vitamin D, are the most important bone-building minerals.

'I used to have . . . '

John developed arthritis at the age of 23. When he turned 40, he couldn't sleep at night from the pain and had to go upstairs on his hands and knees. Walking just 100 metres was painful. He was then tested for IgG food allergies and eliminated his food intolerances.

'Life is now pain- and tablet-free and I have complete mobility. I am amazed at the difference in my quality of life simply by making such simple adjustments,' he said.

Ed could barely walk without pain, let alone pursue his passion for golf. He followed my advice and within six months was virtually pain-free.

'I used to have constant pain in my knees and joints. I couldn't play golf or walk for more than ten minutes without resting my legs. Since following your advice, my discomfort has decreased by 95–100 per cent. I would never have believed my pain could be reduced by such a large degree and not return, no matter how much activity I do in a day or week,' said Ed.

Ed is living proof that the body can heal itself if you give it the right nutrients, whatever your age.

Best foods

- Oily fish (salmon, mackerel, herring, kippers, sardines)
- Red onions and garlic
- Turmeric
- Olives
- Berries
- Vegetables (strong colours)

Worst foods

- Sugar and refined carbohydrates (promotes inflammation)
- Dairy products (common allergen)
- Meat (rich source of inflammatory fats)
- Coffee (induces a stress response promoting inflammation)

Best supplements

- 2 × omega-3-rich fish oil capsules (choose products with the most EPA)

- 3 × natural anti-inflammatories providing one or more of quercetin, turmeric (curcumin), hop or olive extracts

- 2 × glucosamine (2–4g a day) and 2 × MSM 500mg (1–2g a day); you can get combined glucosamine and MSM supplements

- 2 × high-potency multivitamin–minerals with antioxidants, providing at least 10mcg of vitamin D, plus 400mg calcium, 150mg magnesium, 10mg zinc and 50mcg boron

- 2 × vitamin C 1,000mg

DIG DEEPER
To find out more on this subject, read *Say No to Arthritis* (Patrick Holford), which includes key referenced studies.

ASTHMA

Good medicine solutions

1. Test for, and avoid, hidden allergies

There are two kinds of allergies: IgE and IgG. IgE reactions are conventional allergies, most commonly associated with peanuts and shellfish (see Allergies on page 31). People with asthma are often found to have higher levels of IgE, making them hypersensitive to certain substances. You can test your IgE sensitivity and identify specifically what you are reacting to from an IgE blood test or skin prick test (see Resources).

Most asthma suffers also have IgG sensitivities to foods. This type of intolerance is not so obvious and may not always precipitate an asthma attack. If they do have such a sensitivity, asthma symptoms may not occur for several hours or even until the next day. Common foods that cause reactions are milk products, gluten (gliadin) cereals (wheat, rye, barley) and yeast. Your doctor is unlikely to offer you an IgG allergy test, but you can organise this yourself via a home test kit (see Resources).

Once you know what you are reacting to, you need to avoid your allergens. IgE sensitivities last for life; however, it is possible to 'unlearn' IgG sensitivities if you avoid the allergens strictly for at least four months.

Not all allergens are easy to avoid. If, for example, you are allergic to pollen, you won't be able to avoid it completely. (See Hay Fever on page 180 for more on how to prevent symptoms.)

If you are allergic to house-dust mites, which live in mattresses and carpets, you'll need to go to war on these critters by changing your bedding frequently and by following the other measures below. House-dust mite allergy has increased hugely since most homes have central heating, because these bugs love moisture and don't like large temperature changes. Either buy a new mattress or put yours outside to sunbathe on a couple of extremely hot days. Then cover it in a house-dust mite-proof cover, which you can buy from most major department stores. Also get some house-dust mite-proof pillowcases and covers. Wash your sheets and pillowcases frequently in hot water and dry well. Invest in a bed base that allows the bed to air properly. Don't make your bed in the morning. Leave it to air by folding back the covers fully and, ideally, let the room air as well. It's best not to have a carpet in the bedroom, and don't leave wet towels lying around. Do your drying in the bathroom and leave the towels in there. All these actions will also reduce exposure to moulds (which can also trigger an allergic reaction).

2. Increase antioxidants and natural anti-inflammatories

There's no doubt that increasing your intake of antioxidants reduces asthma severity. Numerous studies have shown that a high intake of fresh fruit and vegetables reduces asthma severity and the strong implication is that it is the high antioxidant nutrient content of fruits and vegetables that does this. The antioxidant nutrients that come out top are vitamins C and E, beta-carotene and bioflavonoids, which are found in especially large amounts in berries.

From a dietary point of view, this means eating lots of broccoli, peppers, berries, citrus fruit, apples (which are all rich in vitamin C), carrots and tomatoes (rich in beta-carotene and lycopene), and seeds and fish (rich in vitamin E). One UK survey of 1,500 asthma sufferers found that people who ate at least two apples per week faced a 22–32 per cent lower risk of asthma than those who ate fewer.

The actual constriction of the airways, known as bronchiols, happens because of an inflammatory reaction. Most anti-asthma drugs are acting as anti-inflammatories, the most powerful mimicking the body's own hormone, cortisol. Nature's most powerful anti-inflammatories are omega-3 fats, curcumin, ginger, quercetin and MSM, which is a form of sulphur.

Ginger and turmeric, as well as garlic and pepper, turn off inflammation. While we await human trials, animal studies show that curcumin, which is the active ingredient in turmeric, has proven highly effective in reducing asthma symptoms. I recommend the liberal use of ginger and turmeric in cooking, and taking concentrated supplements.

Omega-3 fats in oily fish switch off inflammation. A number of studies have found lower rates and less severity of asthma in fish eaters. Children with a higher omega-6 to omega-3 fat ratio in their diet also have worse asthma. Meat, dairy, margarine and sunflower oil are all high in omega-6, whereas flax, chia and pumpkin seeds, walnuts and oily fish are high in omega-3. I'd certainly recommend a diet low in meat and dairy and high in fish, as well as supplementing omega-3-rich fish oils. Choose supplements that have the most EPA, which is the most anti-inflammatory fat.

3. Improve your breathing with the Buteyko method

Hyperventilation, or over-breathing, often plays a significant role in the onset of asthma symptoms. Healthy breathing during rest should be unnoticeable and silent, through the nose and making use of the diaphragm.

There is a simple technique, taught in classes but also through DVDs and books, called the Buteyko method, which encourages this, and it has proven highly effective in reducing asthma symptoms. In most studies, learning the Buteyko method cut the need for medication by half. It is certainly an avenue worth exploring, especially if you have exercise-induced asthma, which has very similar dynamics to hyperventilation.

The basic idea behind Buteyko is that asthma sufferers are breathing too fast – more than 12 breaths a minute – causing them to breathe out too much carbon dioxide. This is important, because even though we tend to think of CO_2 as just a waste gas, it is also vital for the proper functioning of nearly all body chemistry. A drop in CO_2, for example, causes blood vessels and airways to narrow.

The first step in the Buteyko method is learning how to unblock the nose using a breath-hold exercise and switching to nasal breathing on a permanent basis. The patient is then taught to become more aware of their breathing and to relax the muscles involved in respiration in order to create a tolerable need for air. Through mental commands, the aim is to reduce breathing volume by about 30 per cent. Over time, with continued observation, this practice resets the respiratory centre to tolerate a higher pressure of carbon dioxide, thereby bringing breathing volume to normal levels. Patients are also taught correct breathing during physical exercise and sleeping, and how to stop a hyperventilation attack.

4. Try MSM

Asthma sufferers may get real benefits from taking methylsulfonylmethane (MSM), which is a bio-available form of the mineral sulphur. The sulphur is incorporated into the cells of the bronchial tubes, allowing the cell membranes to become more flexible and enabling the person to breathe more freely. There have been some impressive cases of people being successfully treated with MSM. One asthma sufferer tried 2g twice a day. Within a few weeks her breathing became much easier and she was soon able to stop her medication. However, there's a real need for more research on this harmless and potentially beneficial nutrient. The daily therapeutic dose for MSM ranges from 1,000 to 6,000mg. MSM works better if taken with vitamin C, which is a natural antihistamine.

MSM also provides the intestinal bacteria with building blocks for the manufacture of major anti-allergy, anti-inflammatory sulphur-containing amino acids, such as methionine and cysteine. Cysteine then increases the production of glutathione, low levels of which are associated with inflammation. Onions and garlic are rich in cysteine. Along with vitamin C, cysteine is also needed for the production of collagen, the major component of connective tissue in the lungs. Cysteine itself is very helpful in reducing asthmatic tendencies if supplemented at levels of 400mg or more.

5. Increase your intake of magnesium

Magnesium is a mineral that relaxes the bronchioles: the air tubes in the lungs. It is one of the most deficient minerals in today's diet. Magnesium supplements have been found to reduce symptoms of asthma, and intravenous magnesium, given at the time of an asthma attack, halves recovery time and dramatically reduces severity. Although this is known, it is rarely given in hospital emergency rooms. It could also be taken as an inhaler, but I know of none yet available.

Magnesium is found in green leafy vegetables, nuts, beans, lentils and seeds – especially pumpkin seeds. A small handful of pumpkin seeds (25g/1oz) will give you 150mg of magnesium. If you are also supplementing a high-strength multivitamin, that may provide a further 150mg. If you have asthma attacks quite frequently, it's probably worth supplementing an additional 200mg of magnesium in an easily absorbable form (such as magnesium glycinate, citrate or ascorbate) twice daily.

6. Improve your air quality

Most people with asthma are hypersensitive to changes in air quality and do much better in clean air. It's well worth investing in a decent ioniser for the bedroom or your major living space. Ionisers remove dust, smoke and pollen, and other particulate matter, from the air. Better-quality ionisers replicate the natural ions found in nature that can be absorbed through the lungs into the bloodstream. They are available from larger department stores and online. Research has consistently shown that improved lung capacity and relief from asthma symptoms are achieved quite rapidly by exposure to these types of ions.

'I used to have . . . '

John had suffered from asthma since the age of nine months. He was on medication all his life and had been using inhalers from the age of seven. At 35, John changed his diet dramatically and went on a low-allergen diet, eliminating milk almost completely. He also learnt how to improve his breathing.

'Since I've changed my diet, avoiding foods I'm allergic to, and learnt how to breathe using the Buteyko method, I've managed to stop using my bronchial inhalers almost completely. The trick is to find all the factors that contribute to the problem and gradually eliminate them.'

In John's case, keeping fit and minimising both caffeine and alcohol made a difference. He still carries his bronchial inhalers 'just in case'.

Best foods

- Fruit, especially apples, berries, citrus fruit
- Vegetables, especially carrots, tomatoes, green vegetables
- Chia seeds
- Flax seeds
- Pumpkin seeds
- Ginger
- Turmeric
- Oily fish (salmon, mackerel, herring, kippers, sardines)
- Beans and lentils (pulses)

Worst foods

- Meat
- Dairy products
- Caffeine
- Wheat and other gluten/gliadin foods (if allergic)

Best supplements

- 2 × high-potency multivitamin–minerals providing 150mg of magnesium and extra antioxidants including 100mg of vitamin E

- 2 × vitamin C 1,000mg (ideally with berry extracts and zinc)

- 2 × magnesium 100mg

- 2 × MSM 1,000mg or a combined supplement with quercetin, MSM and vitamin C

- 1 × cysteine 500mg

DIG DEEPER

To find out more on this subject, read *Asthma Free Naturally* by Patrick McKeown concerning Buteyko breathing (also see Resources).

AUTISM

Good medicine solutions

1. Balance your blood sugar

Many children with autism also have symptoms of ADHD/ hyperactivity (see page 19). For these children, improving blood sugar balance is a must by removing all added sugar and following a low-GL diet. (See Chapter 1, Part 2 for details on how to follow a low-GL diet.)

2. Increase your intake of omega-3 fats

Deficiencies in essential fats are common in people with autism. Research has shown that some children with autism have an enzymatic defect that removes essential fats from brain cell membranes more quickly than it should. This means that an autistic child is likely to need a higher intake of essential fats than the average. Supplementing the omega-3 fish oil eicosapentaenoic acid (EPA), which can slow the activity of the defective enzyme, has been shown to improve many of the symptoms of autism.

3. Increase vitamins and minerals

Going back to the 1970s, Dr Bernard Rimland of the Institute for Child Behavior Research in San Diego, California, showed that combinations of vitamins B_6 and C, zinc and magnesium supplements significantly improved symptoms in children with autism. More recent studies confirm that many children with autism benefit from extra amounts of these nutrients. Many of them have excess levels of pyrroles, tested in the urine, which deplete zinc and vitamin B_6.

Another critical nutrient is vitamin A, retinol, vital for building healthy cells in the brain and also essential for vision. Without sufficient amounts of this vitamin, the black and white light receptors in the eye don't work efficiently. Given that there are more colour receptors in the centre of the field of vision, and more black and white receptors in the peripheral field, those with this deficiency may rely more on peripheral vision, which would explain why some people with autism don't look you in the eye. Vitamin A is also important for gut integrity, and a lack of it may also increase the risk of gut-related problems and allergies.

The best dietary sources of vitamin A are breast milk, organ meats, milk fat, fish and cod liver oil. Since some autistic children react to dairy products, fish is probably the best source. Synthetic retinyl palmitate, often used in supplements, may not work as well as natural retinol, which is found, for example, in cod liver oil.

4. Test for and avoid any food allergies

There is substantial evidence that many people with autism have food allergies or intolerances. The strongest evidence of a food–autism link exists for wheat and dairy products, and the specific proteins they contain – namely, gluten and casein. These proteins are difficult to digest and, especially if introduced too early in life, may result in an allergy. Fragments of these proteins, called peptides, can have negative impacts on the brain. They can act directly on the brain by mimicking the body's own natural opioids (called endorphins), and so are sometimes called exorphins ('ex' meaning from outside). Researchers at the Autism Research Unit at Sunderland University have found increased levels of these peptides in the blood and urine of children with autism.

Exorphin peptides are derived from incompletely digested proteins, particularly food containing gluten and casein.

There are many anecdotal reports of dramatic improvements in children with autism from parents who have removed casein (milk protein) and gluten (the protein in wheat, barley, rye and oats) from their diet. It is best to test for food allergies (see page 31) and work with a nutritional therapist to identify, and then slowly remove, potential allergens.

5. Improve the digestion

Many parents of children with autism report that their child received repeated or prolonged courses of antibiotic drugs for ear or respiratory infections during their first year, before the diagnosis of autism. The gut is strongly linked to the brain, and changes in gut integrity, which is maintained by having a healthy balance of gut bacteria and sufficient nutrients, such as vitamin A (retinol), may have repercussions on brain function. Broad-spectrum antibiotics kill good as well as bad bacteria in the gut and can exacerbate bowel irregularities.

A lack of sufficient zinc and vitamin B_6, both of which are essential for the production of stomach acid and for protein digestion, may also contribute towards poor digestion.

To help restore and maintain a healthy gut, take a digestive enzyme supplement with probiotics to restore the balance of good gut bacteria. For those with gut problems, 1 teaspoon of glutamine powder in a glass of cold water, taken last thing at night on an empty stomach, helps to improve gut integrity and thus reduce allergic sensitivity.

Best foods

- Oily fish (salmon, mackerel, herring, kippers, sardines)
- Fresh fruit
- Vegetables
- Nuts and seeds
- Beans (pulses)
- Whole, gluten-free grains, such as rice, quinoa

Worst foods

- Gluten- and gliadin-rich grains (wheat, rye, barley, oats*)
- Dairy products
- Sugar

*Oats are rarely a problem, but are best excluded during the first month of a trial gluten-free diet.

Best supplements

- 2 × high-potency multivitamin–minerals providing at least 20mg of vitamin B_6, 10mg of zinc and 100mg of magnesium
- 2 × vitamin C 500mg
- Cod liver oil (rich in vitamin A) 500–2,000mcg and omega-3 EPA 300–500mg
- Digestive enzymes and probiotics with each meal (some supplements contain both)

Optional

1 teaspoon glutamine powder in a glass of cold water before bed on an empty stomach (for one month only). These amounts are appropriate for children from the ages of 8 to 14. For younger and older children, scale down or up the nutrient levels accordingly, or as guided by the supplement instructions of your nutritional therapist. As a rough guide, for younger children, give half the dose.

CAUTIONS

Children with autism are often almost addicted to allergy-provoking foods, so their removal can be tricky. It is best to work with a nutritional therapist when testing and removing potential food allergens, and to ensure the allergy-free diet is nutritionally balanced.

Very rarely, a child will become over-stimulated by glutamine powder. If this happens, stop giving them glutamine.

DIG DEEPER

To find out more on this subject, read *Optimum Nutrition for the Mind* or *Optimum Nutrition for Your Child* (Patrick Holford and Deborah Colson), which include key referenced studies.

BIPOLAR DISORDER

General information

Bipolar disorder, previously called manic depression, is characterised by episodes of deep depression followed by mania. The depression phase responds best to nutritional therapy. Exactly why a person has phases of mania is not known, although they are linked to hyper-stressed states. It is important, during those phases, to ensure that the person has enough sleep (see Insomnia on page 236) and keeps stress levels low (see Chapter 6, Part 2). It is not uncommon for depression to be misdiagnosed as bipolar, allowing for the prescription of anti-psychotic drugs, which can be extremely difficult to stop taking. (Due to the overlap with depression, see also the recommendations for Depression on page 132.)

Good medicine solutions

1. Increase your omega-3 intake

The richest dietary source of omega-3 fats is from fish, specifically carnivorous cold-water fish, such as salmon, mackerel and herring. A lower intake of fish is linked to a higher risk of bipolar disorder.

In one of the first trials of an omega-3 fish oil supplement, high in eicosapentaenoic acid (EPA), Dr Andrew Stoll from Harvard Medical School gave 40 bipolar patients in the depressive phase either omega-3 supplements or a placebo and found a highly significant improvement in the former group. A more recent trial gave an EPA supplement or a placebo to 26 people with bipolar disorder and again found a significant improvement in the EPA group.

EPA appears have the most potent antidepressant effect of all omega-3 fats. Most trials show an effect when given 1,000mg of EPA a day. Fish oil supplements vary in the amount of EPA they contain, with the most potent providing about 500mg per capsule, so you'll need at least two a day for a therapeutic effect.

A serving – 100g (3½oz) – of oily fish (salmon, mackerel, herring, kippers, sardines) provides about 500mg of EPA. If you eat oily fish three times a week and supplement at least 600mg of EPA, perhaps in two fish oil supplements, that provides a daily average of 1,000mg.

2. Balance your blood sugar

There is a direct link between mood and blood sugar balance. All carbohydrate foods are broken down into glucose, and your brain runs on glucose. The more uneven your blood sugar supply, the more uneven your mood. This is why it's absolutely essential to eat a low-GL diet to help even out mood and energy. This is especially important during a manic phase, at which time it is also important to avoid stimulants such as caffeine and nicotine which, together with sugar, are a recipe for fluctuating mood. (See Chapter 1, Part 2 for details on how to follow a low-GL diet. Also, see Depression on page 134 to find out about the potential benefit of supplementing chromium, if you have the symptoms of 'atypical' depression.)

3. Increase your intake of magnesium

Magnesium is a mineral that helps to maintain normal muscle and brain function. Some indications of magnesium deficiency are: muscle tremors or spasm, muscle weakness, insomnia or nervousness, high blood pressure, irregular heartbeat, fits or convulsions, hyperactivity and depression. Magnesium is interesting in bipolar disorder because of its chemical similarity to lithium (the drug most commonly used as a mood stabiliser). In fact, there is some evidence that lithium may attach to the same receptor sites in the brain, producing a calming effect. Studies have found that people with bipolar disorder tend to have lower levels of magnesium and that giving them magnesium improved their symptoms or reduced the frequency of their manic phases. Magnesium also helps to support good sleeping patterns.

Foods rich in magnesium include greens, seeds and nuts. Almonds, chia seeds and pumpkin seeds are particularly good sources; however, I recommend supplementing 300mg of magnesium every day if you have bipolar disorder, in both the depressed and manic phases.

Best foods

- Oily fish (salmon, mackerel, herring, kippers, sardines)
- Chia seeds
- Almonds
- Pumpkin seeds
- Green vegetables

Worst foods

- Sugar
- Caffeinated drinks
- Alcohol

Best supplements

- 2 × high-potency multivitamin–minerals providing 100mg of magnesium
- 2 × vitamin C 1,000mg
- 2 × magnesium 100mg (giving a total of 300mg with your multivitamin)
- 2 × high-potency omega-3-rich fish oil capsules (giving about 600mg of EPA, or EPA, plus DPA)

CAUTIONS

Don't change your medication without speaking to your doctor or health-care provider.

DIG DEEPER

To find out more on this subject, read *The Feel Good Factor* (Patrick Holford), which includes key referenced studies.

BLOATING

see **IRRITABLE BOWEL SYNDROME (IBS)**

BREAST CANCER

General information

As well as following the general advice for Cancer (see page 74), there are some dietary factors that specifically relate to breast cancer.

Good medicine solutions

1. Control the factors that stimulate growth

Cancer cell growth is influenced by hormones and growth factors. Eating too much sugar and refined carbohydrates promotes high insulin levels, which stimulate the growth of breast cells. High-sugar diets also lead to weight gain – another risk factor for breast cancer. Both healthy and cancerous breast cells have receptors for insulin. Once insulin has attached to the receptor, it encourages the cell to divide and multiply, encouraging the tumour to grow. Losing weight and eating less sugar can make a big difference to breast cancer survival, as does taking regular exercise and staying relaxed. The best way to lose weight is to follow a low-GL diet. Essentially, that means: (a) eating plenty of complex, unrefined carbohydrates, such as whole grains (oats, brown rice, barley, wholegrain bread and pasta, millet), pulses (lentils, soya beans, kidney beans, and so on) and lots of vegetables; (b) you should always combine carbohydrates with protein, for example by eating fish with brown rice, or an apple with some almonds; and (c) cut out all refined carbohydrates, such as white bread, white pasta and rice, cakes, biscuits, sweets and any foods containing added sugar. (See Chapter 1, Part 2 for details on how to follow a low-GL diet.)

Another major promoter of insulin, which is strongly linked to breast cancer, is milk. Milk is naturally high in oestrogen, as well as growth factors such as insulin-like growth factor (IGF-1). IGF-1 has been found to directly stimulate the growth of cancer cells. It also stops overgrowing cells from committing suicide (called apoptosis). If you have breast cancer, I recommend the complete avoidance of dairy products. If you don't have cancer, keep your intake of dairy products low; that is, below 300ml (10fl oz/½ pint) a day and ideally less than 1.2 litres (2 pints) a week. Try rice milk, oat milk or soya milk instead. I would also recommend avoiding red meat.

Other growth promoters can come from excess hormone disruptors, which are carcinogens found in some pesticides, cosmetics and cleaning products. Follow the guidelines given for the general Cancer advice (page 74) to see how to switch to alternatives.

2. Increase your intake of phytoestrogens

Phytoestrogens in beans, especially soya beans, but also in chick-peas, lentils, nuts, seeds and rye, help to block oestrogen receptors from powerful hormone-disrupting chemicals that mimic oestrogen, such as PCBs, dioxins and some pesticides. Much attention has focused on soya due to its high levels of phytoestrogens; however, the other pulses mentioned above have high levels too. Eat at least some beans, lentils, rye, alfalfa, raw nuts or seeds every day. When you do have soya, try fermented soya products such as miso, natto or tempeh. Fermenting breaks down digestion inhibitors, making the protective components (isoflavones) more available. Of the seeds, flax and pumpkin are the best anti-cancer types.

I recommend you aim for about 15,000mcg (15mg) of phyto-estrogens a day. This is easily achieved by having a small portion of tofu: a 100g (3½oz) serving provides 78,000mcg. Alternatively, a 100ml (3½fl oz) glass of soya milk or soya yoghurt provides 11,000mcg and a portion of chickpeas, perhaps prepared as hummus, contains 2,000mcg. Supplements of isoflavones made from fermented soya are another option.

The liver is the main organ responsible for removing excess hormones from the body. Eating cruciferous vegetables (including broccoli, kale, cabbage, cauliflower and Brussels sprouts), which are rich in di-indolylmethane (DIM), helps the liver to do this. Growth hormones stop cancer cells from committing suicide; DIM switches this suicide signal back on. Making cruciferous vegetables part of your daily diet, therefore, is essential. You might also think about boosting your levels of DIM by taking supplements.

3. Increase your intake of vitamin D

Numerous studies show an association between higher levels of vitamin D and a lower risk of developing and/or surviving cancer. It has long been known that women who live in sunnier countries are less likely to develop breast cancer than women who see little sunshine, but it has also been found that women who develop cancer but who also have high levels of vitamin D are more likely to survive it. Interestingly, a high-meat-protein diet and high-calcium diet, which is what you get from dairy products, blocks the ability to create active vitamin D. Testing for vitamin D levels is the only way we can really know how much we have in our bodies. Family doctors will often test for this, and there are home test kits available, or you could visit a nutritional therapist who can do it for you.

There are three ways to increase your blood level of vitamin D: eat it, supplement it or expose yourself to sunlight. The best dietary sources are oily fish and eggs, but to reach optimum levels you'll need to supplement, especially if you are not exposed to much sunlight. Better-quality high-potency multivitamin–minerals should give you 600iu (15mcg). During the winter months this is certainly not enough, so it's worth supplementing an additional 1,000iu (25mcg), and possibly more.

4. Take high-dose vitamin C and salvestrols

Also consider taking high-dose vitamin C and salvestrols. (See Cancer on page 74 for more on this.)

Best foods

- Whole grains (oats, brown rice, barley, wholegrain bread and pasta, millet)
- Beans (lentils, soya beans, kidney beans, chickpeas)
- Fermented soya products (miso, natto, tempeh)
- Cruciferous vegetables (broccoli, Brussels sprouts, cabbage, cauliflower, kale)

Worst foods

- Sugar
- Alcohol (strongly linked to cancer)
- Red meat and dairy

Best supplements

- 2 × high-potency multivitamin–minerals
- 2 × high-potency omega-3-rich fish oil capsules (choose products with the most EPA)
- 5,000mg or more vitamin C
- 2 × antioxidant complex (containing beta-carotene, vitamin E and selenium, plus other antioxidant nutrients, such as glutathione, alpha lipoic acid, co-enzyme Q_{10} (CoQ_{10}) and resveratrol)
- 2 × salvestrol 2,000 units for recovery; 350 units for prevention
- 1 × 1,000iu (25mcg) vitamin D

CAUTIONS

Many chemotherapeutic drugs are oxidants. It may therefore not be a good idea to take lots of antioxidants while undergoing certain types of chemotherapy. (Vitamin C in high doses acts as a pro-oxidant, so it should not interfere.) Please check with your oncologist if you are undergoing chemotherapy.

It is wise to seek the advice of a nutritional therapist if you wish to undertake an extensive nutritional strategy.

CANCER

Good medicine solutions

In most cases, cancer is caused by not just one factor but a number of factors. For prevention to be effective, then, it has to respect the fact that the cancer process is multi-factorial. If a person has cancer, or early stage cancer risk, such as pre-cancerous cells, these prevention factors have to be applied more aggressively; for example, by using higher amounts of anti-cancer nutrients and practising strict avoidance of all cancer growth promoters such as dairy products.

If you are currently receiving cancer treatment, please check whether any additional supplements, as recommended here, are incompatible with that treatment. It is also best to get advice from a nutritional therapist, because different cancers have different causative factors to consider. The following general advice is also useful for anyone wanting to minimise their risk.

1. Reduce your exposure to carcinogens

There is no doubt that a significant contributor to cancer is our increased exposure to carcinogens. Although it is impossible to avoid them all, there are many changes you can make to your diet and lifestyle that can substantially decrease your exposure. For many factors, such as smoking, the necessary action is clear: don't! With food carcinogens, eating organic foods instantly minimises your exposure to herbicides and pesticides. I would also avoid processed meats (sausages, ham, smoked foods and bacon), which can contain nitrates. Any burned or browned food – which means the food has been oxidised – adds to the carcinogenic load of the meal. This applies as much to fast food, such as French fries, charred burgers, fried fish and crispy pizzas. The reality is that anything crispy, browned or burned, or cooked or processed using high heat, may be bad for you. The bottom line is to eat more raw foods and steam-fry (where you cook in a very small amount of oil plus a little stock) or boil food, rather than using high-heat cooking.

What is more, I recommend minimising your intake of any fatty foods exposed to soft plastics, including packaged meals. This is because some chemicals that keep plastics flexible easily pass out of the plastic into fatty food, such as cheese.

Other powerful carcinogens come from pollution, for example from traffic, radiation, and even what we put on our skin or use in the home. Regarding your exposure to radiation, there are naturally occurring radioactive materials in the air, our food and water. The more forms of radiation we are exposed to (for example, from the sun or mobile phones), the more free radicals are likely to be generated that can harm body cells. Apart from the effects of sunlight, the largest natural source of radiation is radon, a naturally occurring gas, present in some areas because of their underlying geology. If you suspect you live in a high-radon area, check with your local environmental health office and make sure your house is well ventilated.

Sunlight is necessary for 30 minutes per day, but avoid long exposure with unprotected skin. With respect to cosmetics and cleaning products, many health-food shops stock alternatives that are less chemical-laden than those generally on sale.

2. Increase your intake of antioxidants

Antioxidants are substances that remove or disarm potentially damaging oxidising agents in the body, which are created like 'exhaust fumes' when our cells turn food into energy. Of all the dietary factors, increasing your intake of fruit and vegetables provides the greatest protection from cancer – and certain foods appear to be especially protective. Among these are carrots; some studies have indicated that eating the equivalent of one carrot a day could cut cancer risk by a third. Tomatoes share similar properties to carrots – both are high in antioxidant nutrients.

Most research has been carried out on the amount of vitamins A, C and E in foods. Although these are important in treating cancer, there are literally hundreds of active compounds in plants, collectively known as phytonutrients. Many of these active compounds are cancer-protective antioxidants.

Others, such as salvestrols, harness the power of nature's defence mechanisms. The key feature of salvestrols is that they are initially inert. They are activated only inside the cancer cells, which they arrest or kill. Although some salvestrols can be obtained by eating lots of organic fruit and vegetables, extra virgin olive oils and unfiltered juices, it is difficult to get enough from diet alone. Since the salvestrol concentration in foods varies enormously, to obtain higher amounts you will need to take supplements. This could be as an antioxidant formula containing salvestrols in the form of resveratrol, or a vitamin C supplement containing black elderberry and bilberry extracts – both are rich sources. If you have cancer, however, you may benefit from higher therapeutic doses of salvestrols.

Phytonutrients are especially helpful in countering oxidant, or free-radical, damage in the body. Generally speaking, where you find the most colour and flavour in a food (such as blueberries, raspberries and strawberries) you will also find the highest antioxidant levels. Eat plenty of fruit and vegetables – seven or more servings a day and organic whenever possible. Heating destroys antioxidants, so aim to eat mostly raw, or lightly cooked or steamed. In addition, an all-round antioxidant supplement may be appropriate for people with cancer. (How to increase your intake of antioxidants is explained in more detail in Chapter 2, Part 2.)

3. Improve your liver's detoxification potential

One of your key lines of defence is your own body's ability to detoxify harmful chemicals. If your liver is compromised, either as a result of over-exposure to toxins or due to an underlying imbalance, this makes you more sensitive to carcinogens. Avoid alcohol, sugar and processed and deep-fried food as much as possible. The better your diet and intake of antioxidant nutrients and fibre, the more efficient your liver will be. Particularly important are the liver-friendly foods, such as onions, garlic, artichokes, watercress and rocket.

Garlic is especially important. Not only does it help to protect against the formation of tumours, including metastases, but it also inhibits the growth of established tumours, strengthening the immune system and detoxifying the liver. These effects can be achieved by eating a garlic clove or two a day. Cooking decreases the potency of the garlic, so it's even better to crush and stir in just before serving. If you really don't like the taste or smell, you can take a garlic capsule instead.

Other liver helpers are di-indolylmethane (DIM) and indole-3-carbonol (I3C), the substances in cruciferous vegetables that help to detoxify excess oestrogens and hormone-disrupting chemicals, such as PCBs and dioxins, as well as some herbicides and pesticides. I recommend a serving of cruciferous vegetables daily – these include broccoli, Brussels sprouts, cabbage, cauliflower, kale, radish and mustard. Turmeric has been shown to inhibit the growth of cancer. It also disarms a wide range of carcinogens. Adding this spice to your food helps both your liver and your immune system.

4. Boost your immune system

It is the immune system's job to identify pre-cancerous cells and put them out of action. If a person's immune system is weak, cancerous cells can multiply. Certain things have a suppressive effect on the immune system, including cigarettes, sugar, coffee, alcohol, stress, a negative attitude, and a lack of sleep and natural sunlight. Stress, sugar and stimulants not only suppress the immune system but they also rob the body of B vitamins, which are vital for activating your immune defences. As well as B vitamins, the immune system depends on a whole host of nutrients. Most important are vitamins A, C, D and E, selenium and zinc.

Vitamin C, in high doses, is supported by good evidence for preventing cancer. An intake of above 5,000mg a day (the equivalent of 100 oranges) substantially increases the life expectancy of cancer patients. Whereas supplementing 1–5g vitamin C may be helpful to take to prevent some cancers, those who have cancer are most likely to benefit from 10g or more a day. These higher levels are best taken with the guidance of your health-care practitioner. The best way to do this is to buy pure ascorbic acid (vitamin C) powder, dissolve it in some juice and water, and drink it throughout the day, thereby keeping the body permanently saturated in this powerful immune-boosting nutrient. An alternative way of achieving very high levels is through intravenous vitamin C therapy. A number of cancer specialists are providing this (see Resources).

Vitamin D is also vital for strong immunity. People living in the northern hemisphere are almost all deficient, especially in winter, since vitamin D is made in the skin in the presence of sunlight. The best dietary sources are oily fish and eggs, but to reach optimum levels you'll need to supplement. Better-quality high-potency multivitamin–minerals should give you 600iu (15mcg) but I recommend supplementing an additional 1,000iu (25mcg) and possibly more. As well as vitamins, other powerful immune-boosters are mushrooms: reishi, shiitake and maitake have all been shown to have anti-cancer effects. All these mushrooms are also available as powders. Many are also included in natural remedies designed to support healthy immunity. Shiitake mushrooms are also sold fresh or dried in most supermarkets. They are delicious and, as a regular part of your diet, will add to your immune strength. Often used in conjunction with these mushrooms is the herb astragulus, which has been well proven to increase immune function and protect from radiation and harmful chemicals, including chemotherapy.

5. Take salvestrols

The holy grail of chemotherapy has been to find a way of targeting only cancer cells, leaving healthy cells untouched. More than a decade ago it was discovered that cancer cells have an active enzyme, called CYP_1B_1 (pronounced sip-one-B-one), which differentiates cancer cells from healthy cells. The discovery that many plants contain compounds called salvestrols, which are converted by the CYP_1B_1 enzyme into a compound that kills cancer cells, is a major conceptual breakthrough for cancer treatment. By flooding the body with harmless salvestrols, theoretically, cancer cells should self-destruct.

This is exactly what happens in the laboratory when you expose cancer cells to salvestrols. Although we lack human clinical trials, more and more cases of successful cancer treatment are being reported with high-dose salvestrols (see Resources). (Salvestrols are measured in relation to their comparative effect against cancer cells, in points, rather than in milligrams.)

The discovery of CYP_1B_1 also opens up another possibility: CYP_1B_1 blood tests to screen for the presence of cancer cells before a cancer mass is detected. This would then be a strong indication for high-dose salvestrol treatment.

6. Lower inflammation

Inflammation is a key component of tumour progression. Cancer needs inflammation to grow. A pro-inflammatory diet can lead to cell damage and DNA mutations. It is best to reduce your intake of inflammatory saturated fats (principally from meat and dairy products) and processed or damaged fat (from fried and processed foods). Ideally, avoid dairy altogether, if you have cancer. The fat in meat, if burned, generates powerful oxidants and carcinogens. If you are going to eat red meat, limit your intake to a maximum of 300g (11oz) a week, which equates to two small servings twice a week (roughly the amount that would fit into the palm of your hand). Choose organic lean meat, especially game, and avoid burned and processed meat, whether grilled, fried or barbecued.

There is growing evidence that an increased intake of omega-3 fats may reduce the risk of cancer. It is well documented that these fats help to reduce inflammation, and it is thought that they prevent the expression of genes that promote cancer. Those omega-3s derived from fish oils appear to be the most protective. Fish is also a rich source of many nutrients, including vitamin B_{12}, selenium, zinc and vitamin D, all of which have anti-cancer properties. The best sources are salmon, mackerel, herring including kippers, sardines and anchovies. Vegetarian sources include seeds (chia, flax, pumpkin) and nuts (walnuts) or their cold-pressed oils.

Meat and dairy are bad news, not just because of their inflammatory properties but also because they contain growth factors. Two key growth factors for cancer cells are oestrogen and IGF-1 (insulin-like growth factor). IGF-1 is made in the body, but it is also found in milk. Another key growth promoter is too much insulin. Eating too much sugar and refined carbohydrates promotes high insulin levels, which stimulate the growth of cancer cells. High-sugar diets also lead to weight gain – another risk factor for cancer. (See Chapter 1, Part 2 for details on how to follow a low-GL diet.)

Best foods

- Brightly coloured fruit and vegetables (cherries, berries, beetroot, carrots, tomatoes)
- Cruciferous vegetables (broccoli, Brussels sprouts, cabbage, cauliflower, kale, radish, mustard)
- Turmeric
- Garlic
- Oily fish (salmon, mackerel, herring, kippers, sardines)
- Shiitake, reishi and maitake mushrooms

Worst foods

- Alcohol
- Sugar
- Meat and dairy

Best supplements

- 2 × high-potency multivitamin–minerals
- 2 × high-potency omega-3-rich fish oil capsules (choose products with the most EPA)
- 5,000mg or more vitamin C (ascorbic acid powder)
- 1 × antioxidant complex (containing beta-carotene, vitamin E, and selenium, plus other antioxidant nutrients, such as glutathione, alpha lipoic acid, co-enzyme Q_{10} and resveratrol)
- 1 × 1,000iu (25mcg) vitamin D
- 2 × salvestrol 2,000 units for recovery; 350 units for protection

> **CAUTIONS**
>
> It is wise to seek the advice of a nutritional therapist if you
> wish to undertake an extensive nutritional strategy so that it
> can be tailored to your particular kind of cancer.
>
> Many chemotherapeutic drugs are oxidants. It may
> therefore not be a good idea to take lots of antioxidants
> while undergoing certain types of chemotherapy. (Vitamin
> C in high doses acts as a pro-oxidant, so it should not
> interfere.) Please check with your oncologist if you are
> undergoing chemotherapy.

CANDIDA/THRUSH

General information

One of the most common gut infections of all is an overgrowth
of a kind of yeast called *Candida albicans*. The infection is technically called candidiasis. This is what is meant by a yeast infection.
The name *Candida albicans* means 'sweet and white', suggesting something delicate and pure, but in reality *C. albicans* is a
minute microbe, a yeast, which multiplies, migrates and releases
toxins. All of us have some *Candida* present as part of a normal
balanced gut ecology; however, when it overgrows, it can afflict
us with countless symptoms, both physical and mental: bowel
problems, allergies, extreme fatigue, hormone dysfunction, skin
complaints, joint and muscle pain, thrush, infections and emotional disorders, many of which mimic other diseases and are
frequently misdiagnosed.

To find out whether you are likely to have *Candida* you can
complete an online checklist (see Resources). If you find you have
a high score, you should see your health-care practitioner who can

run a diagnostic test for it. A reliable test is the *Candida* antibody test (saliva or blood tests for IgG and IgA antibodies). It is important to confirm that you do have candidiasis before following a restrictive anti-*Candida* diet as recommended in the next section.

Good medicine solutions

1. Follow an anti-*Candida* diet

The aim of an anti-*Candida* diet is to cut off the *Candida*'s sugar supply. This should quickly improve your digestive symptoms and will stop fuelling the *Candida*'s growth. All forms of sugar must be strictly avoided, including lactose (milk sugar), malt and fructose (fruit sugar). Refined carbohydrates add to the glucose load in the body, so it is essential to use only wholegrain flour, rice, and so on. The simplest way is to follow a low-GL diet, as this ensures that you will omit sugar and eat only slow-releasing complex carbohydrates. (See Chapter 1, Part 2 for details on how to follow a low-GL diet.)

Other substances to be avoided are yeast (bread, gravy mixes, spreads), fermented products (alcohol, vinegar), mould (cheese, mushrooms), and stimulants (tea, coffee).

Candidiasis often brings on cravings for its favourite foods; at these times steely determination is needed to keep to the diet. Even when *Candida*-related symptoms have completely disappeared, the diet should be maintained for several months to consolidate the newly corrected balance of gut flora. Before long, a 'sweet tooth' disappears, making it easier to stay on a sugar-free diet. I recommend you read Erica White's *Beat Candida Cookbook* for recipes, which shows that mealtimes can still be an enjoyable experience.

2. Take immune-boosting supplements

A supplement programme is important to boost your immune system so that it can play its role in keeping the *Candida* under control. It is also important to correct imbalances in blood sugar and to detoxify the body, because *Candida* generates its own toxins. This means increasing vitamin C and other antioxidants. I also recommend you take an all-round comprehensive supplement programme, plus a supplement specifically designed to improve digestion, with both enzymes and probiotics and, ideally, glutamine – an amino acid that helps heal the gut – during the first month.

3. Take anti-fungal supplements

As surprising as it may sound, one of the best supplements to tackle *Candida* is itself a yeast, called *Saccharomyces boulardii*. It's a non-colonising yeast, which means that it will never take up residence in your gut. As it passes through, it stimulates your gut's production of an immune component called secretory immunoglobulinA (SIgA). Greater amounts of this immunoglobulin make it increasingly difficult for the *Candida* to stick to your gut wall. Some people with *Candida* may be hypersensitive to all yeast, including *S. boulardii*, so taking it could make you feel worse. In which case, you should wait until you've cut all yeast out of your diet for about four weeks to reduce your hypersensitivity and then introduce the *S. boulardii* at very low doses and increase very gradually. This may mean starting with as little as 1 billion organisms (½ capsule) once daily before building up to the full dose of about 10 billion organisms a day. *S. boulardii* also helps to make the environment of your gut more hospitable to friendly bacteria, thereby enhancing their chances of taking up residence.

Other effective anti-*Candida* agents are caprylic acid (a fatty acid that occurs naturally in coconuts), oregano and olive leaf extract. These additional anti-fungal supplements work directly to kill off *Candida* overgrowth. They can be taken while you are taking the *S. boulardii*, but should be taken several hours apart so as not to kill off the *S. boulardii* as well. It's generally best not to start any of these additional supplements until you've been on the anti-*Candida* diet and have been taking the *S. boulardii* for about a month in order to minimise the 'die-off' reaction (see below).

Caprylic acid is one of the most useful anti-fungal agents. Its great advantage is that it does not kill off your friendly gut flora. When taken as calcium/magnesium caprylate, it survives the digestive processes and is able to reach the colon, where the *Candida* resides.

Oregano oil is another excellent anti-fungal agent. It also has the advantage of crossing the gut wall into the body, so it may be the better choice if you have fungal symptoms elsewhere in the body, such as athlete's foot.

Olive leaf contains an active ingredient named oleuropein, which helps to kill *Candida*. It is also an antioxidant.

Artemisia is a herb with broad-spectrum anti-fungal properties, which is useful against a wide variety of pathogens without disturbing friendly flora. If you have a high score on the *Candida* questionnaire and a history of illness that originated in a hot climate, these are sufficient reasons to suspect you may have a parasite other than *Candida* and to use a broad-spectrum anti-fungal agent such as artemisia.

4. Re-inoculate the gut with probiotics

Supplements are needed to carry the beneficial bacteria into the intestines and re-establish a colony of healthy bacteria. The role of these bacteria is to increase acidity by producing lactic acid and acetic acid, and to inhibit undesirable micro-organisms that would compete with them for space.

Lactobacillus acidophilus is the major coloniser of the small intestine and *Bifidobacterium bifidum* inhabits the large intestine and vagina; *B. bifidum* also produces B vitamins. Other helpful bacteria are the transient *Lactobacillus bulgaricus* and

Streptococcus thermophilus, which also produce lactic acid as they pass through the bowel. These friendly bacteria are contained in yoghurt, which is therefore a helpful food provided you don't have an intolerance to dairy foods. In yoghurt, the lactose (milk sugar) content has largely been converted into lactic acid by enzyme-producing bifidobacteria, which accounts for the sharpness of its taste.

To ensure safe passage of these bacteria through the gastric juices, it is necessary to take them in a capsule supplying large numbers of viable organisms in freeze-dried form. Two capsules should be taken daily, at breakfast and dinner.

An acidophilus cream is a beneficial aid for a vaginal fungal infection.

5. Deal with die-off

Thriving *Candida* releases a minimum of 79 known toxins. Dead and dying *Candida* releases even more. A general feeling of toxicity includes aching muscles, fuzzy head, depression, anxiety, nausea and diarrhoea. In specific areas where *Candida* has colonised, there can be an apparent flare-up of old symptoms, such as a sore throat, thrush, painful joints, eczema, and so on. This unpleasant situation is known as 'die-off', or formally as Herxheimer's reaction.

The art is to destroy *Candida* slowly but surely, so that it is not being killed off faster than the body can eliminate the toxins. Initial die-off is usually triggered by the diet, and by vitamins and minerals as they boost the immune system to fight it. These first two points of the four-point plan usually cause more than enough die-off for most people to cope with, and anti-fungal agents should not be added to the regime until this phase is over. By the end of a month, the majority of people claim that they feel better than they have for years! This is the time to add the anti-fungal and probiotic supplements to the programme.

Most people on caprylic acid should be able to start with one medium-strength capsule (about 400mg) daily, without too much difficulty. If, after five days, you are not battling with die-off symptoms, the dose can be increased to 400mg × 2, and so on, up to 6 capsules daily. After this, you can graduate to a higher-strength capsule (about 700mg) three times daily and increase again if necessary.

The climb up is seldom straightforward, however, and at some stage there might come a surge of die-off reaction necessitating a drop to a lower level, or even a complete break, while the body eliminates the toxins. This should not be regarded as a setback, but simply as a necessary part of the process. Drinking plenty of fluid and taking good levels of vitamin C and the B vitamins will speed up detoxification. Eventually, caprylic acid will accomplish its job. You can monitor this by rescoring yourself on the *Candida* check mentioned on page 449.

Best foods

- Vegetables
- Fish
- Nuts, seeds, beans (pulses)
- Whole grains

Worst foods

- Sugar
- All fast-releasing carbohydrates
- Yeast-rich and fermented foods (bread, gravy mixes, yeast-based spreads, alcohol, vinegar)

Best supplements

- 2 × high-potency multivitamin–minerals with antioxidants, providing at least 10mcg of vitamin D, 10mg of zinc, plus B vitamins and antioxidants

- 2 × vitamin C 1,000mg

- 1 × digestive enzymes, probiotics and glutamine capsule with each meal

- 1–5 × *Saccharomyces boulardii* (1 billion viable organisms)

- 2 × Acidophilus and bifidobacteria (5 billion viable organisms), taken twice a day away from the following anti-fungal agents:

    1–6 × caprylic acid 400mg

    Or/and 2–6 drops of oregano oil

    Or/and 2–6 olive leaf extract 500mg (20 per cent oleuropein)

    Or/and 2–4 capsules of artemisia (350mg), or 10–20 drops of artemisia extract

---

CAUTIONS

Don't follow this restrictive diet unless you've been clinically tested to confirm candidiasis. Insufficient quantities of the anti-*Candida* agents will be ineffective but too much can make you feel worse while the *Candida* dies off. It is best to follow the suggestions above under the supervision of a nutritional therapist who can advise you on the correct supplements to take at each stage of your recovery.

CHRONIC FATIGUE

General information

There are many potential causes of feeling tired for much of the time. These include nutritional deficiencies (for example, a lack of B vitamins), blood sugar problems and adrenal fatigue as a consequence of prolonged stress. All these potential contributors should be explored and corrected. True chronic fatigue syndrome (CFS) is something different. People with CFS often talk about becoming exhausted after eating, rather than energised, and after exercise or any mildly strenuous activity. This is often due to liver detoxification issues (explained below).

Good medicine solutions

1. Balance your blood sugar

The most common cause of general fatigue is blood sugar problems, or a lack of nutrients, especially the B vitamins and vitamin C, which are vital for converting food into energy. If you experience pronounced energy dips when you haven't eaten, and you crave sweet foods, it is particularly important to start following a low-GL diet and to supplement a good-quality, high-potency multivitamin–mineral, with extra vitamin C. (See Chapter 1, Part 2 for details on how to follow a low-GL diet.)

Another condition associated with blood sugar problems is adrenal fatigue, which is often linked to the overuse of stimulants. Reducing your stress levels is also an important step in combating fatigue (see Chapter 6, Part 2).

A nutritional therapist can check for adrenal fatigue by running a stress hormone test that measures levels of adrenal hormones in saliva over a 24-hour period.

2. Check your thyroid

Another common cause of CFS is an underactive thyroid gland, which produces the hormone thyroxine – vital for keeping good energy levels. The classic symptoms are fatigue, low sex drive, low body temperature, weight gain, poor memory, dry skin and constipation. Your thyroid function can be tested by your doctor. For nutritional advice on how to improve thyroid function see Underactive Thyroid on page 371.

3. Check for digestion problems or hidden food allergies

Many CFS sufferers complain of digestion-related problems, such as bloating, indigestion and abdominal pain. Often CFS relates to poor liver detoxification (see below), but such problems usually start in the gut, which is the barrier between your food and your bloodstream. The epithelial cells that make up your digestive tract form a barrier that is less than half the thickness of a piece of paper. This barrier is easily damaged by alcohol, food allergens and antibiotics, but most of all by painkillers, of which the average person takes 373 a year!

As a consequence, incompletely digested food particles can cross the barrier. When this happens, the immune system reacts, resulting in the development of a food intolerance or allergy. If your CFS comes and goes, or improves when you are eating a very different diet, perhaps on holiday abroad, it may be that you have developed hidden food allergies or intolerances. This is something worth checking for. How to do this is explained in Allergies on page 31.

In the meantime, it is worth supplementing a combination of digestive enzymes, which help to break down your food completely, plus beneficial bacteria to re-inoculate the gut, and glutamine, which helps to repair and rejuvenate healthy epithelial cells in the gut wall, thus reducing your allergic potential.

Increased intestinal permeability, also known as 'leaky gut syndrome', can be tested by drinking a test substance and collecting a urine sample. A nutritional therapist can arrange this for you. The more permeable the intestinal wall, the more work the liver has to do in detoxifying the blood. The remedy for leaky gut syndrome is to remove food allergens and to supplement glutamine, taken as a powder, one to two teaspoons (4–8g) a day in cold water on an empty stomach.

Another common cause of CFS and digestive problems is an overgrowth of the *Candida albicans* yeast, known as candidiasis. (See *Candida*/Thrush on page 82 to see if this fits with your symptoms.)

4. Check your liver detoxification potential

Poor liver detoxification is a common cause of fatigue, because the liver has to break down and dispose of the by-products, or the 'exhaust fumes', of our normal metabolism, as well as any other toxic substances we consume. You can get a good indication of your detox potential from your 'detox' score when you complete my 100% Health Check online (see Resources).

Alternatively, complete the following detox check below.

Score one point for every symptom you occasionally have, and two for those you have frequently.

Head – headaches, faintness, dizziness, insomnia.

Eyes – watery or itchy eyes, swollen, red or sticky eyelids, bags or dark circles, blurred vision.

Ears – itchy ears, earache, ear infection, drainage from ear, ringing in ears, hearing loss.

Nose – stuffy nose, sinus problems, hay fever, sneezing attacks, excessive mucus formation.

Mouth – chronic coughing, gagging, frequent need to clear throat, hoarseness, loss of voice, swollen or discoloured tongue, gums or lips, canker sores.

Skin – acne, hives, rashes, dry skin, hair loss, flushing or hot flashes, excessive sweating.

Digestion Nausea or vomiting, diarrhoea, constipation, a bloated feeling, belching, passing gas, heartburn, intestinal/stomach pain.

Heart Irregular or skipped heartbeat, rapid or pounding heartbeat, chest pain.

Lungs Chest congestion, asthma, bronchitis, shortness of breath, difficulty breathing.

Joints/muscles Joint/muscle aches or pain, arthritis, stiffness or limitation of movement, feeling of weakness or tiredness.

Weight Binge eating/drinking, craving certain foods, excessive weight, compulsive eating, water retention, underweight.

Energy Fatigue, sluggishness, apathy, lethargy, hyperactivity, restlessness.

Mind Poor memory, confusion, poor comprehension, poor concentration, poor physical coordination, difficulty in making decisions, stuttering or stammering, slurred speech, learning disabilities.

Emotions Mood swings, anxiety, fear, nervousness, anger, irritability, aggressiveness, depression.

Score:

Above 25: suspect a detox problem and clean up your diet.

Above 50: your detox potential is under par.

Above 75: you are well advised to seek the help of a nutritional therapist.

Some people with CFS are 'pathological detoxifiers'. This means that the first phase of liver detoxification works very well, but the second phase doesn't. For these people, taking lots of antioxidants – which largely drive the first phase – can make matters worse. Feeling worse after taking supplements can be a sign of liver detoxification problems, and a sign that it's worth having a liver detoxification test, which a nutritional therapist can also arrange. This involves ingesting a mixture of substances, and collecting a urine sample. By analysing what is excreted it is possible to identify which biochemical pathways are functioning properly, and which ones aren't.

The second phase of liver detoxification depends on four main processes. One is called glycine conjugation, another glutathione conjugation. These amino acids are attached to toxins (conjugation means attachment) and escorted out of the body. If they aren't working, a nutritional therapist will give you either glycine or glutathione – or N-acetyl cysteine (NAC), its precursor – to get the pathway working again.

Another critical process is called sulphation, and the highly absorbable form of sulphur, methylsulfonylmethane (MSM), helps in these cases. There is then glucoronidation, which is helped by glucosinolates, found in cruciferous vegetables. And finally there is methylation. If a person is poor at methylation (described below), their homocysteine level is high.

(Homocysteine is a toxic amino acid that can directly damage the arteries and heart.)

5. Check homocysteine and improve methylation

There are about a billion methylation reactions in your body every few seconds, and they are vital for mental and physical energy, and dependent on a host of nutrients, mainly the B vitamins; for example, your ability to make stress hormones or insulin depends on methylation. Without sufficient adrenalin or functioning insulin your energy goes down. Faulty methylation is therefore another common cause of chronic fatigue. You can test your methylation potential with a blood homocysteine test, either tested at a lab (a health-care practitioner can arrange this) or using a home test kit (see Resources). If your level is high, you'll be given a combination of homocysteine-lowering nutrients (see Chapter 4, Part 2). One not uncommon cause of raised homocysteine is vitamin B_{12} deficiency, often as a result of malabsorption of that vitamin. This is more common later in life, but some people are just very bad absorbers of B_{12} and only start to feel better when given very large supplemental amounts, or B_{12} injections.

'I used to have . . .'

Ten years ago, Amanda-Jane had a bad car accident, and her health had declined ever since. She was suffering with CFS, and had her homocysteine level checked. She was shocked when she found her result was 25.9 units (the ideal level is below 7). To address this, Amanda-Jane followed a homocysteine-lowering diet, eating lots of greens and beans, and took a supplement containing therapeutic doses of vitamins B_6, methylB_{12} and folic acid, plus tri-methyl-glycine (TMG) and zinc.

Almost immediately, her sleep improved, and within four weeks she had much more energy. Two months later, Amanda-Jane re-tested her homocysteine level and found it had dropped to 9.4 units. That's a 64 per cent decrease. Here's what she told me:

'I feel much better. I'm very busy right now, but in the past I
would feel overwhelmed and not able to cope, both mentally
and physically, but now I feel great. My mood is very positive – no panic or depression. I feel buoyant, energetic and
enthusiastic. I haven't had any colds or infections. I'm sleeping
much better and my PMS [pre-menstrual syndrome] has disappeared. I experienced no breast tenderness, mood swings
or tearfulness during my last period. I am really delighted.'

Best foods

- Vegetables, especially greens and cruciferous vegetables
  (broccoli, Brussels sprouts, cabbage, cauliflower, kale)
- Fish, especially oily fish (salmon, mackerel, herring,
  kippers, sardines)
- Gluten-free grains such as brown rice, quinoa, oats
- Berries
- Raw nuts and seeds
- Red onions and garlic

Worst foods

- Sugar
- Processed food
- Burned fat and meats
- Dairy products
- Wheat
- Yeast

Best supplements

- 2 × high-potency multivitamin–minerals providing B
  vitamins, zinc 10mg and magnesium 100mg
- 2 × vitamin C 1,000mg
- 1 × digestive enzymes, probiotics and glutamine with each meal

Optional

To pursue if the basic recommendations above don't improve your energy:

- 2 × MSM (sulphur) 1,000mg
- 2 × N-acetyl cysteine 500mg
- 1–3 × homocysteine-modulating formula (if your homocysteine score is high – see Chapter 4, Part 2)

CAUTIONS

It is well worth seeing a nutritional therapist to be given the correct diagnosis, guidance and support if these changes to your diet, plus additional supplementation, make little difference. There are many potential causes and contributors to CFS and it is rarely caused by just one imbalance or deficiency.

COELIAC DISEASE

General information

Coeliac disease is a permanent disease of the small intestine, caused by an allergic toxicity to the gliadin protein found in gluten cereals. Where the condition is present, the lining of the small intestine is mercilessly attacked by gliadin, even in extremely small amounts – less than 0.5g a day. The lining becomes damaged and loses its ability to absorb nutrients from food.

Good medicine solutions

1. Screen for and diagnose coeliac disease

People with coeliac disease used to be diagnosed only by means of a gut biopsy showing atrophy (that is, damage) of intestinal villi (the cells that line the intestine). Although a gut biopsy is certainly thorough, it is also expensive and inconvenient. Many doctors and their patients are understandably reluctant to have it performed unless there is a very good reason for doing so.

If you have not been diagnosed already, but are suspicious about whether or not you have coeliac disease, testing whether you are producing antibodies to gliadin is a useful place to start, since gliadin appears to be the key offending protein to which coeliac sufferers react. Often, people with coeliac disease produce anti-gliadin IgA antibodies, along with anti-gliadin IgG antibodies. When you have an IgG food allergy test (see Allergies on page 31), one of the hundred or so foods you'll be tested for will be gliadin, so you'll get this information with your results.

There is a problem with relying on just an IgG gliadin test, however. If you don't have coeliac disease, you can still test positive. You may be gliadin sensitive, but not have coeliac disease. Also, if you've strictly avoided all sources of gluten/gliadin for several months, you may not test positive.

The answer to the dilemma is a test called IgA anti-transglutaminase (IgA-TGA). It measures anti-transglutaminase, a key enzyme that is targeted when you have coeliac disease. In a recent study, all coeliac sufferers (100 per cent) were found to react positively to this test; also, the greater the level of reactivity, the greater was the level of damage to gut mucosa. The test, therefore, confirmed not only whether or not the person was sensitive, but also the degree of sensitivity. This test is available as an inexpensive home test kit, which gives immediate results (see Resources).

2. Avoid all gluten- or gliadin-containing foods

The only known effective therapy for coeliac disease calls for the complete, life-long elimination of gluten and gliadin from the diet. This means no wheat, rye or barley, in any form. Initially, I also recommend the avoidance of oats; however, if an IgG food allergy test does not show the presence of oat antibodies, then you can try reintroducing uncontaminated (gluten-free) oats and monitor any symptoms. Eight in ten coeliac-disease sufferers can tolerate oats, which do not contain gliadin. If this kind of diet is strictly followed, a dramatic resurgence of health should occur. The following are the gluten and non-gluten grains:

Gluten Wheat, rye, barley, oats, spelt, kamut

Non-gluten Rice, corn (maize), buckwheat, millet, gram (chick-pea flour), amaranth

3. Heal your digestive tract with glutamine

Regardless of whether or not you have coeliac disease, your 'inner skin' – your digestive tract – works hard to digest and deal with the mountains of food you eat and, as a consequence, it can easily become damaged. If the gut's immune system is reacting against gliadin, damage will result.

Although most of your body's organs are fuelled by glucose, your digestive tract is a different story. It's a vast and highly active interface between your body and the outside world (and actually measures the same size as a small football pitch when stretched out). Your digestive tract needs a lot of fuel to work properly day in and day out, and it runs on an amino acid called glutamine – thus sparing vital energy-giving glucose for use by your brain, heart and the rest of your body.

Not only does glutamine power your gut but it also heals it as well. The endothelial cells, which make up the inner lining of your digestive tract, replace themselves every four days and are

your most critical line of defence against developing food allergies or getting infections.

If you have been diagnosed with coeliac disease, you need to
take glutamine for at least a month, ideally together with digestive enzymes and a probiotic supplement. Some supplements
provide all three in one (see Resources).

These don't provide enough glutamine for rapid healing,
however. For concentrated repair during the first month, take
4–8g of glutamine a day, the equivalent of one to two heaped
teaspoons of glutamine powder, which is much cheaper and
more convenient than capsules. (Capsules usually contain
500mg, so you'd have to take between 8 and 16 of those.) This
will provide your gut with all the glutamine it needs to heal and
rejuvenate. Glutamine is best taken last thing at night or first
thing in the morning, when your stomach is empty, in a glass
of cold water. Heat destroys glutamine, so don't have it in a hot
drink. Do this every day for a month to accelerate gut healing
after avoidance.

4. Get the correct balance of beneficial bacteria

Inside your body are more bacteria than living cells. Thriving bacteria flourish in a healthy digestive tract and die off in an unhealthy
one. Once you've improved your digestion, 're-inoculating'
your digestive tract with probiotics (the name for these beneficial strains of bacteria) makes a big difference. These are called
'human strain' acidophilus and bifidus bacteria and work much
better than dairy-derived strains found in normal yoghurt. If you
do eat yoghurt, it's best to choose those that use acidophilus and
bifidus strains of bacteria.

These friendly bacteria are not only good for your digestive
tract but also for your immune system and overall health. Once
you've got the optimum bacterial balance in your gut, feeding
them the right food helps to maintain the gut's perfect bacterial
balance. Taking a capsule, or powder, of probiotics for up to 30
days is all you need to get your inner flora flourishing.

What our two main beneficial bacterial species – *Lactobacillus acidophilus* and bifidobacteria – need us to eat is a diet rich in the fibre found only in fresh, unprocessed fruit, vegetables and grains. These foods contain 'prebiotics' – factors that nourish gut bacteria. Especially good foods in this respect are vegetables, especially chicory and Jerusalem artichokes; beans and lentils (pulses), especially soya; and seeds, especially chia and flax.

Some probiotics also contain digestive enzymes and glutamine, covering three bases in one. The addition of digestive enzymes helps to promote digestive health, especially in those people who may have difficulty digesting particular food groups. A good digestive-enzyme supplement will contain glucoamylase and alpha-galactosidase, which help to digest greens and beans.

Best foods

- Rice
- Corn
- Buckwheat
- Quinoa
- Oats (for some)
- Flax and chia seeds
- Vegetables, especially chicory and Jerusalem artichokes, beans, including soya, lentils
- Fish (unbreaded)

Worst foods

- Wheat
- Rye
- Barley
- Oats (only for a minority)
- Alcohol
- Deep-fried foods

Best supplements

- 2 × high-potency multivitamin–minerals
- 2 × vitamin C 1,000mg
- 1 × probiotic supplement containing acidophilus and bifidobacteria (at least 1 billion viable organisms) ideally with digestive enzymes for a month
- 1–2 teaspoons glutamine powder, dissolved in a glass of cold water on an empty stomach for a month after diagnosis

Optional

- 2 × digestive enzymes, probiotic, glutamine supplements, one taken with each main meal, or when foods you find hard to digest are eaten

CAUTIONS

Some oat products are contaminated with wheat by virtue of being processed in a factory using wheat. Be careful to pick uncontaminated oats.

DIG DEEPER

To find out more on this subject, read *Hidden Food Allergies* (Patrick Holford and Dr James Braly), which includes key referenced studies.

COLDS AND FLU

General advice

When your immune system is fighting off an infection, it needs energy, so it's important to rest and avoid stress. Also, the immune system works more efficiently when you are hotter – this is why the body produces a fever to fight off an infection – so keep warm and take warm baths. Eat well, but don't eat too much; conserve your energy for fighting the infection.

Act fast. Viruses survive by breaking into your body's cells and reprogramming those cells to make more viruses. By acting quickly in the first 24 hours, you can stop that happening. Don't wait until it's too late.

There's some evidence that those who supplement probiotics on a regular basis recover from colds faster.

Good medicine solutions

1. Take high dose vitamin C

Taking 1,000mg or 2,000mg of vitamin C every day will shorten the duration, and lessen the symptoms, of a cold or flu if you catch one, but what really works is to increase your blood level of vitamin C dramatically, and keep it high until the cold or flu has gone. This means taking 2,000mg immediately you get the first symptoms, then 1,000mg an hour until the cold has gone (usually within 24 hours and often within 12 hours). You could take 2,000mg every two hours, or even 3,000mg every three hours (during the night, for example, the latter is more practical). The point is to keep drip-feeding enough vitamin C into your bloodstream to keep the level consistently high. Vitamin C passes out of the body in four to six hours.

The effectiveness of vitamin C is increased when it is taken with other antioxidants and immune-boosting nutrients. It also has fewer side effects.

The trick is to start taking vitamin C as soon as you get the first hints of the symptoms of a cold – perhaps a sore throat or feeling blocked up. If you wait too long, it is less effective. In a study of students, those given 1,000mg of vitamin C every hour for six hours during the first day of a cold reported 85 per cent fewer cold symptoms than those taking decongestants and painkillers.[1]

Vitamin C, in high doses, has been well proven to be non-toxic in both adults and children even if taken over many years; however, it does cause loose bowels. The best dose is the level just below 'bowel tolerance', which means the maximum level you can take before it causes loose bowels. Everyone is different in this respect, so it's best to just try it and find your own way. There is no harm in having high doses for a few days. When all the cold or flu symptoms have gone, don't suddenly cut it out completely. Have, for example, 4,000mg spread over the next day, then reduce to 2,000mg a day, one in the morning and one in the afternoon.

Some vitamin C tablets contain other immune-friendly nutrients for extra effect. You can use effervescent vitamin C, but this becomes expensive at high doses. You can also buy pure ascorbic acid powder and mix it with water and a little juice for taste, then drink it throughout the day. There is a form of lipospheric vitamin C which enables you to absorb a little more before reaching 'bowel tolerance'. If you are very sensitive to vitamin C, this would be worth trying.

It is also important to increase your intake of foods that are high in antioxidants, such as carrots, berries and cherries.

2. Increase your intake of zinc

Zinc is an essential mineral that most of us are relatively deficient in. It is found in the 'seeds' of things – from eggs to nuts, seeds and beans. It is also high in meat and fish. (The immune system also needs more protein when under attack.) The ideal intake is about 15mg a day. Most people achieve half of this from diet. Thus a good daily multivitamin and mineral supplement should provide an additional 10mg to help ensure an optimal intake every day.

Zinc, in much higher doses of 50–100mg a day, has also proved to be significantly anti-viral.[2] It is available in lozenges for coughs and colds which help to shorten the duration of the symptoms. Supplementing this amount of zinc has been shown to make the body's T cells much more effective, hence boosting immunity. Some vitamin C supplements contain a small amount of zinc, so if, for example, one contains 1,000mg of vitamin C and 3mg of zinc, and you take 1,000mg an hour, you will be taking close to 50mg zinc over 24 hours. This is effective.

3. Take black elderberry extract

Viruses get into body cells by puncturing their walls with tiny spikes made of a substance called haemagglutinin. According to research by virologist Madeleine Mumcuoglu (working with Dr Jean Linderman, who discovered interferon), an extract of elderberry disarms these spikes by binding to them and preventing them from penetrating the cell membrane. Mumcuoglu found a significant improvement in symptoms – fever, cough, muscle pain – in 20 per cent of patients within 24 hours, and in a further 73 per cent of patients within 48 hours. After three days, 90 per cent had complete relief of their symptoms compared to another group on a placebo, who took at least six days to recover. In another double-blind controlled trial, elderberry extract cut recovery time in those with influenza by four days.[3]

4. Take echinacea

This root of the plant *Echinacea purpurea* is probably the most widely used immune-boosting herb. It possesses interferon-like properties, which are part of the body's natural defence against infections, and is an effective anti-viral agent against flu and herpes. It contains special kinds of polysaccharides, such as inulin, which increase macrophage production, which are the immune cells that destroy bugs. Echinacea is best taken either as capsules of the powdered herb (2,000mg a day), or as drops of a concentrated extract (usually 20 drops three times a day).

5. Increase your vitamin D level

Keep your vitamin D level up, especially during the winter. Vitamin D is a very important immune-boosting vitamin. Although some foods contain vitamin D, such as oily fish and eggs, it is primarily made in the skin in the presence of sunlight. If you rarely go outside, exposing your skin to direct sunlight, your body won't make any vitamin D. During the winter, most people's vitamin D levels drop quite substantially, leaving their immune systems vulnerable. In one study of 19,000 people, those with the lowest average levels of vitamin D were about 40 per cent more likely to have had a recent respiratory infection, compared to those with higher vitamin D levels.[4]

The minimum level needed for optimal health is about 30mcg a day, although some experts in vitamin D say this is too low. If you expose your body to moderate sunlight for 30 minutes a day, and eat eggs and, especially, oily fish such as mackerel, you might achieve 15mcg. There is, therefore, a good case to supplement 15mcg, especially if you live in the UK or equivalent. The recommended daily allowance (RDA), which is desperately out of date, is a mere 5mcg.

There are two forms of vitamin D: D_3 is the natural form, found in foods such as fish and eggs, and made by the skin when exposed to sunlight. It is the more effective form. D_2 is derived from plants and can substitute for D_3 in the human body, although not as effectively. In the winter, if you live in northern Europe, for example, it is worth boosting your vitamin D intake with one or two vitamin D drops a day. These should provide 25mcg per drop. Taking 50mcg a day for a month should build up your vitamin D stores for the winter. Then cut back to one drop,

25mcg. A good multivitamin can provide 15mcg. You will need more if you rarely get outdoors with your skin exposed, and/or have dark skin, and/or live far north (or south) during the winter months when the angle of the sun means less intensity.

'I used to have . . . '

'I used to get colds all the time, and would often take more than a week to recover. Since following your recommendations I haven't had a single cold all winter, even though many people in my office have. If I get the first signs of a cold, I just increase my intake of vitamin C,' says Mary.

Best foods

- Ginger (use in juice and teas and to soothe sore throats)
- Carrots and carrot juice
- Water (drink lots)
- Berries
- Montmorency cherry juice (Cherry Active)
- Fish/beans (pulses) for protein
- Raw nuts and seeds

Worst foods

- Dairy products (often mucus forming)
- Sugar and refined foods
- Too many carbs, such as lots of bread and cereals

Best supplements

- 1,000mg vitamin C every hour (ideally one with zinc and berry extracts)
- 10 drops of echinacea every 2 hours
- 1 teaspoon, or equivalent, of black elderberry extract every 2 hours

- 1 × high-potency multivitamin–mineral with 15mcg of vitamin D and 10mg zinc
- 1 × 1,000iu (25mcg) vitamin D a day during the winter (for immune protection rather than immediate effect)

> **CAUTIONS**
>
> Vitamin C, in high doses, can cause loose bowels, or even diarrhoea. This is not dangerous as such, as long as you keep hydrated. It is, however, ideal to consume less than the amount that gives you extremely loose bowels. This also means you will need to decrease your daily dose down to 1,000–2,000mg a day once you are better.

DIG DEEPER

To find out more on this subject, read *How to Boost Your Immune System* (Patrick Holford and Jennifer Meek), which includes key referenced studies.

COLITIS AND DIVERTICULITIS

General information

Colitis means inflammation of the large intestine. Diverticulitis is a condition of the small and large intestine, in which pockets in the intestinal wall, called diverticula, become distended and are then more likely to become infected and inflamed. The condition, probably the result of not enough fibre and exercise, is rarely seen in primitive cultures.

A more serious form of colitis is called ulcerative colitis, which is thought to be autoimmune in nature (see Crohn's Disease and Ulcerative Colitis on page 114).

Good medicine solutions

1. Increase the gentle fibres

Both colitis and ulcerative colitis often result from eating low-fibre foods and foods that irritate the gut. These include alcohol, wheat and coffee. Fibre absorbs water, making the faecal matter less hard, more bulky and easier to pass through the body.

Best in this respect are soluble fibres, which are found in very high amounts in oats, but also found in flax seeds. Small seeds can get stuck in the extended diverticula, so any seeds eaten should be ground and soaked. Making porridge with ground seeds is a good way to increase soluble fibres. Vegetable fibres are also important to include in the diet, by either steaming the vegetables or making them into soup. Stay away from wheat bran. Insoluble fibres, principally in wheat and wheat bran, are not so effective, despite their reputation for being so.

One of the most absorbent fibres is glucomannan fibre, from the konjac plant (see Resources). Fibre powders based on glucomannan (which are taken with a large glass of water, or added to water to start the absorption process) can help restore normal gut peristalsis, the muscular action that passes faecal matter along the digestive tract.

2. Ease your digestion

Bloating, creating pressure in the inflamed colon, can be caused by certain foods or other triggers, such as an unidentified food allergy (see Allergies on page 31) or a lack of particular digestive enzymes. The enzyme glucoamylase, for example, helps digest carbohydrates in vegetables, whereas alpha-galactosidase helps to digest carbohydrates in beans and lentils. It is very helpful to supplement a digestive enzyme formula that contains both of these, especially if certain foods trigger bloating or discomfort. Digestive enzymes should be taken at the start of a meal.

3. Re-inoculate the gut with beneficial bacteria

The health of the digestive tract is dependent on having a healthy colony of beneficial bacteria. The two main families of essential bacteria are *Lactobacillus acidophilus* and bifidobacteria. It is worth supplementing these for a month to establish a healthy colony, then following a good diet will 'feed' the bacteria, removing the need to continue supplementation ad infinitum. Some yoghurts use these essential strains of bacteria, but most don't. Be wary of yoghurt as a source of bacteria if you suspect you may be dairy intolerant and choose only plain, unsweetened yoghurt.

Some digestive enzyme supplements also contain beneficial bacteria as well as glutamine, an essential amino acid that helps to heal the gut. In the early stages of gut healing taking 1 teaspoon of glutamine powder in cold water last thing at night on an empty stomach for two to four weeks helps to heal the gut.

3. Increase essential fats

Both omega-3 and omega-6 fats are important for gut healing and reducing inflammation. Omega-3 fats are found in oily fish whereas omega-6 fats are richest in evening primrose and borage oil. Combination supplements providing omega-3s from fish oil and omega-6 from evening primrose oil and borage oil are best.

The best vegetarian sources of omega-3 fats are chia and flax seeds, but these should be ground and soaked, especially during the early stages of recovery.

4. Consider a shot of aloe vera

Aloe vera juice is very good for digestive health. It contains mucopolysaccarides and acemannan, which help to reduce inflammation in the gut and may accelerate healing. Having a shot of aloe vera juice a day is a good option for digestive health.

5. Lose weight, exercise and deal with stress

The digestive tract is surrounded by muscles that help move every-thing along with a snake-like motion called peristalsis. If you do no exercise, you will lose abdominal muscle strength, gain weight and have a distended gut – this is a recipe for disaster. If you cannot do a sit-up, then you have weak abdominal muscles.

Exercises such as yoga and pilates, or any exercise system that helps build abdominal muscles, can help digestion. In yoga the exercise called 'udiyama', which involves pumping the stomach muscles in and out after an exhale (with no air in the lungs), is particularly good.

Following a low-GL diet is one of the most effective ways to lose weight, and it is naturally high in soluble fibres. (See Chapter 1, Part 2 for details on how to follow a low-GL diet.)

Stress also shuts down proper digestive peristalsis. For this reason, it is important not to eat when you are stressed. Chapter 6, Part 2 gives you practical solutions for reducing stress.

Best foods

- Oats
- Ground flax and chia seeds
- Steamed or puréed vegetables, as in soup
- Puréed beans (pulses), as in soup (provided they don't cause bloating)
- Oily fish (salmon, mackerel, herring including kippers, sardines)

Worst foods

- Fibreless refined foods (sugar, white flour)
- Wheat bran
- Burned meat, and meat in excess

Best supplements

- 2 × high-potency multivitamin–minerals

- 2 × essential omegas with fish-oil-derived omega-3, plus omega-6 from borage or evening primrose oil

- 2 × vitamin C 500–1,000mg (if you are sensitive to vitamin C, choose a formula that provides ascorbate, the non-acidic form of vitamin C)

- 1 × digestive enzyme formula with each main meal

- 1 × probiotic containing acidophilus and bifidobacteria (for one month)

- 1 teaspoon or 3 capsules of glucomannan fibre or PGX (see Resources) with a large glass of water with each main meal

- 1 shot of aloe vera juice

DIG DEEPER

To find out more on this subject, read *Improve Your Digestion* (Patrick Holford), which includes key referenced studies.

COLORECTAL CANCER

General information

Cancers of the colon or rectum are some of the most common cancers, particularly in the Western world. They are strongly linked to diet, and there is little doubt that dietary carcinogens, caused by putrefying food, and created by micro-organisms in an unhealthy gut, play a large part. As well as following the general advice for Cancer (see page 74), some dietary factors specifically relate to colorectal cancer.

Good medicine solutions

1. Follow a high-fibre diet

Dietary fibre has a protective effect on the development of colorectal cancer, and diets rich in vegetables and high-fibre grains have shown significant protection against fatal colorectal cancer. There are a number of mechanisms by which fibre can help. The gut bacteria produce several chemicals, including butyrate from fibre. This creates a condition where tumours are less likely to grow, causing them to die off. Fibre also increases the weight of the stools and the frequency of bowel movements, reducing the contact time between the bowel and carcinogen exposure. It also minimises the formation of carcinogens, which occur if the food passes through slowly. There is little doubt that the modern diet – high in alcohol, sugar and fat, and low in fibre – wreaks havoc with the digestive tract and disturbs the gut-associated immune system. The best way to increase your fibre intake is to eat whole foods, such as whole grains, pulses (lentils, beans), nuts, seeds and vegetables, all of which contain fibre. Some of the fibre in vegetables is destroyed by cooking, so you should also eat something raw every day.

2. Avoid red and processed meat

Compelling evidence suggests a strong association between red meat and fat intake and colorectal cancer. It is not just the naturally occurring hormones, growth factors and pro-inflammatory chemicals in meat that are the problem, it is also how the meat is cooked. Cooking meat at high temperatures, such as frying or barbecuing, produces chemicals called heterocyclic amines. These can damage DNA and increase the incidence of cancer. Some processed meat contains chemicals called nitrites. In the bowel, nitrites are converted into carcinogenic chemicals. I recommend limiting your intake of red meat and avoiding processed meat ('red meat' includes beef, pork, lamb and goat; 'processed meat' refers to meat preserved by smoking, curing or salting, or with chemical preservatives added to it). If you do eat red meat, you should eat less than 300g (11oz) a week. This equates to a 150g (5½oz) serving (roughly the size of your palm), twice a week. Choose organic lean meat, especially game, in preference to red meat or meat from domesticated animals. Avoid, or rarely eat, burned meat, whether grilled, fried or barbecued. Although high consumption of animal fat is positively associated with colorectal cancer, consumption of fatty fish and low fat intake may lower risk.

3. Take probiotics

Probiotics help us maintain a healthy digestive system by maintaining a balance between the harmful and beneficial bacteria. They also support the friendly bacteria in our intestinal tract by secreting certain chemicals that can break down carcinogens. This in turn can help reduce inflammation that can lead to cancer. The body's two main beneficial bacterial species – lactobacilli and bifidobacteria – need us to eat a diet rich in the fibre found only in fresh, unprocessed fruit, vegetables and grains. These are the hard-to-digest carbohydrates known as prebiotics. Other favourite bacterial foods include flavonoids and lignans, found in vegetables, pulses and seeds, such as flax seeds. Foods rich in prebiotics include chicory, Jerusalem artichokes, leeks, asparagus, garlic, onions, oats and soya beans. You can also get prebiotic supplements, which can be especially useful for those not getting enough fruit and vegetables. You need to be careful about taking too much, though. One of the best prebiotics is fructo-oligosaccharides (FOS). Five to eight grams (or capsules, or the equivalent of 1 heaped teaspoon) of FOS should be enough – more than that can lead to bloating, flatulence and intestinal discomfort. Prebiotics can also be useful combined with probiotics if your beneficial bacteria are likely to be under attack. The best probiotic supplements include some FOS in the capsules. That way you are giving the good bacteria population a boost along with an added food supply. Look out for the common-est two strains – lactobacilli and bifidobacterium – because more research has been carried out on them. Sub-strains from these families, most commonly recognised as safe, include: *Lactobacillus acidophilus, L. rhamnosus, L. plantarum, L. casei; and Bifidobacterium bifidum, B. infantis* (for babies) and *B. longum*; among others.

4. Look into high-dose vitamin C and salvestrols

Also consider high-dose vitamin C and salvestrols. (See Cancer on page 74.)

Best foods

- Fibre (whole grains, lentils, beans – pulses – nuts, seeds and vegetables)
- Oily fish
- Chicory, leeks, onions, oats, Jerusalem artichokes
- Live yoghurt

Worst foods

- Alcohol
- Red and processed meat
- Sugar

Best supplements

- 2 × high-potency multivitamin–minerals
- 2 × high-potency omega-3-rich fish oil capsules (choose products with the most EPA)
- 5,000mg or more vitamin C
- 1 × antioxidant complex (containing beta-carotene, vitamin E and selenium, plus other antioxidant nutrients such as glutathione, alpha lipoic acid, co-enzyme Q_{10} and resveratrol)

■ 2 × salvestrol 2,000 units for recovery; 350 units for prevention

■ 1 × 1,000iu (25mcg) vitamin D

■ 1 × probiotic (containing FOS and at least 15 billion micro-organisms)

CAUTIONS

Many chemotherapeutic drugs are oxidants. It may therefore not be a good idea to take lots of antioxidants, including vitamin C, while undergoing certain types of chemotherapy. Please check with your oncologist if you are undergoing chemotherapy.

It is wise to seek the advice of a nutritional therapist if you wish to undertake an extensive nutritional strategy.

CROHN'S DISEASE AND ULCERATIVE COLITIS

General information

Crohn's disease and ulcerative colitis are the two major types of what is known as inflammatory bowel disease (IBD), involving abnormal immune system responses, possibly allergies, intestinal permeability and genetic factors.

Whether a person is diagnosed with Crohn's or ulcerative colitis depends on the location and type of inflammation, as well as the symptoms. Ulcerative colitis causes inflammation of the lining of the colon only. Classic symptoms are passing blood and mucus, pain before defecation, a general feeling of tiredness and, in more severe cases, diarrhoea. Crohn's disease can affect any part of the bowel, usually the last part of the small intestine (the ileum), in a more severe way, thickening the intestinal wall, often with normal bowel in between inflamed sections.

Good medicine solutions

1. Switch off autoimmunity

Your immune system is designed to react to unwelcome substances from the outside world, such as viruses, harmful bacteria, pathogens and food allergens, and to misbehaving cells such as cancer cells. But sometimes the immune system can attack healthy cells. This results in autoimmune diseases such as Crohn's disease and ulcerative colitis.

Many people think, incorrectly, that because the immune system seems to be overreacting, anything that might 'boost' it, for example, vitamin C, could make matters worse. But autoimmune diseases are a 'system-control' problem and many of the foods and nutrients that help an immune system to work make matters better, not worse.

Coeliac disease, an extreme form of wheat allergy (see page 95), is very common among sufferers of Crohn's and ulcerative colitis and should always be screened for. This is an extreme reaction to gluten, and usually the gliadin protein, which is in wheat, rye and barley, but not in oats (80 per cent of those with coeliac disease don't react to oats). It is important also to find out if your body is producing IgG antibodies or IgE antibodies, indicating an intolerance to certain foods. (See Allergies on page 31 to find out how to test for and eliminate allergies.) The theory is that if the immune system becomes hyper-alert against foods, it 'cross-reacts' against certain body tissues. The goal, therefore, is to eliminate the food and lessen the immune system's belligerent attitude.

Oats are not only gliadin-free but also a rich source of beta-glucans, which help to lower cholesterol and promote healthy blood sugar balance. Beta-glucans may help lessen autoimmunity and improve general health in a counter-intuitive way. One of the prevalent theories as to why autoimmune diseases are on the increase is that we live in too clean environments and therefore don't have enough exposure to bugs and bacteria early on in our lives. Most such microbes have beta-glucans present in their cell walls, and the beta-glucans consequently stimulates the immune system and helps to build up normal, strong immunity. Many known immune-enhancing foods and herbs – such as shiitake mushrooms and echinacea – are rich sources of beta-glucans. Beta-glucans appears to act as an immune-system modulator and may also help autoimmune diseases. As well as eating more oats and shiitake mushrooms, you can take supplements of purified beta-glucans. Choose those that contain the following, written as: (1–3) (1–6) beta-d-glucans.

Sugar is another potential trigger for autoimmunity, because having sugar levels that are too high leads to proteins in the body becoming damaged – known as glycosylation – in such a way that they may start to misbehave, or are no longer recognised by the body's immune system as a friend but, rather, as a foe. These damaged proteins are called AGEs (advanced glycation end-products) and the more you have the more your immune system is likely to react. Particularly bad is fructose (fruit sugar), which the body finds harder to burn or turn directly into fat than glucose. If you follow my low-GL diet you will naturally be limiting your fructose intake to healthy levels. (See Chapter 1, Part 2 for details on how to follow a low-GL diet.)

Another successful diet approach for autoimmune diseases is to follow a Paleo diet, or a Stone Age diet. Before we became peasant farmers (about 12,000 years ago for Europeans), humanity lived on lean meat, seafood, plants, fruit and nuts with just small amounts of seeds and grains. We weren't yet eating grains or dairy products in large quantities. The Paleo and Stone Age diets are based on the evolutionary diet that existed before agriculture, as the theory is that our digestion hasn't evolved to eat grains, especially in large quantities. Although dairy may have been eaten before animals were domesticated, it would also have been consumed in much smaller amounts. Many people with autoimmune diseases report great improvements eating an essentially grain- and dairy-free diet. A Paleo or Stone Age diet is also naturally high in omega-3 fats.

Another difference between modern living and Paleo living is vitamin D exposure. Given that we are originally designed to be naked, outdoors and living in Africa, our intake of vitamin D, primarily made in the skin in the presence of sunlight, has drastically declined. Even though people from the northern hemisphere evolved to have pale skin to increase their ability to absorb vitamin D, most pale-skinned people do not get enough sunlight on their bodies during the year. Vitamin D deficiency is linked to an increasing risk of autoimmune diseases. Smaller amounts of vitamin D are found in oily fish, but we need at least 30mcg a day. Eating oily fish and exposing your face and arms for 30 minutes a day might give you 15mcg, so it's best to supplement at least another 15mcg a day. There is some evidence that higher amounts, say 50mcg a day, may help switch off autoimmunity.

2. Heal the gut

The cells that make up the inner wall of the digestive tract can easily become damaged and hence more permeable, allowing incompletely digested food particles through. Studies show that those with Crohn's have greater increased gut permeability, which thereby increases the chances of developing allergies because when food proteins cross through the gut wall the immune system reacts against them. Having a highly nutritious diet, but with low-allergenic foods, helps to both heal the gut and lessen symptoms. The most common offending foods are wheat, milk and yeast, although the ideal diet varies from person to person.

The first step therefore lies in identifying offending foods and eliminating them. (See Allergies on page 31 to find out how to identify IgE- and IgG-based allergens and how to build an allergy-free diet.)

The next step is to correct dysbiosis and re-inoculate the digestive tract with beneficial bacteria. There is some evidence that the wrong balance of bacteria may generate toxins that then damage the intestinal wall. The wrong bacterial imbalance can also affect immune function, leading to increased inflammation in the digestive tract, so balancing this is important.

The amino acid glutamine is especially important in healing the digestive tract as the epithelial cells that make up the gut wall are regenerated by it. Look for supplements that combine digestive enzymes with probiotics and glutamine, but also take 1 heaped teaspoon (5g) in a glass of cold water last thing at night on an empty stomach to accelerate gut healing.

3. Increase nature's anti-inflammatories

The main medical treatment is the use of anti-inflammatory drugs to calm down the inflammation, or medication to turn off the body's immune reactions. Inflammation, however, is the body's way of saying that something is wrong. Inflammation is a systemic problem, not just a localised phenomenon, in which the body's physiology is shifted into an 'alarm state'. Simply taking anti-inflammatory drugs fails to address the underlying causes.

There are several factors that set the scene for inflammation, and then there are those that trigger the manifestation of symptoms. These triggers are important and may include a trauma, an allergy, an infection, a toxin or exposure to too many oxidants. All these factors need to be considered to restore health.

A diet high in meat and milk, rich sources of the pro-inflammatory fat arachidonic acid encourages inflammation. A diet high in omega-3 fats, however, found in flax seeds and chia seeds (which must be ground or soaked to avoid any potential for gut irritation) and oily fish, switches off inflammation. Fish oils high in the omega-3 family of fats, particularly EPA, are well known for fighting inflammation. Most inflammatory disease responds best to about 1,000mg of EPA. This means taking two high-strength omega-3 fish oil capsules a day.

There are also a number of natural anti-inflammatory agents found in common foods. These include:

Turmeric Curcumin, the active ingredient in the yellow curry spice turmeric, works as well as anti-inflammatory drugs, but without the side effects.

Olive extracts The first is hydroxytyrosol, a very powerful anti-oxidant (called a polyphenol) with anti-inflammatory effects. Another key ingredient is oleocanthal, which is chemically related to ibuprofen, although it has none of the negative side effects. Studies on olive pulp extract have shown that it reduces levels of two inflammatory messengers called TNF-alpha and interleukin-8.

Hops An extract from hops, called iso-oxygene, is one of the most potent natural COX-2 inhibitors (COX is an enzyme that promotes pain) and one of the most effective natural painkillers of all. It works just as well as painkilling drugs, but it doesn't cause gut damage.

Quercetin This potent anti-inflammatory is found in red onions, and in lesser amounts in berries and greens. One red onion, or a cup of berries, or three servings of greens provides about 10mg of quercetin. When taken in doses of 50 times this amount – 500mg a day – quercetin becomes a potent anti-inflammatory inhibiting the production of the pro-inflammatory prostaglandins (type-2 prostaglandins) and also inhibiting the release of histamine, which is involved in inflammatory reactions.

Look for supplements containing concentrates of these natural anti-inflammatory agents.

4. Choose soluble fibres

Crohn's and colitis sufferers are rightly wary of eating high-fibre food, which can irritate the gut, and are often advised to avoid fibre to help heal the gut. But soluble fibres are different. These are found in foods such as oats, chia seeds and flax seeds; they absorb water and partially dissolve, as in porridge. These soluble fibres are much more gentle on the digestive tract and help to move the faecal matter along, which is essential for gut health. If you grind and/or soak the oats, flax seeds or chia seeds, or saturate them in water, as in porridge, all the better. Oats are a rich source of beta-glucans.

5. Improve your methylation

One of the key 'control' mechanisms of the body is methylation, which is vital for mental and physical energy, and dependent on B vitamins and other 'methyl' nutrients. If a person is poor at methylation, they have high levels of a toxic amino acid, called homocysteine, in their blood. It is not surprising to find that those with autoimmune diseases are much more likely to have a raised homocysteine level.

Your homocysteine level can be easily tested using a home test kit. If you find that it is high, there are specific nutrients – vitamins B_2, B_6, B_{12}, folic acid, tri-methyl-glycine (TMG), N-acetyl-cysteine (NAC) and zinc – that you need to take in specific quantities to normalise your homocysteine level. The correct amount to take, depending on your homocysteine level, is explained in Chapter 4, Part 2.

Best foods

- Oily fish (salmon, mackerel, herring, kippers, sardines)
- Ground and soaked flax and chia seeds
- Soaked oats, as in porridge (use soft oats)
- Berries and soft fruits
- Steamed vegetables
- Rice (white during the healing phase)
- Quinoa

Worst foods

- Sugar
- Wheat
- Dairy products
- Yeast
- High insoluble-fibre foods: wheat, corn, nuts (during the healing phase)

Best supplements

- 2 × vitamin C 1,000mg
- 2 × vitamin D 1,000iu (25mcg) for up to 3 months
- 2 × (1–3) (1–6) beta-d-glucans
- 1 × combination supplement with digestive enzymes, probiotics and glutamine with each meal
- 2 × omega-3-rich fish oil capsules to achieve 1,000mg of EPA
- 1 heaped teaspoon glutamine in a glass of cold water last thing at night on an empty stomach for 1–2 months
- 3 × combination formulas providing turmeric (curcumin), olive and hop extracts and quercetin

---

CAUTIONS

Although high-fibre foods are good for the digestion during the healing phase, be wary of including too much whole grains, nuts, seeds and raw vegetables. If foods are ground, soaked or steamed, some of the plant fibres break down and become gentler on the digestive tract.

CYSTITIS

General information

Cystitis is a common condition where the lining of the bladder becomes inflamed, making urination painful. Most of the time the inflammation is caused by a bacterial infection, in which case it may be referred to as a urinary tract infection (UTI). Common symptoms include an urgent and frequent need to pass urine (often with little or no urine being passed) and a burning sensation and/or a sharp pain when passing urine. Other possible symptoms include blood in the urine, backache, loin pain, lower abdominal aches and generally feeling unwell.

Good medicine solutions

1. Take probiotics and increase alkalinity

If there is evidence of infection – for example, with *Escherichia coli* (*E. coli*) bacteria – you will probably be prescribed antibiotics. If so, make sure you also take probiotics, but not at the same time as taking the medication, and continue for two weeks after completing the antibiotic course.

Some people find relief by taking alkalising agents such as potassium citrate, which you can buy in a pharmacist. Alternatively, mix 1 teaspoon of bicarbonate of soda with 300ml (10fl oz/½ pint) of water. Creating a more alkaline environment in the urine makes it harder for certain pathological bacteria to survive. Vegetables are particularly alkaline, so taking vegetable juices for one day may also help.

The presence of vitamin C in the urine also makes it harder for bacteria to colonise. The ascorbate form of vitamin C, available more often in vitamin C powders, is also alkaline.

2. Check for candidiasis or food intolerance

The cause of cystitis can be confirmed by a urine analysis, although bacteria are not always found. It can also be caused by *Candida albicans* (see *Candida*/Thrush on page 82) or a food intolerance.

If there is no evidence of infection, you may be diagnosed with 'interstitial' cystitis, a condition where there is inflammation of the bladder for reasons unknown, but possibly related to allergy or autoimmune-type reactions (see Allergies page 31).

3. Try cranberry and D-mannose

Some people report relief from drinking cranberry juice, which is a rich source of D-mannose, a natural sugar. Cranberries also contain hippuric acid, which is known to prevent bacteria clinging to the bladder wall and urinary tract. Unfortunately, most processed cranberry juice contains added sugar, which is not so good because sugar feeds bacterial infections. If the taste of unsweetened cranberry juice is too tart, add a little xylitol – a sugar alcohol that also prevents bacteria from taking hold.

Alternatively, you can supplement the naturally occurring simple sugar D-mannose (found in peaches, apples, berries and some other plants). It is a harmless, natural sugar and is safe for anyone to take, including young children and pregnant women. It is absorbed in the upper part of the gastrointestinal tract and never reaches the intestines; it doesn't affect the normal bacterial growth in that area. Although small amounts of D-mannose are made by our bodies, if we consume large amounts it is promptly excreted into the urine, which is the reason why taking D-mannose helps to heal and maintain a healthy bladder. Also, due to the speed at which it is excreted in the urine, it can be safely be taken by diabetics. Make sure you buy pure D-mannose with no fillers, additives or preservatives.

Research has shown that *E. coli* likes to attach to the

D-mannose produced naturally as part of the walls of cells. D-mannose is present in the bladder and the urinary tract, providing ideal docking ports for the *E. coli*. In this way, the *E. coli* can bury themselves into the bladder wall, making them very difficult to get rid of, and this can lead to repeated attacks of cystitis. The theory is that providing a richer supply of D-mannose in the urine can encourage the *E. coli* to attach to the free mannose instead of the mannose in the cell walls.

General advice

- Always wipe from front to back after going to the toilet, to prevent bacteria from entering the urethra.
- Use only white unscented toilet paper, to avoid potential dye reactions.
- Avoid potential irritants, such as perfumed soaps, bath oils and vaginal deodorants at all times, as chemicals are strongly implicated in this condition. Don't douche.
- Urinate as soon as possible after sex, to stop the transmission of bacteria into the bladder, and always wash before and after sex.
- If symptoms are acute, avoid intercourse for at least one week, as bacteria can be passed from one partner to another.
- Wear cotton underwear and loose clothing. Avoid tight-fitting jeans, especially in hot weather.

Best foods

- Vegetables
- Fish
- Nuts, seeds, beans (pulses)
- Whole grains
- Filtered or bottled water – 8 glasses a day
- Cranberries and unsweetened cranberry juice
- Live, unsweetened yoghurt

Worst foods

- Sugar
- All fast-releasing carbohydrates
- Yeast-rich and fermented foods

Best supplements

- 2 × vitamin C 1,000mg, ideally in the ascorbate (alkaline) form
- 2 × high-potency multivitamin–minerals providing at least 50mcg of biotin – check it is yeast-free
- 1 teaspoon (3g) D-mannose every 3 hours when experiencing cystitis – comes in powder form (can be mixed into drinks), or capsule form, usually 500mg, so you'll need to take 6 capsules at a time
- 1 × *Lactobacillus acidophilus* and bifidobacteria, at least 10 billion viable organisms, for at least 6 weeks – especially important following antibiotics

> **CAUTIONS**
>
> A bladder infection can be painful and annoying, and can become a serious health problem if the infection spreads to your kidneys. For this reason, you should consult your doctor immediately if your symptoms are accompanied by fever, blood in the urine, loin pain, or lower backache – all these can be signs of a kidney infection.

DEMENTIA AND ALZHEIMER'S DISEASE

General information

The earlier you screen for potential memory loss, and then take the actions below, the better. The earliest diagnosed condition is called 'mild cognitive impairment', although you can have signs of decreasing memory before this stage. The next level is 'dementia', which can be diagnosed on the basis of symptoms and results from cognitive function tests. Alzheimer's disease involves the degeneration of specific areas of the brain, and is thus only identifiable from a brain scan. About three in four cases of dementia are Alzheimer's, with most of the remainder being 'vascular' dementia, which relates to blocked arteries and poor circulation of blood to the brain (see Angina on page 38 and High Blood Pressure on page 195). All the advice given here is also applicable for prevention of memory loss.

Good medicine solutions

1. Get early screening and take preventive action

The average time between the first signs of losing your memory and Alzheimer's is thought to be at least 30 years, and it is therefore essential to test your memory and cognitive abilities objectively, certainly from the age of 50. The Food for the Brain Foundation (see Resources) offers a free cognitive function test, which is a reliable screening test. Although it cannot diagnose as such, it can generate a letter for your doctor advising further investigation and that you test your homocysteine level, if your score suggests this might be necessary (see below). Please note that you can get a false poor score because, for example, you may have been distracted; however, if your cognitive abilities are not good, your score will not be good either. It is then essential to test your homocysteine level, and take the following advice seriously.

2. Test and lower your homocysteine

Homocysteine is a toxic amino acid that accumulates in the blood when your intake of certain vitamins is low, and as a result of other diet and lifestyle factors. A blood level below 7mmol/l is ideal. Above 9.5mcmol/l is associated with accelerated brain shrinkage and memory loss. Homocysteine is thought to damage the brain directly, leading to the formation of amyloid plaque, and also to damage the arteries. It is therefore important to lower homocysteine levels in cases of vascular dementia.

Your homocysteine is not only a reliable predictor of risk but also when you lower it by taking B vitamins it has been shown to halt accelerated brain shrinkage and further memory loss. It is, therefore, well worth testing, because there is something you can do about high levels. In some countries you can go directly to a laboratory for testing. In others you need to request a test through your doctor. (See Resources for more details about testing.) Always take the test on an empty stomach, such as first thing in the morning.

If your homocysteine level is raised, you will be recommended to supplement additional vitamins B_6, B_{12} and folic acid. In fact, B_2, zinc and tri-methyl-glycine (TMG) also help to lower homocysteine. Most supplement formulas designed to normalise homocysteine contain all these nutrients, but it is vital to get the dose right and this depends on your personal score. Exactly what to take is explained in Chapter 4, Part 2.

3. Increase omega-3-rich fish and fish oils

Although the evidence is not nearly as strong as for B vitamins, having a high intake of fish or fish oils is associated with a lower risk of memory loss and Alzheimer's. There is also some evidence that supplementing docosahexaenoic acid (DHA), a type of omega-3 fat found in fish that is used to build brain cells, can improve memory in those with memory decline. Therefore, it is worth eating more fish, especially oily fish, and taking fish oil supplements containing DHA. Studies that have shown benefits have usually involved taking in excess of 500mg of DHA, which means taking two high-potency omega-3 fish oil supplements a day.

All fish, not just oily fish, also contains phospholipids – important nutrients that build the brain – as well as vitamin B_{12}.

Walnuts, flax and chia seeds are also high in omega-3; however, eating them has a limited effect in raising DHA.

4. Increase antioxidants and eat a low-GL diet

You can increase your intake of antioxidants by eating lots of fruit, vegetables, herbs and spices. Go for the strong colours, such as blackberries, blueberries, broccoli, butternut squash, carrots, cinnamon, kale, mustard, red cabbage, sweet potato, tomatoes and turmeric. (See Chapter 2, Part 2 for more on increasing your antioxidant intake.) Eating these kinds of antioxidant-rich foods is associated with a lower risk of Alzheimer's, as is drinking tea (not coffee) and eating dark chocolate. Coffee consistently raises homocysteine levels.

A small study found that giving people a daily shot of blueberry juice improved mood, blood sugar control and, if given in the afternoon, memory and work performance.

There is some evidence that certain antioxidants, especially in combination, may enhance memory and protect against memory decline. These include N-acetyl cysteine (NAC), alpha lipoic acid and vitamin C, in combination with vitamin E.

Following a low-GL diet by eating slow-releasing carbohydrates with more protein is also associated with less risk. (See Chapter 1, Part 2 for details on how to follow a low-GL diet.)

5. Keep active

There are a number of lifestyle factors that are associated with keeping your memory sharp. These include:

- Keeping physically fit by taking some exercise every day, preferably outdoors to get exposure to the sun so that you can make vitamin D.
- Keeping socially active; staying in touch with friends and family.
- Keeping mentally active by learning new things and challenging your mind. If you don't use it you will lose it.
- Keeping your stress levels down. (See Chapter 6, Part 2 for more on this.)

6. Consider coconut oil

Although largely anecdotal at this stage, there are hundreds of reports of people with dementia who have made remarkable recoveries, or slowed down the rate of cognitive decline, by taking coconut oil.

Virgin, cold-pressed coconut oil is a rich source of medium-chain triglycerides (MCTs), a type of fat that the body converts into ketones and burns for energy. It appears that switching your metabolism away from glucose (sugar) – for example, by eating a low-GL diet – and adding 1 teaspoon of virgin, cold-pressed coconut oil three times a day may increase ketones and help dysfunctional brain cells to work better.

Although trials are needed, this may be worth trying, especially if you already have significant memory decline. There is no evidence yet to suggest that daily coconut oil guards against memory decline in those not yet affected.

'*I used to have . . . '*

Chris felt very unwell, with constant tiredness, worsening memory and concentration, and little zest for life. He was depressed, had no sex drive and felt brain-dead. His homocysteine score was 119. He changed his diet and took homocysteine-lowering nutrients and, within three months, his homocysteine level dropped to 19. After six months it had dropped to 11. He cannot believe how well he now feels. His memory and concentration are completely restored. He has boundless energy from 6.00 a.m. until 10.00 p.m. He now exercises for an hour every day and has lost weight.

'You have saved my life, or at least made it worth living again. I'm a new man and my love life has perked up,' says Chris.

Best foods

- Fish, especially oily fish (salmon, mackerel, herring, kippers, sardines)
- Beans (pulses)
- Vegetables, especially greens
- Raw nuts and seeds
- Coconut oil
- Fruit, especially berries, and particularly blueberries
- Tea
- Dark chocolate

Worst foods

- Coffee
- Alcohol (in excess)
- Sugar

Best supplements

- 2 × high-potency multivitamin–minerals providing 10mcg of B_{12}, 200mcg folic acid, 20mg B_6, 10mg of zinc

- X* × homocysteine-normalising B vitamin formula (*dose and need dependent on your homocysteine score, as explained in Chapter 4, Part 2)

- 2 × high-potency omega-3-rich fish oil capsules (choose products with the most EPA)

- 2 × antioxidant formulas providing NAC, ALA, vitamins E and C

- 2 × vitamin C 1,000mg

CAUTIONS

There is some evidence that a high intake of supplemental folic acid may increase the risk of colorectal cancer in those with pre-cancerous cells, which is more common in less well-nourished elderly people. For this reason, I do not recommend supplementing more than 200mcg of folic acid without first testing your homocysteine level.

DIG DEEPER

To find out more on this subject, read *The Alzheimer's Prevention Plan* (Patrick Holford with Deborah Colson and Shane Eaton), which includes key referenced studies.

DEPRESSION

General information

There are many factors that can contribute to the development of depression. There might be underlying biochemical or psychological issues that predispose an individual; there might be a trigger, such as a stressful event, a bereavement, loss of a job, or the break-up of a relationship. Counselling can be very helpful, or even essential, in these circumstances.

Good medicine solutions

1. Increase your omega-3 fats

Surveys have shown that the more fish the population of a country eats, the lower is their incidence of depression. There are two key types of omega-3 fats, eicosapentaenoic acid (EPA) and docosahexaenoic acid (DHA), and the evidence suggests that it's the EPA that seems to be the most potent natural antidepressant, and this is most concentrated in oily fish. EPA is thought to boost serotonin, the brain's feel-good neurotransmitter.

Many studies have shown that taking fish oil supplements high in EPA improves mood more than antidepressant drugs, but without the side effects. You need to take in the region of 1,000mg of EPA for a significant mood boost, which means taking two high-potency EPA-rich fish oil supplements a day. These can be prescribed by your doctor.

2. Increase your intake of B vitamins

People with either low blood levels of the B vitamin folic acid or high blood levels of the amino acid homocysteine (a sign that they are not getting enough B_6, B_{12} or folic acid) are more likely to be depressed and less likely to have a positive result from anti-depressant drugs. Supplementing extra B vitamins also helps antidepressants to work better.

Women with a high level of homocysteine – a toxic amino acid found in the blood – will have double the odds of developing depression. For reasons unknown, the association is not so strong for men; however, it is still advisable for men to test their homo-cysteine level. The ideal level is below 7, and certainly below 10. The average level is 10–11. Your homocysteine level indicates how good you are at 'methylation', a critical biochemical process in the brain and body. Folic acid is one of seven nutrients – the others being B_2, B_6, B_{12}, zinc, magnesium and tri-methyl-glycine (TMG) – that help normalise homocysteine and improve methylation. Deficiency in vitamins B_3 and B_6, folic acid, zinc and magnesium has been linked to depression, so it makes sense to eat whole foods, fruits, vegetables, nuts and seeds, which are high in these nutrients, and also to supplement a multivitamin–mineral with good levels of these B vitamins. (See Chapter 4, Part 2 for more details on testing and lowering your homocysteine level with B vitamins.)

S-adenosyl methionine (SAMe) is an amino acid that greatly improves methylation. Known as the 'master tuner' it is a highly effective antidepressant. In some countries you can buy it over the counter or on the internet. In the EU it is classified as a medicine. You therefore either need to obtain it on pre-scription or buy it for your own use, which is perfectly legal, from a country where it is available over the counter. Many people buy it from the US over the internet. You need 200–400mg a day, ideally first thing in the morning on an empty stomach, to benefit.

3. Boost your serotonin

The feel-good neurotransmitter, serotonin, is made in the body and brain from an amino acid called tryptophan. Tryptophan is converted into another amino acid called 5-hydroxytrypto-phan (5-HTP), which in turn is converted into the neurotransmitter serotonin. Tryptophan can be found in the diet; it's in many protein-rich foods, such as meat, fish, beans and eggs. High levels of 5-HTP are found in the African griffonia bean, but this bean is not a common feature of most people's diet. The foods richest in 5-HTP are seafood, meat and eggs.

When you fail to have enough tryptophan you are likely to become depressed; indeed, people taking part in studies who have been fed food that is deficient in tryptophan have become depressed within hours.

Both tryptophan and 5-HTP have been shown to have an antidepressant effect in clinical trials, although 5-HTP is more effective – there have been 27 studies, involving 990 people, to date, most of which proved its efficiency. Start by taking 100mg 5-HTP a day, in two doses of 50mg, then build up to a maximum of 300mg a day.

Exercise, sunlight and reducing your stress level also tend to promote serotonin.

4. Balance your blood sugar and try chromium

There is a direct link between mood and blood sugar balance. All carbohydrate foods are broken down into glucose, and your brain runs on glucose. The more uneven your blood sugar supply, the more uneven your mood. A high sugar intake has been implicated in aggressive behaviour, anxiety, fatigue and depression.

Lots of refined sugar and refined carbohydrates (meaning white bread, pasta, rice and most processed foods) are also linked to depression, because these foods not only supply very little in the way of nutrients but they also use up the mood-enhancing B vitamins: turning each teaspoonful of sugar into energy requires B vitamins.

The best way to keep your blood sugar level even is to eat a low-GL diet. (See Chapter 1, Part 2 for details on how to follow a low-GL diet.)

Chromium is vital for keeping your blood sugar level stable, because insulin, which clears glucose from the blood, can't work properly without it. People classified with 'atypical' depression (with symptoms of daytime sleepiness and grogginess, carbohydrate cravings, weight gain and an inclination to be very emotional) have been shown to benefit from supplementing high-dose chromium, many experiencing relief in a matter of days. This is well worth a try if these symptoms relate to you.

5. Get enough sun exposure, exercise and vitamin D

Vitamin D is known as the 'sunshine vitamin'. About 90 per cent of the body's vitamin D is synthesised in the skin by the action of sunlight. Vitamin D deficiency is implicated in depression, particularly if you feel worse during the winter.

You are most at risk of vitamin D deficiency if: you are elderly (because your ability to make it in the skin reduces with age); you are dark skinned (because you require up to six times more sunshine than a light-skinned person to make the same amount of vitamin D); you are overweight (because your vitamin D stores may be tucked away within your fat tissue); or you tend to shy away from the sun by covering up and using sun-block. Of course, you should never risk your skin health by getting sunburned. Getting sufficient sun exposure, supplementing vitamin D and eating oily fish all help to boost your reserves.

Exercising outdoors gives you the double benefit of getting vitamin D and the mood-boosting effects of the exercise itself.

6. Consider allergies

Sometimes eating a food you are unknowingly allergic to can bring on feeling low and tired. (See Allergies on page 31 to explore this further, especially if you have other symptoms that could be related to food allergies.)

Best foods

- Oily fish (salmon, mackerel, herring, kippers, sardines)
- Chia seeds
- Almonds
- Pumpkin seeds
- Green vegetables

Worst foods

- Sugar
- Caffeinated drinks
- Alcohol

Best supplements

- 2 × high-potency multivitamin–minerals providing 100mg of magnesium
- 2 × vitamin C 1,000mg
- 2 × magnesium 100mg (giving a total of 300mg with your multivitamin)
- 2 × high-potency omega-3-rich fish oil capsules (giving around 600mg of EPA, or EPA, plus DPA)
- 2 × mood-support formula providing 5-HTP 100mg, chromium 200mcg, B vitamins and/or vitamin D

Or

- 1–2 × SAMe 200mg, on an empty stomach

CAUTIONS

SAMe can be stimulating and should be used with caution in those with bipolar disorder, hyperactivity or schizophrenia.

→

If you are on SSRI antidepressants and also take large amounts of 5-HTP, this could theoretically make too much serotonin. I don't recommend combining the two. Some people get mild nausea when starting 5-HTP. If so, lower the dose. 5-HTP doesn't suit everybody.

Don't change your medication without speaking to your doctor or health-care provider.

DIG DEEPER

To find out more on this subject, read *The Feel Good Factor* (Patrick Holford), which includes key referenced studies.

DIABETES (TYPE-2)

Good medicine solutions

1. Eat a low-GL diet

Type-2 diabetes is the result of having too much sugar in your blood. Glucose – or blood sugar – fuels our brain and body, but it is highly toxic in large amounts. This is because the glucose requires large amounts of the hormone insulin to process it. Your body then becomes insensitive to insulin and therefore makes larger and larger amounts to deal with the glucose. The result of this extra insulin is damaged arteries, brain cells, kidneys and eyes. Glucose also feeds infections, causes chronic inflammation and promotes the formation of blood clots.

The solution to this is to eat a low-GL diet, which avoids the foods that raise blood sugar. Your body then becomes more sensitive to insulin and requires less to keep your blood sugar level stable. Hundreds of studies now prove that a low-GL diet helps to improve blood sugar balance, making you less insulin-resistant, and hence reducing the need for medication.

The basic principles of a low-GL diet are: (a) to eat foods that release their sugar content slowly, such as whole grains, oats, lentils, beans, apples, berries and raw or lightly cooked vegetables; (b) to eat protein with every meal or snack – for example, chicken or fish with brown rice, fruit with nuts or seeds, oatcakes with hummus; and (c) to limit refined or processed carbohydrates found in cakes, white bread and biscuits. (See Chapter 1, Part 2 for details on how to follow a low-GL diet.)

My low-GL diet is naturally high in fibre, the most effective form being the soluble fibres found in oats. The most potent soluble fibre, however, is glucomannan from the Japanese konjac plant. Supplemental glucomannan, taken either by the teaspoon in water or in 3 capsules before each meal, always with a large glass of water, is highly effective at evening out blood sugar.

2. Take daily exercise

Exercise does so much more than burn calories. It actually lowers insulin, helps to stabilise your blood sugar level, and it helps you to burn fat and build muscle. Resistance or strength-building exercise, such as using weights – which is the kind that helps build muscle – makes your body more sensitive to insulin. Also, simply moving about after a meal, such as taking a brisk ten-minute walk, helps get glucose out of the blood into the cells that need it, such as the brain and muscle cells. Ideally, take a combination of aerobic exercise (such as running, swimming or walking) and resistance training throughout the week, starting with at least 20–30 minutes a day.

3. Watch your weight

There's a strong link between being overweight and type-2 diabetes (about 80 per cent of people with diabetes are also overweight). The current thinking for the reason behind this is that fatty acids and proteins released from fat stores – especially the fat around your middle – actively interfere with the messages that normally allow glucose to be stored. It's therefore vital to get your weight under control, which you can do by following the low-GL diet and taking exercise.

4. Take supplements

In addition to following a low-GL diet, a number of supplements can help. Dozens of top-quality studies now confirm that supplementing 400–600mcg of chromium a day, which is more than ten times the average intake in the British diet, for example, helps to stabilise blood sugar. Another important vitamin for people with diabetes is vitamin C. Having a high level of vitamin C in your blood, consistent with that achieved by supplementation and eating a diet high in fruit and vegetables, reduces your risk of diabetes by 62 per cent. The optimal blood level for diabetes reduction is achieved by supplementing 1,000mg a day and eating lots of fruit and vegetables.

An essential-fat supplement will help to reduce inflammation, which promotes insulin resistance. Magnesium, manganese and zinc also help to stabilise blood sugar, and you will get these from a good-quality multivitamin and mineral supplement. Lipoic acid and vitamin E help to reduce the effects of the damage caused by excess blood sugar and these can be found in a good antioxidant formula. For further information, see Chapter 2 (Increase Your Intake of Antioxidants), Chapter 3 (Increase your Intake of Essential Fats) and Chapter 5 (Personalise Your Supplement Programme) in Part 2.

5. Reduce stress

Your blood sugar levels are also affected by the hormone cortisol, which is released into your blood when you are stressed. It instructs your cells to release sugar into your blood for energy in case of the need to take flight or fight – a vital survival mechanism in our distant past. Nowadays, however, stress is normally caused by traffic jams, work overload or family problems, and we often deal with it by taking stimulants such as caffeine or nicotine. This has the effect of releasing yet more cortisol into your blood, more sugar being released and hence more insulin, eventually leading to insulin resistance. The solution, therefore, is to find ways that help to reduce stress, which might include meditation, yoga, walks in the fresh air or deep breathing. (See Chapter 6, Part 2 on effective ways to reduce stress.)

6. Take a spoonful of cinnamon

It's now been found that just ½ teaspoon of cinnamon a day significantly reduces blood sugar levels in people with diabetes, although 1 teaspoon (6g) might be more effective. The active ingredient in cinnamon is called MCHP and can be supplemented in cinnamon concentrate called Cinnulin, which is 20 times more potent. Supplementing 150mg is the equivalent of ½ teaspoon of cinnamon. Some chromium supplements also include Cinnulin.

Best foods

- Oats, rye and barley
- Beans, lentils and chickpeas (pulses)
- Quinoa (a good source of zinc and protein)
- Seeds and nuts, especially chia, flax and pumpkin seeds, walnuts (rich in omega-3) and almonds (rich in magnesium)
- Courgettes, marrows, pumpkins and butternut squash
- Berries, cherries and plums
- Cinnamon

Worst foods

- Refined foods such as white bread, cakes, croissants (anything made with white flour and/or sugar)
- Alcohol
- Tobacco

- Caffeine
- Sugary drinks

Best supplements

▨ 2–3 × chromium picolinate or polynicotinate 200mcg daily. Cut back to 200mcg when you achieve normal blood sugar levels

▨ 1–2g of vitamin C daily

▨ 2 × a good multivitamin and mineral supplement containing at least 150mg magnesium and 10mg zinc

▨ 2 × high-potency omega-3-rich fish oil capsules giving a total of 600mg of combined EPA, DPA and DHA

▨ The equivalent of at least ½ teaspoon of cinnamon or 150mg of cinnamon extract, sometimes included in chromium supplements

Optional

▨ 3g of glucomannan fibre, with water, before each main meal

▨ 1 × antioxidant complex containing alpha lipoic acid, vitamin E as well as glutathione or NAC and co-enzymeQ_{10} (CoQ_{10})

> **CAUTIONS**
>
> I have focused here on type-2 diabetes because it is the more common type and is reversible. Type-1 (insulin-dependent) diabetes is far less prevalent and requires injection of insulin. It usually develops in children whose immune systems mistakenly attack cells in the pancreas that make insulin. Although these people will benefit from following the suggestions above, as they help to decrease the need for insulin, they will still need to inject it. Type-1 diabetes is not completely reversible. →

Bear in mind that your need for medication may decrease, so it is important to monitor your blood sugar levels and inform your health-care practitioner accordingly. If you have type-2 diabetes and follow the above guidelines, there's a good chance that you'll eventually be able to stop your medication. If you have type-1 diabetes, the same recommendations apply, but you'll still need to supplement insulin, although possibly less of it.

DIG DEEPER

To find out more about how to prevent or reverse diabetes, read *Say No to Diabetes* (Patrick Holford).

DIVERTICULITIS

see **COLITIS AND DIVERTICULITIS**

DRY SKIN

Good medicine solutions

1. Stay hydrated

An adequate fluid intake is the first step to improving dry skin, helping cells to stay plumped up and healthy by drawing water out of the bloodstream. Drinking frequently throughout the day will ensure that you don't become thirsty and dehydrated.

If you struggle to do this, try drinking at specific times instead. For example, drink a glass of water first thing in the morning, one 30 minutes after lunch, one when you get home from work, another after dinner and a small glass before you go to bed – that's already five glasses with hardly any effort.

Caffeinated drinks are not ideal, because they act as diuretics, causing you to pee more. The long-term use of diuretic medicine, used to lower blood pressure, also has the same effect and may contribute to dull, scaly, flaky and dry skin. Naturally caffeine-free herbal teas are a better option. Rooibos (red bush) tea contains no caffeine and has a similar taste to black tea; it can be taken with milk or lemon.

2. Encourage sebum production

The amount of natural oils produced by the body is the second factor in dry skin. Normally, the sebaceous glands, which are present in the deeper layers of the skin, produce sebum to lubricate the skin surface and form a barrier preventing the evaporation of moisture from the top layers of the skin. Sebum is comprised of an oily mixture of fats and triglycerides, and other substances, such as squalene and a small amount of cholesterol. It is particularly important to avoid using harsh cleansers on the skin because they will strip the sebum from the skin, leaving it feeling 'squeaky clean' but dry.

When the skin does not produce enough sebum, it becomes underprotected and susceptible to dryness. This condition is more typically seen in young skin. Mature skin that becomes dry, on the other hand, tends to lack both oil and water. Sebum secretion is primarily under the control of androgens, a type of sex hormone, but it has also been shown that calorie-restricted diets can decrease the sebum secretion rate, so it is wise to avoid these. Hormonal deficiency, for example during the menopause (see Menopausal Symptoms on page 261), can also contribute to dry skin. Conversely, eating fats, especially processed or burned 'trans' saturated fats, and carbohydrates has been shown to increase production.

The best carbohydrates to eat are wholegrain and unprocessed foods such as brown rice, brown pasta and pulses. These low-GL options naturally balance your blood sugar levels, thereby reducing stress hormone release which promotes sebum, bringing the added benefit of reducing the inflammatory processes that underlie chronic dry skin conditions such as eczema and psoriasis. (See Chapter 1, Part 2 for details on how to follow a low-GL diet.)

Eat cold-water fish such as sardines and mackerel, as well as flax or chia seeds and their cold-pressed oils to help provide the omega-3 essential fats, linoleic acid, eicosapentaenoic acid (EPA) and docosahexaenoic acid (DHA). Some supplements also provide evening primrose or borage oil for the most beneficial omega-6 fat – gamma-linolenic acid (GLA).

As well as reducing inflammatory processes, these essential fats provide the necessary raw materials for sebum production, helping to form part of the skin's protective fatty layer, and they are also incorporated into the membranes of skin cells, making them more fluid and flexible, thereby helping the skin to retain moisture. Meat and cheese are high in saturated fats, which are more rigid and inflexible, and therefore less useful as components to build cell membranes. Similarly, fats used for frying foods become damaged and are also poor for cell membrane repair.

3. Moisturise and protect cells with antioxidants

Antioxidants provide the greatest skin-nurturing effects when taken as a complex. They minimise free-radical damage in both the lipid- and water-based compartments of skin cells and help to recycle each other, prolonging their antioxidant capabilities. (There's a full explanation of antioxidants and their actions in Chapter 2, Part 2.)

Vitamin E is one of the most well-known skin nutrients, offering both moisturising and protective actions. As a fat-soluble antioxidant, it migrates to the fatty subcutaneous skin layer where it defends cells from oxidative damage. Avocado, almonds, walnuts, olives and wheatgerm are all excellent food sources of vitamin E, and you could also add their cold-pressed oils to your diet.

Vitamin A, beta-carotene and the carotenoids – abundant in carrots, apricots, sweet potatoes and broccoli – are other fat-soluble antioxidants that help to keep the skin cells moisturised. Without them, the skin becomes rough and dry. This is because vitamin A regulates the rate of skin-cell replication and the process of keratinisation. As the skin cells migrate from deeper layers towards the surface, they become harder, flatter and filled with keratin, eventually settling into a regular-shaped, tight-fitting, overlapping configuration, much like the tiles on a roof. This cellular arrangement ensures that moisture remains locked in.

It is worth both supplementing vitamin A and using a skin cream that contains it; however, products vary considerably in the amount of vitamin A used, and manufacturers don't have to declare it on the label, so it's important to choose the best skin-care products (see Resources). Some skin creams also include vitamin C and vitamin E, other important skin-friendly antioxidants.

Vitamin C helps improve circulation and the transport of nutrients to and waste from the skin's cells. Vitamin C is also essential for the synthesis of collagen, the main structural protein in the skin. It is good to eat plenty of vitamin C-rich foods (fruits and vegetables) and to ensure a minimum intake by including a daily 1,000mg supplement.

4. Take vitamin B complex for total skin support

Deficiencies in a single B vitamin can have negative effects on the skin; for example, being low in vitamin B_2 can result in dull skin and dry patches. As a group, the B vitamins support skin health in a variety of ways: encouraging circulation to the outer layers of the skin and enhancing the utilisation of essential fats. To maximise your intake, start by including brown rice and pasta, along with dark green leafy vegetables, such as kale and spinach, and eggs in your diet, and take a high-strength multivitamin or B complex, which will provide you with all eight of the B vitamins.

Best foods

- Water
- Oily fish (salmon, mackerel, herring, kippers, sardines)
- Flax and chia seeds
- Avocado
- Almonds
- Walnuts
- Olive oil
- Wheatgerm
- Eggs

Worst foods

- Caffeine
- Alcohol (associated with poor skin)
- Fried foods
- Refined foods
- Sugar

Best supplements

- 2 × high-potency multivitamin–minerals providing at least 10mg of zinc, vitamins A and E and high amounts of B vitamins

- 1 × essential omegas with fish-oil-derived omega-3, plus omega-6 from borage or evening primrose oil

- 1 × antioxidant complex providing additional vitamin A and beta-carotene, vitamin E, selenium and zinc

- 1 × vitamin C 1,000mg

Use a daily moisturiser containing vitamins A, C and E.

CAUTIONS

If you are pregnant or hoping to become so, do not exceed 3,000mcg (10,000iu) of vitamin A (retinol). Beta-carotene is not a concern.

DIG DEEPER

To find out more on this subject, read *Solve Your Skin Problems* (Patrick Holford and Natalie Savona), which includes key referenced studies.

EATING DISORDERS

General information

An eating disorder is a complex issue involving food and body weight as well as obsessive–compulsive disorder and is best dealt with by a specialised health professional. A good place to start is to contact Beat (formerly the Eating Disorders Association – see Resources). There are, however, some simple steps that can help.

Some people suffer from anorexia nervosa, which is, essentially, self-starvation. One possible reason for so doing is an unconscious desire to suppress hormonal changes in puberty to avoid 'growing up'. Another is to stimulate the release of adrenal hormones, which make the person feel good. Psychologists often say that many people with anorexia are the holders of family secrets so explore family dynamics in case there are any deep-rooted issues that need addressing.

More common today is bulimia – binge eating followed by self-induced vomiting or laxative use. Some people with anorexia are also bulimic, but not all bulimics are anorexic.

The main characteristics of an eating disorder are:

- Recurrent episodes of binge eating (the rapid consumption of large amounts of food in a discrete period of time).

- A feeling of lack of control over eating behaviour during the binges.

- Regular self-induced vomiting, use of laxatives, diuretics, strict dieting, fasting, or exercise in order to prevent weight gain.

- A minimum average of two binge-eating sessions a week.

- Persistent over-concern with body shape and weight.

- An apparent inability to eat anything other than the smallest amounts of food.

Good medicine solutions

1. Supplement zinc to correct deficiency

Many of the symptoms of zinc deficiency mimic those of eating disorders: weight loss; loss of appetite; no periods (or impotence in males); nausea; bad skin; disperceptions (a distorted sense of shape or size); depression and anxiety. A review of all the research concludes: 'There is evidence that suggests zinc deficiency may be intimately involved with anorexia in humans: if not as an initiating cause, then as an accelerating or exacerbating factor that may deepen the pathology of anorexia.' Treatment with zinc supplementation has been shown to double weight recovery.[1] Often, anorexics also choose to become vegetarian, and most vegetarian diets are lower in zinc, essential fats and protein. Many studies have shown that supplementing zinc at a daily dose of 45mg makes a big difference.

Although high levels of zinc supplementation are used in the treatment of anorexia, this does not necessarily mean that the cause of anorexia is zinc deficiency. Psychological issues may, and probably do, bring about a change in the eating habits of susceptible people.

2. Increase tryptophan: the appetite controller

Loss of weight and loss of muscle tissue is an indication of protein deficiency. This can be the result of either insufficient intake, or inadequate digestion, absorption or metabolism. The amino acids valine, isoleucine and tryptophan have been found to be low in people with anorexia. Supplementing valine and isoleucine helps to build muscle, whereas tryptophan is the building block of serotonin, a neurotransmitter that controls both mood and appetite. In fact, the conversion of tryptophan into serotonin is both zinc and B_6 dependent. These three nutrients may all be needed for proper appetite control, as well as a balanced, happy mood.

Supplementing tryptophan – or 5-hydroxytryptophan (5-HTP), which is the most powerful form of tryptophan – plus zinc and vitamin B_6 is the most direct way to address these imbalances in people with eating disorders, but in the long run the goal must be to change the diet. As a person's nutrition improves, so their anxieties and compulsive behaviours decline, and they can see the logic behind making dietary changes.

3. Ensure adequate protein and essential fats

The ideal diet should include foods that are nutrient-dense and easily digested. It is often useful to work with a health-care professional to address issues relating to resistance to eating. Good foods include those containing good-quality protein, such as quinoa, fish and soya. Others are ground seeds, such as chia, lentils and beans, plus fruits and vegetables.

Fish and seeds are especially important because they contain essential fats. Most people with eating disorders go out of their way to avoid fat, and their diets are frequently low in these essential nutrients as a result. Essential fats are vital for the body to make serotonin (the brain's feel-good neurotransmitter) and to receive the serotonin signals that cross between one neuron and another. Often, especially in those with anorexia, supplements (including concentrated fish oils) are more acceptable at first because, unlike food, they contain virtually no calories.

4. Eliminate binge foods

In the case of bulimia, the food a person chooses to binge on can be very revealing; it can be linked to either food sensitivities or blood sugar problems. The most common binge foods are sweet foods, wheat foods or dairy foods. Both wheat and dairy products contain exorphins, chemicals that mimic (and can therefore block) the pleasure-giving endorphins in the brain, and they may influence behaviour. Sweetened foods satisfy a low blood sugar condition, but the cure is to eat foods that keep your blood sugar level even by avoiding sugars. I have often asked people with bulimia to binge as much as they like for the next two weeks, but not on these foods. Often they report that their desire to binge is dramatically reduced. These foods may provoke a change in mood and behaviour in certain people that sets them off on a slippery slope to overeating. It is also possible that a person may be allergic or intolerant to certain foods that they crave.

Best foods

- Quinoa
- Fish, including oily fish (salmon, mackerel, herring, kippers, sardines)
- Beans and lentils (pulses), including soya
- Raw nuts and seeds, especially chia
- Fruits
- Vegetables

Worst foods

- Sugar and refined 'white' carbohydrates
- Caffeinated drinks (these promote excess adrenal hormones)
- Possibly specific binge foods, if food intolerance is suspected

Best supplements

- 2 × high-potency multivitamin–minerals providing at least 10mg of zinc and 20mg of B_6. This, plus the 25–35mg mentioned later, makes 45mg
- 1 × vitamin C 1,000mg
- 1 × zinc 25–35mg, possibly with added B_6
- 2 × 5-HTP 50–100mg
- 1 × high-potency omega-3-rich fish oil capsules (high EPA)

CAUTIONS

See a psychotherapist who has experience of helping people with eating disorders to achieve full recovery, and also consult a nutritional therapist with some experience of working with eating disorders.

Don't supplement 5-HTP if you are taking antidepressant drugs.

ECZEMA

General information

Eczema is an inflammatory skin condition that produces painful, red and itchy skin. The nutritional approach to eczema is based on the idea that a sufferer's total environmental 'load' – that is, how much pollution, stress and poor nutrition they are dealing with – has exceeded their capacity to adapt to it. Although there may be a specific trigger, such as an emotional crisis, drinking too much coffee or eating a food allergen, these can be experienced by the body as the final straw rather than the root cause. The goal therefore becomes to increase a person's adaptive capacity and to lessen the total load. Anti-inflammatory drugs, which are routinely prescribed for the treatment of eczema, by contrast, merely suppress the symptoms.

Good medicine solutions

1. Identify, and avoid, hidden allergies

There are two main types of allergy, IgE and IgG, which refer to different kinds of antibodies produced by your immune system. IgE, or immunoglobulinE, antibodies cause the more severe and immediate reactions.

You can test your IgE sensitivity by a blood test or a skin-prick test to identify specifically what you are reacting to. You may already have been tested routinely as an eczema sufferer, but if not, ask your doctor or arrange it yourself (see Resources).

Most eczema sufferers, however, also have IgG-based allergies to foods. These allergies are less obvious, and are sometimes called food intolerances or hidden allergies, because they don't cause immediate or severe reactions. ImmunoglobulinG (IgG) allergies are rarely tested for by doctors. (See Allergies on page 31 for more details.)

In a study involving 183 eczema sufferers, of those who were tested and then avoided the identified foods, 83 per cent reported a moderate, high or considerable benefit, with their symptoms usually resolving in three weeks.[1] The most common food allergy that can provoke eczema, especially in children, is an allergy to milk, followed by eggs.

2. Increase antioxidants

It is known that inflamed tissue results in more oxidants. Oxidants are formed, rather like exhaust fumes, whenever our cells turn food into energy. They are also created when something is burned, whether cigarettes or fried food or the petrol in cars. Oxidants have to be disarmed by antioxidants because the damage they cause in the body, oxidation, is harmful. It's sensible to increase your intake of antioxidants to counter the inflammation of eczema. Numerous studies have shown that a high intake of fresh fruit and vegetables – which boost antioxidant levels – reduces the severity of eczema.

Antioxidants are found in abundance in greens, especially broccoli, as well as peppers, berries, citrus fruit, apples (all rich in vitamin C), carrots and tomatoes (rich in beta-carotene and the powerful carotenoid, lycopene, which have been shown to be particularly important for the skin), seeds and fish (rich in vitamins A and E and selenium).

Vitamin C is a natural antihistamine; a histamine is the chemical that prompts inflammation during an allergic reaction. This means that vitamin C can give you instant relief from an eczema flare-up, as long as you take enough. A dose of 1,000mg of vitamin C reduces blood histamine by approximately 20 per cent, and 2,000mg reduces histamine by over 30 per cent.[2] There is also evidence that people supplementing 1,000mg of vitamin C a day are able to reduce their need for corticosteroids.

3. Apply transdermal vitamin A and C

Eczema sufferers may have a lot of skin damage caused by oxidants, so using creams is important. Cortisone creams, if used frequently, thin the skin, whereas vitamin A helps to thicken the outer layer, the epidermis, providing protection from sun damage, for example. Alternatives to the problematic cortisone creams are products containing the powerful antioxidant vitamins A, C and E. These have proven to be highly beneficial in trials.

Topical vitamins A and C are the most potent skin healers. In cream form, vitamin A effectively treats the negative side effects of steroids, encouraging the skin to produce a better water-proofing barrier and significantly reducing the dry skin that arises with eczema. The gentle retinyl palmitate form of vitamin A should be used in preference to the acid form.

It is important, though, to start with relatively low levels that are nevertheless effective. If a skin cream provides less than 100iu (33mcg) of vitamin A per gram, for example, it's not worth using. On the label, look for retinyl palmitate, or acetate, or retinol. On rare occasions, however, starting with too high a concentration of vitamin A – for example, double or triple this amount – can further aggravate the skin. Begin with smaller amounts of A and C cream on the skin; for example, using a product once a day for the first week, then twice a day thereafter, plus you will be taking in vitamin A from the high-strength multivitamin I recommend later, then gradually increase the amount. Some skin-care products have graded strengths of vitamin A to allow you to build up the dose gradually. If your skin does react by becoming red, lower the daily dose. This is, however, best done with the guidance of a skin-care therapist who is used to applying vitamin A-based creams.

4. Understand about omega fats

Meat and dairy products are high in arachidonic acid, a type of omega-6 fat that can promote inflammation, whereas flax seeds, chia seeds and oily fish are high in omega-3 essential fat, which is anti-inflammatory. Another anti-inflammatory fat is a type of omega-6 fat called gamma-linolenic acid (GLA), which is found in evening primrose and borage oil.

A number of studies have found that supplementing evening primrose oil reduces the itching, redness and swelling of eczema, with benefits appearing after four to eight weeks. Increasing omega-3s may help too. A study in Japan found that children who ate more omega-3-rich fish had less risk of eczema,[3] while another study gave supplements to pregnant women and reported a lower incidence of eczema in their babies.[4]

I would certainly recommend a diet low in meat and dairy, and high in oily fish such as sardines, herrings and mackerel (that is, three times a week). It's a good idea, too, to have 1 tablespoon of ground flax seeds or chia seeds and a daily supplement of 600mg of EPA, 400mg of DHA and 200mg of GLA as the ideal balanced intake.

5. Increase intake of natural anti-inflammatories

Natural anti-inflammatories include omega-3 fats, methylsulfonylmethane (MSM), quercetin, zinc, magnesium, ginger and turmeric.

MSM is a non-toxic, highly usable form of sulphur, which is part of the chemical make-up of both the skin and collagen, the intracellular 'glue'. MSM also provides the intestinal bacteria with building blocks for the manufacture of the major anti-allergy and anti-inflammatory sulphur-containing amino acids, such as methionine and cysteine.[5] Cysteine goes on to increase the production of glutathione, low levels of which are associated with inflammation.

Onions and garlic are rich in cysteine. Along with vitamin C, cysteine is also needed for the production of collagen, the major component of connective tissue. MSM helps to bond collagen fibres together, giving elasticity to the skin; it is also very effective in helping the repair of damaged or scarred skin.

The daily therapeutic dose for MSM ranges from 1,000 to 6,000mg and it is a very safe supplement to take in high doses. It works better if taken with vitamin C. A reduction in inflammation is usually seen within one to three weeks.

Quercetin is a potent anti-inflammatory found in red onions. It reduces the activity of mast cells, which release inflammatory chemicals such as histamine, certain prostaglandins, and the inflammatory 'messengers', leukotrienes.[6]

For most people, the effective therapeutic dose of quercetin is 500mg in combination with approximately 125mg of bromelain (a digestive enzyme found in pineapples) and 250–500mg vitamin C, taken before meals two to three times a day.

Ginger and turmeric have long been known to help inflammatory diseases. Exactly why they work has only recently been discovered. In inflammatory diseases, an inflammation-promoting protein known as nuclear transcription factor kappa B is produced. Ginger and turmeric, along with garlic and pepper, turn this protein off, thereby reducing inflammation.[7] I recommend the liberal use of both ginger and turmeric if you suffer from eczema. They're both tasty additions to curries and relishes, and fresh ginger is also delicious with red lentils, sliced into stir-fries or used to make tea.

Zinc and magnesium are also natural anti-inflammatories. Zinc also helps heal the skin.

'I used to have . . .'

Liza used Betnovate cream (a corticosteroid cream) for her eczema almost every day. She then took an IgG food intolerance test, which showed that she was reacting to dairy products and mildly sensitive to gluten (the protein found in wheat, rye, barley and oats) and egg white. She avoided those foods and stopped drinking coffee (there is a strong link between stimulants and stress exacerbating inflammation), took supplements and applied vitamin A cream to her skin.

One month later, Liza said:

'I feel so much better – nothing like as tired. My skin is a lot better. I have no sores or cuts. The vitamin A cream really works very well.'

Three months later, Liza was still eczema-free and had not needed to use the Betnovate cream once since she had begun her allergy-free diet.

Best foods

- Oily fish (salmon, mackerel, herring, kippers, sardines)
- Free-range eggs
- Turmeric
- Ginger
- Red onions
- Garlic
- Fresh fruits, especially berries
- Vegetables, especially greens
- Flax seeds and chia seeds

Worst foods

- Sugar and refined 'white' foods (promote inflammation)
- Caffeinated drinks
- Alcohol (promotes inflammation)
- Dairy products (for many people)
- Meat

Best supplements

- 2 × essential omegas with fish-oil-derived omega-3, plus omega-6 from borage or evening primrose oil providing about 600mg of EPA, 400mg of DHA and 200mg of GLA
- 2 × high-potency multivitamin–minerals providing at least 1,500mcg of vitamin A, 10mg of zinc, 100mg of magnesium
- 2 × vitamin C 1,000mg
- 2 × anti-inflammatory formulas containing a combination of quercetin, MSM, vitamin C, bromelain

Or

- 2 × MSM 1,000mg

- 2 × N-acetyl cysteine (NAC) 500mg

Apply vitamin A and C skin creams daily

CAUTIONS

Gradually increase the concentration of vitamin A in skin creams to avoid initial irritation.

DIG DEEPER

To find out more on this subject, read *Solve Your Skin Problems* (Patrick Holford and Natalie Savona), which includes key referenced studies.

EYESIGHT DETERIORATION

General information

As you get older you are encouraged to have regular eye checkups, partly to make any adjustments to your spectacles prescription but also to check for the three most common eye conditions that can lead to blindness: cataracts (clouding of the lens in the eye), glaucoma (a dangerous rise in the pressure in the eye) and age-related macular degeneration (a loss of the sharp-focusing area at the centre of the retina). The following advice can help to protect you from these eye problems and slow down eyesight deterioration.

Good medicine solutions

1. Increase your intake of vitamin A and other antioxidants

Vitamin A is the most important nutrient for eyes. It is a key part of the chemical process that turns photons of light into the electrical nerve impulses that travel from the eye to the brain. It also maintains the mucous lining of the eye; supports tear production; protects the eye from the harmful effects of bright sunlight; and prevents night blindness. Vitamin A can only be obtained from the diet, and comes in two forms. One is the readily absorbed, fat-soluble vitamin retinol, found in animal tissues; the other is known as beta-carotene and is obtained from plants, particularly apricots, cantaloupe melons, carrots, pumpkins, sweet potatoes, spinach, squashes and broccoli. Beta-carotene is converted into retinol in the liver.

If your eyesight is deteriorating, you would need to be supplementing at least 10,000iu (3000mcgRE) vitamin A a day.

Oxidants are created in our cells when something is burned, whether cigarettes or fried food or the petrol in cars. They have to be disarmed by antioxidants because the damage they cause in the body, oxidation, is harmful. Oxidants are also created by ultraviolet rays from the sun. The antioxidants that help protect against these oxidants include vitamins C and E, as well as co-enzyme Q_{10} (CoQ_{10}) and some rather more specialised compounds: acetyl-l-carnitine, n-acetyl-cysteine and alpha lipoic acid. One large study of over 3,000 people found that a combination of antioxidants (vitamins C and E and beta-carotene, plus zinc), could slow down the progression of age-related macular degeneration (AMD) by 25 per cent and reduce vision loss by 19 per cent.[1] The higher your vitamin C intake, the lower your risk of cataracts and glaucoma. CoQ_{10} has been shown to help prevent both cataracts and AMD. It is naturally present in the eye, but the amount declines by about 40 per cent between youth and old age.

These nutrients are often provided in antioxidant and eye-support supplements and are well worth taking to protect your eyes as you get older.

2. Eat more green vegetables, red onions and brightly coloured fruits

Carrots are an especially rich source of a group of nutrients called carotenoids. Two carotenoids present in the macula of the eye – lutein and zeathanthin – are powerful antioxidant pigments. The richest sources of these are found not in carrots but in green leafy vegetables and brightly coloured fruits, as well as egg yolks. Lutein and zeathanthin appear to protect the retina and help prevent age-related diseases such as AMD and cataracts. The more you eat, the lower your risk. Lutein and zeathanthin are also worth supplementing and are often found in eye-support formulas.

Lutein is an oil-soluble nutrient found in vegetables. If you add a splash of olive oil or a little butter to your vegetables you will actually absorb the lutein better from them than if you eat them without any fat.

Red onions are particularly high in quercetin, a potent antioxidant and anti-inflammatory, which has been shown to protect against cataract formation.[2] In an animal study, onions have been shown to prevent cataract formation.[3]

3. Check your homocysteine level and supplement B vitamins

Studies have found that patients with AMD have higher levels of the damaging amino acid homocysteine, but those who took a combination of B vitamins (which brings down homocysteine) had a lower chance of developing it. As a minimum, to keep homocysteine levels lower, take a multivitamin that provides 20mg of vitamin B_6, 200mcg of folic acid and 10mcg of vitamin B_{12}, which are the most important B vitamins for keeping your homocysteine level healthy. Ideally, check your homocysteine level. (See Chapter 4, Part 2 for more on this.)

4. Eat fish, supplement fish oil and get enough vitamin D

Omega-3 fats are essential for the eyes, because the retina naturally contains high levels of docosahexaenoic acid (DHA), which is a type of omega-3 fat that is also part of the brain's structure.[4] Abnormalities in the tear film, which keeps the eye moist, result from a lack of omega-3 oils, which are obtained in the diet from oily fish and seeds such as flax and chia. Combining omega-3 fats with antioxidants is particularly protective.

Another important nutrient to supplement, especially if you live in northern Europe, is vitamin D. High levels of vitamin D in the blood are associated with a decreased risk of developing AMD.

5. Protect your eyes with a low-GL diet

Eating white rice, pasta and bread increases your odds of developing AMD, because these foods disrupt blood sugar levels, leading to weight gain. In turn, obesity immediately puts you at a greater risk of developing cataracts, glaucoma and AMD, because high levels of blood sugar, which tend to go with obesity, can lead to diabetes and can also cause damage to the blood vessels of the eye. If you're carrying extra weight, you should aim to bring it down. The best way to do this is by following a low-GL diet, which keeps blood sugar levels stable. A low-GL diet will also help to keep your blood pressure down (see page 195), which is also important for eye health. (See Chapter 1, Part 2 for details on how to follow a low-GL diet.)

General advice

Here are some ways to protect your eyes from degeneration:

- Only wear sunglasses in very strong sunlight – your eyes need certain wavelengths of sunlight to remain healthy.

- Sleep in total darkness to allow the rods and cones in the retina to replenish.

- Trayner pinhole glasses can help with focusing problems, such as far- and near-sightedness, computer strain, eye strain, headaches and presbyopia (difficulty reading small print). Regular use of the Trayner glasses builds up the eye muscles and reshapes the eyes.

- If you spend a lot of time on the computer, make sure that you sit squarely facing the computer and aim to position the screen so that it's a little below your eye level. Blink very regularly to rest and lubricate the eyes. Take a short break every hour and use the palming technique from the Bates Method to increase eye responsiveness: place your palms over your eyes, relax and breathe deeply until all you see is black.

- The lighting of your work area should be equal to the computer screen.

'I used to have . . . '

Daisy, 82, had been suffering from AMD for six years and could no longer go shopping or enjoy her garden, because she had tripped over several times and hurt herself quite badly. She was keen to try supplements to see if she could at least stop the disease progressing. Daisy took a broad-spectrum antioxidant capsule, a B complex, and an omega-3 essential fat supplement, and then made some changes to her diet as recommended here. Her eyesight and overall health have improved considerably.

Best foods

- Green vegetables and broccoli
- Orange-coloured vegetables
- Oily fish (salmon, mackerel, herring, kippers, sardines)
- Chia and flax seeds
- Raw nuts, especially walnuts (a rich source of omega-3)
- Red onions
- Eggs
- Brightly coloured fruits
- Tomatoes

Worst foods

- Vegetable oils (except olive oil)
- Sugar and refined 'white' food
- Dairy products (if allergic or if you have sinus problems)

Best supplements

- 2 × high-potency multivitamin–minerals providing optimal levels of B vitamins, plus vitamin A (at least 1,500mcg), beta-carotene (at least 500mcg) and vitamin D (at least 15mcg)

- 2 × vitamin C 1,000mg

- 2 × essential omegas with fish-oil-derived omega-3, plus omega-6 from borage or evening primrose oil

- 2 × antioxidant or eye support formula* including as many of these as possible: vitamins A, C and D, lutein, zeathanthin, CoQ_{10}, alpha lipoic acid and acetyl-l-carnitine. *Aim for a total intake of vitamin A of at least 3,300mcg (10,000iu), if not twice this amount

> ### CAUTIONS
>
> High doses of vitamin A in the animal form of retinol (about 10,000iu (3,000mcg) a day), is not recommended during pregnancy.

DIG DEEPER

For more information on the Bates Method, read the book *Improve Your Eyesight – A Guide to the Bates Method for Better Eyesight without Glasses* (Jonathan Barnes).

FIBROMYALGIA

General information

Fibromyalgia (FM) is a debilitating condition, characterised by chronic musculo-skeletal pain that doesn't respond to anti-inflammatory drugs. It is often accompanied by chronic, disabling fatigue; many very tender spots on the neck, shoulders, back and hips; constant aches; general stiffness; sleep disturbances; and depression. As such, it is similar in a number of ways to chronic fatigue syndrome (see page 88), but with the addition of muscular pain.

True fibromyalgia does not arise from inflammation. Rather, research indicates that the painful muscles are caused by decreased energy production and the reduced ability of muscles to relax.[1] This has been linked to a deficiency in the energy molecule adenosine-5 triphosphate (ATP) which is normally produced in each cell of the body to provide the fuel for its functions.[2] Without ATP, the cells (and consequently the muscles) cannot function optimally. In the case of FM, the muscles fail to relax properly once they have contracted. One factor contributing to ATP deficiency is poor oxygen supply to cells. Insufficient oxygen (called hypoxia) results in low energy production and compromised cellular function in general.

Good medicine solutions

1. Boost magnesium and energy vitamins through supplements and food

Research has shown that a deficiency in magnesium can lead to an increased perception of pain.[3] This, in turn, increases stress, which stimulates the release of stress hormones. One effect of these is to push magnesium out of the cells, further depleting stores of this vital mineral[4] and worsening muscular pain. The way out of this vicious cycle is to supplement both magnesium and malic acid as magnesium malate, which is required for the proper function of muscle cells (malic acid is found in apples and apple cider vinegar).[5] This can reduce pain within days. Other nutrients that are particularly necessary for the efficient production of ATP are B vitamins, manganese and co-enzyme Q_{10} (CoQ_{10}). Indeed, symptoms of a deficiency in B vitamins, particularly B_1, resemble those of fibromyalgia. Manganese is also needed for various hormonal processes that lead to thyroxine output, a lack of which can result in an overall decline in metabolism and energy production.

It is also wise to eat nutrient-rich foods such as green vegetables, raw nuts and seeds, especially pumpkin and chia seeds, fresh fruit, oily fish and other whole foods such as beans and lentils (pulses). Avoid nutrient-empty foods such as sugar, processed and refined foods, as well as damaged fats in burned meat.

2. Supplement 5-HTP

The disrupted sleep patterns experienced by many FM sufferers can contribute to further exhaustion and anxiety. Studies taken in France found that people diagnosed with FM have low levels of serotonin in the brain.[6] Serotonin is a neurotransmitter that is partly responsible for bringing about restful sleep. It is made from the amino acid tryptophan. Supplements of 5-hydroxytryptophan (5-HTP), in doses of 200mg one hour before bedtime, can help restore restful sleep (see Insomnia on page 236).

5-HTP can also help to reduce muscular pain.[7] According to Professor Federigo Sicuteri from the University of Florence, an expert in this area of research, 'In our experience, as well as in that of other pain specialists, 5-HTP can largely improve the painful picture of primary fibromyalgia'.[8] This is especially useful to try if you have either sleep or mood problems.

3. Check for, and lower, your homocysteine

A team of researchers headed by Dr Bjorn Regland at the Institute of Clinical Neuroscience at Sweden's Göteborg University ran a battery of tests on fibromyalgia sufferers, including testing for homocysteine. Homocysteine is a toxic amino acid that is linked to a number of health issues. It accumulates if you have an insufficient intake of B vitamins (B_2, B_6, B_{12}, folic acid). By far the most significant finding was that every single person with fibromyalgia also had high homocysteine. The researchers also found a direct correlation between the participants' B_{12} status and the severity of their reported symptoms.[9] Fibromyalgia sufferers should routinely test for homocysteine and, if high, immediately start on a homocysteine-lowering programme, including high-dose vitamin B_{12} (see Chapter 4, Part 2).

4. Reduce stress; take gentle exercise and stretch

Massage and exercise help to increase the supply of oxygen to tissues by stimulating the blood flow. These do not, however, address the underlying cause of the energy deficiency and pain.

Indeed, some people feel worse after having a massage, and many feel unable to take any exercise while they are exhausted and in pain, so I suggest you proceed with caution.

Reduce your stress levels and learn how to relax (see Chapter 6, Part 2). Other relaxation methods, such as yoga, t'ai chi and breathing exercises, can also be useful.

Exercise should be gradually increased as your capacity for taking it increases. Posture and overall body structure need to be optimised, perhaps with the help of an osteopath or Alexander Technique teacher. Gentle massage, heat treatment and gentle stretching will also help to improve muscle function and reduce pain.

Best foods

- Green vegetables
- Raw nuts and seeds
- Pumpkin and chia seeds
- Fresh fruit
- Whole foods
- Oily fish (salmon, mackerel, herring, kippers, sardines)

Worst foods

- Sugar
- Processed and refined 'white' food
- Burned fat and meats

Best supplements

- 2 × high-potency multivitamin–minerals providing optimal levels of B vitamins, vitamin D, manganese and magnesium

- 2 × vitamin C 1,000mg

- 2 × essential omegas with fish-oil-derived omega-3, plus omega-6 from borage or evening primrose oil

- 2 × magnesium malate giving 300mg of elemental magnesium
- 2 × 5-HTP 50–100mg

Optional

- 2 × CoQ$_{10}$ 30–50mg

CAUTIONS

Make sure you have the correct diagnosis. Some people with vitamin D deficiency, which can cause muscle aches, have been wrongly diagnosed with fibromyalgia. It is worth checking your vitamin D status and supplementing accordingly.

DIG DEEPER

To find out more on this subject, read *Say No to Arthritis* (Patrick Holford), which includes key referenced studies.

GASTROENTERITIS (STOMACH BUGS)

General information

A severe stomach bug is called gastroenteritis, which means inflammation of the gastrointestinal tract. This can be caused by a viral or bacterial infection. Other parasitical organisms can cause similar symptoms to gastroenteritis.

Good medicine solutions

1. Take essential probiotics

There are different causes of acute stomach bugs and gastroenteritis, all of which can result in abdominal pain, diarrhoea and vomiting. If the symptoms are acute, and the cause is thought to be bacterial, the appropriate treatment is antibiotics. These, however, can often make diarrhoea worse because they irritate the gut.

Taking probiotics – bacteria that are beneficial to the digestive system – during infection has been shown to halve the recovery time from diarrhoea. Also, if you have been taking a course of antibiotics, these disturb the normal gut bacteria that keep you healthy. Supplementing probiotics for a few weeks after an infection, or during and after taking antibiotics, will greatly accelerate the recovery of the gut by repopulating it with normal, healthy gut bacteria.

The two main strains of bacteria that are resident in the human gut are *Lactobacillus acidophilus* and *Lactobacillus bifidus* (bifidobacteria). There is also another strain called *Lactobacillus rhamnosus* (sometimes called *Lactobacillus GG*) and a type of yeast called *Saccharomyces boulardii* (or *S. boulardii*), all of which have been shown to speed up recovery from diarrhoea.

Lactobacillus acidophilus and *Lactobacillus bifidus* are the better strains for recovery of healthy gut bacteria after taking antibiotics. Although yoghurt, containing bacteria, is good, you need about 5–10 billion active organisms for an effect. To achieve this, you need supplementation. These are best taken on an empty stomach, because stomach acid will destroy only a proportion, but not all, of these bacteria when taken this way. Stomach acid is released when you eat protein-rich foods.

2. High-dose vitamin C helps

Vitamin C is both antibacterial and anti-viral, but is most effective against viruses. Many cases of gastroenteritis are caused by viruses, such as the rotavirus and norovirus. High-dose vitamin C can help to speed up recovery, but it is a double-edged sword because too much can induce diarrhoea. The optimal dose is the amount that you can take that is just below that which causes loose bowels (known as bowel tolerance).

Because vitamin C is in and out of the body in a few hours, the best results are achieved by taking 500–1,000mg every one or two hours during infection. Pure vitamin C is ascorbic acid. A gentler, alkaline form is called ascorbate. Dehydration is the major problem to watch out for when you have a stomach bug (see below), and a recommended way to take high-dose vitamin C is to mix sodium ascorbate powder with water and a little juice, then to sip it regularly.

Vitamin C also helps antibiotics to work and aids recovery from *Helicobacter pylori*, a bacterial infection that causes stomach ulcers (see page 356).

3. Use high-dose vitamin B₃ to kill super-bugs

Super-bugs, such as the antibiotic-resistant *Staph.* infections, are becoming a real problem, killing thousands of people worldwide. Now, researchers from the Linus Pauling Institute have found that high-dose vitamin B₃ can increase the ability of immune cells to kill *Staph.* bacteria by 1,000 times.[1] The work was done both in laboratory animals and using human blood. The vitamin, given in the form of niacinamide, boosted natural immunity, dramatically increasing the number and efficacy of neutrophils, a specialised type of white blood cell that can kill and eat harmful bacteria. In human blood, clinical doses of vitamin B₃ appeared to wipe out the *Staph.* infection in only a few hours. Although full human trials are yet to be carried out, it suggests that high-dose niacinamide – 1,000–3,000mg – could make a big difference to fighting bacterial infections. There is no known harm from taking this dose of niacinamide, especially for short term use. The recommended daily allowance (RDA) for vitamin B$_3$ is 18mg, so the supplemented quantity is way beyond any amount that could be achieved through diet.

4. Keep well hydrated

The major danger for anyone suffering from gastroenteritis is becoming chronically dehydrated. If you have acute diarrhoea, with a dry mouth and sunken eyes, and you are feeling extremely weak and not peeing much at all, it is vital to see a doctor, who will give you some hydration salts added to water. The salts are essential because if the body loses too much liquid through acute diarrhoea, vital minerals, including sodium (salt), get depleted.

For this reason, it is important to keep drinking. You can buy rehydration salts, to add to water, in any pharmacist.

5. Choose the right foods and drinks

Food poisoning is usually the result of staphylococci, salmonella or campylobacter infection, all of which can be treated with the appropriate antibiotics. Many gastric illness incidents happen after eating food from restaurants that do not practise food safety, such as re-freezing thawed food. The same cautions apply when you prepare and eat at home.

Niacinamide (see above) has been shown to be highly effective against staphylococci infections, however.

The most common foods to cause food poisoning are undercooked meat and chicken, unfresh fish (especially tuna), shellfish and eggs, and leafy greens that have been exposed to animal manure or contaminated water.

You can reduce your risk by:

- Eating fresh food, ideally grown locally and organically. Always wash unpeeled fruit and vegetables thoroughly and wash meat, poultry and fish before preparing.

- Only eating free-range fresh eggs, discarding those with broken shells, and cooking thoroughly.

- Only having raw fish when you know it is fresh and of good quality.

- Only eating shellfish and crab when you know it is fresh and of good quality.

- Only drinking bottled water or boiled water in areas with a high risk of contaminated water.

Although you may not feel like eating, the immune system needs protein to stay strong. Eating soups made with beans, lentils or a meat stock is a gentle way to keep nourished and hydrated.

6. Try natural protection

Garlic contains allicin, a pungent oily liquid that is anti-viral, anti-fungal and antibacterial. Rich in sulphur-containing amino acids, it also acts as an antioxidant. Allicin is undoubtedly an important ally in fighting infections. Consider taking a garlic clove daily, particularly if you are travelling in regions where food poisoning is more common.

Grapefruit seed extract is a powerful antimicrobial agent. The great advantage, however, is that it doesn't adversely affect the beneficial bacteria in the gut. It is bought as drops and can be swallowed or used to gargle with. As it is antiseptic, it can also be used as nose drops or ear drops, depending on the site of infection. This is a good all-rounder to have if you are travelling. You need about 20 drops two or three times a day if you have an infection, or 10 drops or a capsule a day as a preventative.

Glutamine is an amino acid (a basic protein building block) that helps the gut recover when taken after or during an infection.

Antibiotics also take their toll on the gut, and glutamine helps healthy cells in the intestinal wall to regenerate after antibiotic use. You need 5–10g, which is 1–2 heaped teaspoons, of glutamine powder, in a glass of cold water last thing at night or first thing in the morning on an empty stomach.

Zinc, one of the most important immune-boosting minerals, is found in high quantities in nuts and seeds as well as seafood and eggs. Make sure your supplement gives you at least 10mg a day, although up to 30mg a day can help your body fight a variety of infections. Some vitamin C tablets contain zinc. These are ideal during an infection.

Best foods

- Water
- Bean, lentil and vegetable or meat stock soups (such as consommé)
- Vegetable juices
- Oat porridge with ground seeds

Worst foods

- Under-cooked meat, chicken and eggs
- Unfresh fish, especially tuna, or shellfish
- Uncooked vegetables in areas known to have a high risk of infection
- Sugar (feeds pathogenic bacteria)

Best supplements

- 2 × high-potency multivitamin–minerals providing at least 10mg of zinc

- 4–10 × vitamin C 1,000mg, ideally with zinc, up to 'bowel tolerance' or the equivalent of 10g a day of ascorbate dissolved in water, or more up to 'bowel tolerance'

- 2 × *Lactobacillus acidophilus* and bifidobacteria giving 5–10 billion active organisms, ideally away from food or before meals

- 1–2 teaspoons (5–10g) of glutamine powder in water, away from food

Optional

For bacterial infections, especially *Staph.*:

- 2–3 × niacinamide (B_3) 500mg (note: not 'niacin' – a form of B_3 that makes you blush when taken in high doses)

> ## CAUTIONS
>
> If you are not better within a few days, or if your symptoms are acute or you have any signs of dehydration, it is very important to seek immediate medical attention. It is better not to take iron supplements, or a multivitamin with iron, at the same time as antibiotics, as the iron reduces the absorption of some antibiotics.

GOUT

Good medicine solutions

1. Reduce your levels of uric acid

Ideally, your uric acid levels should be 6.0mg/dL or lower, as there is a 90 per cent chance of having an acute attack of gout when levels rise above 9.0mg/dL. Uric acid is not normally harmful; it's actually a potent antioxidant (a substance that removes potentially damaging oxidising agents in the body) with almost as much activity as vitamin C. Problems arise when there are high levels of uric acid, which solidifies into needle-shaped crystals, jabbing their way into the joints, causing the pain and inflammation typically associated with gout.

About 70 per cent of gout sufferers produce too much uric acid, so reducing the foods that promote the production of this acid is a good place to start.

There are several ways for you to do this. Start by limiting alcohol, fried foods, roasted nuts, rich cakes and pies made with refined flour, as these foods either promote production of or decrease your ability to eliminate uric acid. Meat and organ meat have a high uric acid content, so eliminate these from your diet.

I also recommend removing foods that are rich in purines. Purines are metabolised in the body to produce uric acid, so if you regularly eat these foods you're just adding fuel to the fire. During an acute attack, limit your purine intake to between 100mg and 150mg per day.

Purines are present in all of the body's cells and almost all foods; however, recent research indicates that the effect of purines on the body and their impact on gout risk are dependent on the food source. Purines from protein foods such as meat and fish increased gout risk, whereas purines from vegetables didn't change the risk and those from dairy foods appeared to lower the risk.[1]

High-purine foods[2]

The amount in parentheses gives the mg quantity of purine per 100g (3½oz) of food

Theobromine (2,300mg) (between 2 and 10% in cocoa powder)	Mushrooms (488mg) (except chanterelles)
Brewer's yeast (1,810mg)	Sardines (480mg)
Sweetbreads (1,260mg)	Anchovies (239mg)
Smoked sprats (804mg)	Herring (210mg)
Baker's yeast (680mg)	Mackerel (145mg)
Offal (500mg)	Shellfish (118mg)

My advice would be to reduce your intake of fish and meat, limit dairy and focus on fresh vegetables and fruits. Foods with the lowest purine content are listed below:

Low-purine foods[3]

The amount in parentheses gives the mg quantity of purine per 100g (3½oz) of food

Cheddar cheese (6mg)	Lettuce (13mg)
Sweet cherries (7.1mg)	Onion (13mg)
Cucumber (7.3mg)	Radish (13mg)
Yoghurt (min. 3.5% fat) (8.1mg)	Sauerkraut (16mg)
Cottage cheese (9.4mg)	Chanterelle mushrooms (17mg)
Tomato (11mg)	Endive (17mg)
Pear (12mg)	Potato, skin on (18mg)
Rhubarb (12mg)	

2. Eat sour cherries

Sour cherries are particularly beneficial for the reduction of gout. Anecdotal evidence suggests that sour cherries were effective in reducing the frequency of attacks and for alleviating pain. This has since been confirmed with studies showing that consumption of sour cherries reduces uric acid levels and inhibits inflammatory pathways. Generally, it is now recognised that cherries are an effective remedy for gout.

In a 2003 study by the US Department of Agriculture (USDA), University of California at Davis researchers found that eating 280g of cherries (that's about two servings), after an overnight fast lowered uric acid levels by about 15 per cent. In the authors' words: 'The decrease in plasma urate after cherry consumption supports the reputed anti-gout efficacy of cherries.'[4]

The reduction in pain is believed to stem from the high content of anthocyanins, the pigments that give cherries their deep red colour. Anthocyanins have the strongest antioxidant actions of this class of compounds. They also inhibit the inflammatory COX-1 and COX-2 pathways that are typically targeted by painkillers such as aspirin and ibuprofen.

Plums, sweet cherries and berries are also beneficial to eat, but it is sour cherries in particular that provide the strongest benefits. The Montmorency cherry contains the highest concentrations of anthocyanins I and II – about 30–40mg per 100g (3½oz) of fruit – significantly more than sweet cherries. Or, even better, take Cherry Active, a more concentrated form of Montmorency cherry, which gives you 280mg of anthocyanins in three capsules or a single 30ml shot. Take three capsules or one shot each day.

3. Reduce your intake of fructose and follow a low-GL diet

When you drink fruit juices you get a huge hit of fructose, because the fibres from the fruit have been removed, leaving the fruit sugars (fructose) behind. Most fizzy drinks are very high in high-fructose corn syrup (HFCS), which is the worst kind of sugar of all. The problem is that fructose cannot be directly used for energy by the body and has to be converted into glucose by the liver, a process that creates uric acid, and hence promotes gout.

Several studies looking at adolescents and adults have confirmed this link. Levels of uric acid increase when more sweetened drinks are taken. Drinking two or more sweetened drinks a day, drinking fruit juice and eating fructose-rich fruits such as oranges and apples increases the risk of gout in healthy individuals. The best thing is to remove fructose and HFCS from your diet – drinking just one serving a day of sugar-sweetened drinks may increase gout risk by 74 per cent.

You can go further by following a low-GL diet, which is the most rapid way to stabilise blood sugar levels and will, naturally, reduce the amount of both fructose and uric acid in your system. Eating a low-GL diet also improves your resistance to insulin – which is the hormone you produce to process sugar – and this helps to support healthy kidney function, which is particularly important because the kidneys excrete uric acid. When you eat a low-GL diet you will almost certainly find that your gout goes away, along with unwanted fat. This is the best diet to follow if you're reducing your weight to reduce your gout risk, since fasting or severely restricted diets can raise uric acid levels. (See Chapter 1, Part 2 for details on how to follow a low-GL diet.)

A low-fructose/low-GL diet is naturally anti-inflammatory. Essential fats and the supplements quercetin and bromelain will also reduce inflammation. Take a fish oil supplement, add chia seeds to your food or use a cold-pressed organic flax seed oil to obtain your healthy essential fatty acids. These are all rich in the omega-3 fat eicosapentaenoic acid (EPA), which will limit leukot-riene production, thereby reducing tissue damage and inflam-mation, and will also promote tissue repair and healing in the affected joints. (You will find a full explanation of the effects of inflammation on the body in Chapter 3, Part 2.)

You can also supplement quercetin and bromelain. The bio-flavonoid quercetin inhibits both uric acid production and the production of inflammatory compounds. Bromelain, an enzyme primarily found in the stalk of unripe pineapples, is anti-inflam-matory and works synergistically with quercetin. Take these together, 125–250mg of each, preferably between meals.

4. Cut back on alcohol and drink more water

Moderate your alcohol intake, as the more alcohol you drink, the greater your gout risk. It's common to think of gout sufferers as older men, eating rich diets, drinking port and red wine; how-ever, a recent large-scale study published in the *Lancet* found that although drinking alcohol is linked with an increased risk of developing gout, the consumption of beer had the strongest association, followed by spirits, then wine.[5]

Make sure you also drink plenty of water, which helps to flush out the excess uric acid and improves kidney clearance. Around 30 per cent of gout sufferers have a reduced ability to excrete uric acid, and nine out of ten people with high blood uric acid levels and gout have some level of kidney dysfunction. Distilled water, which has fewer inorganic minerals, is better than tap water.

Best foods

- Vegetables
- Cherries, berries, plums, pear, rhubarb, kiwi
- Water – drink at least eight glasses a day, including hot drinks

Worst foods

- Meat and offal
- High-purine foods (see chart on page 175)
- High-sugar/GL foods (Chapter 1, Part 2)
- Alcohol
- Fruit juices and sodas

Best supplements

- 2 × high-potency multivitamin–minerals providing 20mg of vitamin B_6, 150mg of magnesium and 10mg of zinc, all of which are essential for good protein metabolism
- 2 × vitamin C 1,000mg
- 3 capsules or 30ml Cherry Active (see Resources)

CAUTIONS

Avoid taking high doses of niacin (vitamin B_3), over 50mg per day, as niacin competes with urate for excretion.

GUM DISEASE

see **TOOTH DECAY and PERIODONTAL (GUM)
DISEASE**

HAY FEVER

Good medicine solutions

1. Supplement vitamin C

Vitamin C is the most important anti-allergy vitamin. It is a powerful promoter of a strong immune system and it immediately calms down allergic reactions. It is also anti-inflammatory. I recommend everyone takes vitamin C at an absolute minimum of 1,000mg (1g) a day, although 2,000mg (2g) or more is optimum for most people, whether or not you have allergies. If you are suffering from allergic symptoms, you might want to take twice this amount on a regular basis. Vitamin C is flushed out of the body within six hours, and for this reason it is best taken in divided doses, either 1,000mg in the morning and 1,000mg at lunch or, if you're taking larger amounts, 1,000mg four times a day. You also can increase your vitamin C intake through food by eating plenty of fresh fruit and vegetables, although you would have to eat an enormous amount to get up to 2g; for example, 100g (3½oz) of peppers contains about 100mg of vitamin C, 100g (3½oz) of broccoli contains 110mg, and 100g (3½oz) of strawberries 60mg – that's assuming they are fresh, of course. Foods that contain vitamin C typically also contain antioxidant bioflavonoids, such as hesperidin, rutin and quercetin, and these bioflavonoids may actually help the body absorb vitamin C – another good reason to eat vitamin-C-rich foods.

2. Increase your intake of omega-3 fats

Omega-3 fish oils are one of nature's best natural anti-inflammatory nutrients, with countless other benefits besides. Although you can, and should, obtain these from eating unfried, unbreaded fish, I also recommend you supplement omega-3 fish oils every day as an insurance policy. To give you a rough idea, I recommend you take in the equivalent of 1,000mg of combined eicosapentaenoic acid (EPA) and docosahexaenoic acid (DHA) a day, or 7,000mg a week (these are the two most powerful omega-3 fats). A 100g (3½oz) serving of mackerel might give you 2,000mg, whereas a similar serving of salmon might give you 1,000mg. If you eat fish three times a week you'll probably achieve 3,500mg a week. To make up the remaining 3,500mg, take an omega-3 fish oil supplement providing 500mg of combined EPA and DHA a day. This is good advice for anyone, even if you're not especially allergic.

3. Supplement other anti-allergy/anti-inflammatory nutrients

Quercetin is bioflavonoid and potent antioxidant that promotes a healthy response to inflammation. Animal studies show that quercetin helps stop excess histamine, which is what causes most of the symptoms in hay fever. One study found that, of all the flavonoids, quercetin was the most effective at inhibiting histamine. The best food sources of quercetin are red onions, apples and berries, but you would be hard pushed to eat more than 20mg a day. Supplementing therapeutic amounts is therefore necessary if you're suffering with allergies. Take 500mg three times a day if your symptoms are severe, then drop down to 500mg once a day once your reaction is under control. This maintenance dose is also effective for reducing your allergic potential. The best results are achieved by supplementing 250mg twice a day, with some bromelain (see below) and vitamin C.

Bromelain is a collection of proteolytic (literally meaning protein breakdown) enzymes found in pineapple stems that have considerable anti-inflammatory and anti-swelling properties. In a double-blind clinical trial, participants given 160mg of bromelain daily experienced significant improvements in nasal drainage and swelling and restored free breathing, compared to those on a dummy treatment. Take up to 300mg daily and if you are having an allergic reaction, or 100mg daily to reduce your allergic potential.

Methylsulfonylmethane (MSM) has so many benefits for allergy sufferers that it's hard to know where to start. In one study, 55 volunteers diagnosed with seasonal allergies were given 1,300mg of MSM twice daily for 30 days. A significant reduction in symptoms of both the upper respiratory tract (including nasal congestion) and the lower respiratory tract (including coughing) was seen. As long as you're still suffering from any allergic symptoms it's well worth supplementing MSM on a daily basis. Although therapeutic intakes go up to 6,000mg a day, I recommend you start with 1,000mg, or half this if taken in combination with the other anti-allergy nutrients.

Glutamine is an essential part of any regime designed to restore healthy mucous membranes quickly and reduce allergic potential. It is also a powerful nutrient for supporting proper immune function and protecting the liver. As part of a daily anti-allergy regime, take 500mg.

Some supplements contain combinations of these anti-inflammatory nutrients, so you can take them all in one pill.

4. Test for, and avoid, other food allergens

If you are eating foods that you are unknowingly allergic to, your immune system will be primed to react allergically, and grass pollen may be the last straw. The most common food allergens are wheat and milk. Wheat is a kind of grass, and cows make milk from grass. Many people have observed that during the hay fever season avoiding milk and wheat greatly reduces their allergic sensitivity. (See Allergies on page 31 to find out how to test for, and avoid, other potential food allergens or intolerances.)

Even if you are not allergic, having large amounts of dairy products tends to be mucus forming.

Alcohol also aggravates any allergic reaction and is therefore best avoided, or minimised, during hay fever season.

Best foods

- Oily fish (salmon, mackerel, herring, kippers, sardines)
- Chia, flax and pumpkin seeds
- Red onions
- Fresh fruit, especially berries
- Vegetables, especially broccoli and peppers
- Ginger (anti-inflammatory)
- Turmeric (anti-inflammatory)

Worst foods

- Wheat
- Dairy products
- Alcohol

Best supplements

- 2 × high-potency multivitamin–minerals
- 2 × vitamin C 1,000mg
- 2 × essential omegas with fish-oil-derived omega-3, plus

omega-6 from borage or evening primrose oil (ten times more omega-3 than -6)

- 2 × anti-inflammatory formula containing a combination of quercetin, vitamin C, glutamine, MSM (sulphur) and bromelain

Or

- (At least) 2 × quercetin 250mg, and double your intake of vitamin C

HEADACHES AND MIGRAINE

General information

Headaches can occur for many reasons, including: intoxication, muscle tension, dehydration, allergic reactions and blood sugar dips. Migraines share similar causes, but have some tell-tale symptoms including: visual disturbance, extreme pulsing pain in the frontal or temple region of the head, nausea and digestive shut-down and, sometimes, vomiting.

Good medicine solutions

1. Avoid blood sugar dips

One of the most common causes of headaches and migraines is a blood sugar dip. Consequently, people with diabetes are more prone to headaches. When blood sugar concentration increases, your body tries to dilute the excess sugar concentration by triggering thirst, so you drink more water. If you ignore this signal, the combination of dehydration and blood sugar peaks and troughs can often trigger a headache. The solution is to eat a diet that keeps your blood sugar level even – and to avoid sugar and refined carbohydrates. This means never skipping breakfast, eating slow-releasing carbs (such as whole grains, brown rice, lentils and beans) with protein, and snacking on fruit that is low on the glycemic index (low GL), such as apples, strawberries and pears. (See Chapter 1, Part 2 for details on how to follow a low-GL diet.)

2. Test for, and avoid, hidden allergies

Another exceedingly common cause of headaches and migraines is a hidden allergy. In fact, headaches are one of the most common symptoms of allergy. If you do suffer from headaches, it is very important to find out what you are allergic to. The most common offenders are wheat, dairy products, citrus foods and yeast. A number of additives have also been found to trigger migraines, including caffeine, monosodium glutamate (MSG) and the sweetener aspartame. For some people, cheese and chocolate are especially bad news. (See Allergies on page 31.)

3. Reduce exposure to pollution and mobile-phone use, and increase intake of antioxidants

Some people find exhaust fumes or gas fumes can trigger a headache. Many years ago I used to commute by car into London, which involved an hour in heavy traffic. I used to get headaches; however, if I went in by train, I was much less likely to get a headache. In the short term it isn't easy to change your exposure to things like exhaust fumes, but in the long term it's worth considering such factors. If you ride your bicycle through traffic to get to work, try to find a less crowded route.

Many people find they are more likely to get headaches when they use their mobile phones frequently. Nobody in the science community or the government seems to be able to make up their mind about whether there is a link between mobile phones and health problems. Research is very conflicting, but there is some evidence showing that antioxidants (substances that remove or disarm potentially damaging oxidising agents in the body) minimise the effects of the electromagnetic radiation you receive from mobile phones; however, no research has really been done on reversing symptoms, such as headaches, caused by over-exposure to mobile-phone radiation. I recommend reducing your mobile-phone use, and pollution exposure, as much as possible and increasing your intake of antioxidants (see Chapter 2, Part 2). Using an air-tube headset with your phone, or having the phone on hands-free, reduces electromagnetic radiation, for example.

If you are exposed to unavoidable pollution, probably the best weapon against oxidants is to drink a watermelon smoothie, which is loaded with antioxidant nutrients. Just put chunks of watermelon into a blender, whizz them up – seeds and all – and you've got a refreshing and healthy drink. Make sure you're drinking at least 1.5 litres (2¾ pints) of filtered water a day, and avoid coffee and alcohol, which are treated as toxins by the body.

3. Take niacin (vitamin B$_3$)

Most people who experience headaches have a number of triggers, and thus, a combination of factors can be all that is needed to finally bring on a headache. By reducing the triggers, you reduce the chances of having a headache or migraine. But what do you do if you have one? Instead of taking one of the more common vasoconstrictive drugs, which constrict the blood vessels, try taking 100mg of niacin, which is a vasodilator. This will cause a 'flushing' sensation, as well as a feeling of increased heat, but it can often stop or reduce a headache in the early stages. Medical studies have shown substantial relief of migraines by supplementing either vitamin B$_2$ or B$_3$ (niacin). In one study, those taking niacin halved their number of migraines by taking 100mg of niacin every day. It is particularly effective in combination with a regular painkiller.

4. Take 5-HTP to help reduce headaches and migraines

Migraine sufferers are often low in serotonin, a vital neuro-transmitter that is intimately involved in the experience of pain, as well as sleep, mood and appetite. Having a low level of serotonin may make it easier for a headache or migraine to be triggered.

Serotonin is made from a naturally occurring amino acid called 5-hydroxytryptophan (5-HTP). If you are low in serotonin, supplementing 100mg of 5-HTP a day may help reduce headache or migraine incidence. Although there are tests for serotonin status, they are not readily available, so it is probably best to try it and see if it helps you.

Some people experience mild nausea when taking 5-HTP, in which case lower the dose or take with food. Note that 5-HTP is not recommended if you are on antidepressants.

5. Check your homocysteine, if you have migraines

Homocysteine is a naturally occurring protein in the blood that can have a profound effect on blood vessels. Migraine sufferers who experience 'aura' symptoms before a migraine (blurred vision, bright spots in their field of vision, muddled or confused thinking, extreme exhaustion, anxiety, numbness or a tingling sensation in one side of the body) are much more likely to have high levels of homocysteine.

Vitamins B_2, B_6 and B_{12} and folic acid might prove enormously helpful for migraine sufferers. In one study, those taking high-dose vitamin B_2 for four months had substantially fewer migraines. It is wise to take a daily multivitamin–mineral, at least, to ensure a good daily intake of these nutrients. If you check your homocysteine level and it is high (above 10 mcmol/l) you will need more of these B vitamins than those that are supplied in a daily multivitamin. (Read Chapter 4, Part 2 for more details on what to take if your homocysteine level proves to be high.)

6. Look for mind and body triggers

Last, but by no means least, don't rule out the physical and psychological causes of headaches. I recommend that anyone who is experiencing headaches or migraines visits a chiropractor or osteopath. Misalignments of the cervical vertebrae in the neck (particularly C2/C3) can trigger headaches and are usually the result of stiffness in the back and shoulders. A chiropractor or osteopath can manipulate these vertebrae back into alignment for you, to give you relief. We spend far too much time sitting and typing at computers, and too little time stretching and strengthening the back. Frequent tension-reducing massage is also highly recommended.

Migraines, in particular, induce a desire to have no sensory input (such as noise or light). Not only does the sufferer want complete sensory deprivation during a migraine attack but the digestive system also shuts down. Therefore, once a migraine is in full bloom, it is advisable neither to eat nor to take nutrient supplements. This sensory shutdown may be your body's way of saying you should take a break, so, if you are pushing yourself beyond your capacity, you may need to reappraise your priorities, especially if you find that emotional upsets can trigger headaches. (See Chapter 6, Part 2 for ways to reduce stress.)

Best foods

- Fresh fruit
- Vegetables
- Whole, unrefined foods
- Water

Worst foods

- Sugar
- Caffeinated drinks
- Alcohol
- Hidden food allergens (wheat and dairy products for some)

Best supplements

- 2 × high-potency multivitamin–minerals providing at least 200mcg of folic acid, 20mg of B_6, 10mcg of B_{12} and 10mg of zinc

- 1 × vitamin C 1,000mg

- 2 × 5-HTP 50mg (take at any time but before bed if you have difficulty sleeping)

At the start of a migraine:
- 1 × niacin (note: not niacinamide) 100mg to induce 'flushing'

> ### CAUTIONS
>
> Don't take 5-HTP if you are on antidepressants.

HEARTBURN

see **INDIGESTION AND HEARTBURN**

HEART DISEASE

see **ANGINA** and **HIGH BLOOD PRESSURE**

HELICOBACTER PYLORI

see **STOMACH ULCERS AND** *HELICOBACTER PYLORI* **INFECTION**

HERPES AND SHINGLES

General information

Herpes can be sub-divided into two different infections: herpes simplex (oral, such as cold sores, and genital herpes) and herpes zoster (or shingles, which is a reactivation of the chicken pox virus). Both forms of herpes remain dormant in the nervous system after initial infection and can reactivate following minor infections, stress or weakened immunity. Despite their differences, the nutritional treatments for both are essentially the same.

Good medicine solutions

1. Increase lysine and limit arginine in the diet

The herpes virus feeds off an amino acid (a protein building block) called arginine found in foods such as chocolate, nuts, seeds, beans (pulses) and soya. Replication of the virus requires the manufacture of proteins rich in arginine, and it is thought that arginine itself stimulates herpes replication. Lysine is an amino acid that the virus can mistake for arginine. High intakes of lysine can fool the virus and effectively starve it. Foods high in lysine include most vegetables, fish, turkey and chicken. I also recommend supplementing 1,000mg of lysine every day, taken on an empty stomach, to keep the virus at bay. When you have an active infection, increase this to 3,000mg, split throughout the day. The goal is to keep lysine levels high and arginine low. To do this you also need to cut right back on the arginine-rich foods. If you follow this dietary advice as soon as you feel a cold sore developing, you can shorten the duration and severity. Continuing with this on an ongoing basis can help to lower the likelihood of an outbreak.

2. Supplement vitamin C

The more stressed you are, the weaker your immune system will become, allowing the virus to become active – which is why many people succumb to cold sores when they're run down. A good way to boost your immune system is to supplement 3,000mg of vitamin C every day. When you feel symptoms developing, increase your intake quickly. Studies show that the effects are most beneficial when initiated at the beginning of the illness. The ideal is 1,000mg (that's 20 oranges' worth) an hour. The amount needed depends very much on the person. Some will experience loose bowels on high doses, but that is all. There's no harm in taking large amounts of vitamin C for a few days. Preferably, take the prescribed amount of vitamin C to just below 'bowel tolerance', which means the maximum level you can take before it causes loose bowels.

Combining supplements with the topical application of vitamin C through a cream increases the rate of healing herpes ulcers and shingles blisters. As vitamin C needs to reach the target tissue to be effective, this approach raises levels directly in the lesions. Research shows that blisters and sores are smaller, less painful, and heal more quickly using topical vitamin C. Cosmetic creams are available, but not all are equal in terms of quality. Look for products that contain at least 10 per cent or more ascorbic acid (which appears on labels as L-ascorbic acid, ascorbyl palmitate or ascorbyl phosphate). I recommend Environ C-boost (see Resources). Apply the cream as soon as symptoms begin and continue at least three times daily until the symptoms have gone. To make your own vitamin C paste, mix 1 teaspoon (5g) ascorbic acid with 5 teaspoons (25ml) warm water and stir until dissolved. You can apply this with cotton wool to the lesions. This dries out quickly on the skin, so you need to apply it more frequently than the cream.

3. Increase your zinc intake

Although zinc directly inhibits herpes virus replication, its main action is probably its role in enhancing cell-mediated immunity. Zinc is an essential mineral found in the 'seeds' of things – from eggs to nuts, seeds and beans. It is also found in high amounts in meat and fish. The ideal intake is about 15mg a day, but most people achieve only half this amount from their diet. In times of illness much higher doses (50–100mg a day) have been shown to make the body's immune-responsive T cells much more effective, hence boosting immunity.

Supplementing 50mg of zinc a day has been shown in clinical studies to be effective in reducing the frequency, duration and severity of herpes and shingles. Taking zinc lozenges (containing 15–20mg zinc) every three hours for up to three days while suffering an outbreak may work even better. After this time, you must discontinue, as long-term use can cause an imbalance of other nutrients in the body. Topical zinc can also be used to prevent the virus from spreading and can inhibit recurrences. A study using 4 per cent zinc sulphate in water stopped the pain, tingling and burning completely in all participants within the first 24 hours. You can buy zinc creams or make a paste by mixing zinc gluconate or sulphate powder with water.

Another reason zinc may be helpful when you have an infection is because it helps vitamin A, which is stored in the liver, to be used. To fight infections, you need to have sufficient vitamin A in your body. Although you should eat lightly when you have any infection, foods rich in vitamin A help give your immune system a boost. These include dark green vegetables and yellow/ orange fruit and vegetables (carrots, sweet potatoes, squash, apricots, peaches).

4. Take echinacea

Echinacea (*Echinacea purpurea*) is an old Native American remedy for purifying the blood – and that is quite literally what it does. This root of the echinacea plant is probably the most widely used immune-boosting herb. It possesses interferon-like properties and is an effective anti-viral agent against herpes. It contains special kinds of polysaccharides, such as inulin, which increase macrophage production. Echinacea also enhances the movement of immune cells to infected areas. One study on a group of healthy men found that after five days of taking 30 drops of echinacea extract three times a day, their white blood cells had doubled their 'phagocytic' power, allowing them to better destroy viruses. Echinacea is best taken either as capsules of the powdered herb (2,000mg a day), or as drops of a concentrated extract (usually 20 drops three times a day).

5. Apply a lemon balm cream

Lemon balm (*Melissa officinalis*) can effectively treat herpes-family viruses, including those responsible for shingles. Topically, it is one of the most widely used remedies and has been shown to heal lesions and blisters much faster than normal, while also reducing discomfort. Lemon balm has various mechanisms by which it is anti-viral, including preventing the virus from accessing the cells where it can multiply. Research demonstrates lemon balm can prevent recurrences altogether.

Several studies have shown impressive results using a cream containing 1 per cent of a standardised 70:1 extract four to five times a day. The cream used in most studies is called Loma-herpan (formerly LomaBrit) and is available from chemists or online. Alternatively you can use melissa oil or extract, mixed with a carrier oil and applied to the affected area to obtain relief from irritation and pain resulting from shingles.

6. Control your pain from shingles

Many people find, and research suggests, that bathing in chamomile and oatmeal can be particularly soothing to the pain associated with shingles. Colloidal oatmeal is the form to use, which is, essentially, oats ground to a fine powder. It has been shown to relieve the itching, burning and skin inflammation. The compounds in oats can also speed healing time and reduce scarring. Adding chamomile essential oil or chamomile tea bags to the bath further helps soothe pain and inflammation.

Some people find that the pain persists after the acute phase of shingles has passed. In these cases a topical ointment containing capsaicin (a component of cayenne pepper) is recommended, because capsaicin disrupts pain signals in the body. When rubbed into the affected area regularly, it can reduce chronic pain from shingles. Capsaicin creams are available over the counter or on prescription.

General advice

When your immune system is fighting off an infection, it uses energy. It's therefore important to rest. Also, controlling stress is vital to prevent recurrences. Eat well, but don't eat too much. Conserve your energy for fighting the infection.

Act fast. Viruses survive by breaking into your body's cells and reprogramming those cells to make more viruses. You should aim to stop that happening as fast as possible, so what you do in the first 24 hours makes all the difference. Don't wait until it's too late.

Best foods

- Lysine-rich foods (vegetables, fish, turkey and chicken)
- Carrots and carrot juice
- Water (drink lots)
- Montmorency cherry juice (Cherry Active) (low in fruit sugar, which feeds infections)

Worst foods

- Arginine-rich foods (chocolate, nuts, seeds, beans and soya)
- Sugar and refined foods
- Alcohol

Best supplements

- 1 × high-potency multivitamin–mineral with 15mcg of vitamin D and at least 1,500 mcg of vitamin A

- 3 × 1,000mg lysine

- 1,000mg vitamin C (ideally one with zinc and berry extracts) every hour

- 1 × zinc lozenge (15–20mg) dissolved in the mouth every three waking hours for up to three days

- 20 drops of echinacea three times a day

CAUTIONS

Vitamin C, in high doses, can cause loose bowels or even diarrhoea. This is not dangerous as long as you keep hydrated.

HIGH BLOOD PRESSURE

Good medicine solutions

1. Increase magnesium

Increasing magnesium intake, especially if you don't normally eat lots of vegetables, nuts and seeds, has an immediate effect on lowering blood pressure. It works by relaxing the muscles in the arteries. When the magnesium in muscle cells goes up in relation to calcium, your muscles relax. One kind of hypertension drug is called a 'calcium channel blocker', and it lowers blood pressure by lowering calcium, but there are side effects.

Magnesium not only lowers blood pressure but it also lowers anxiety and insomnia. Magnesium is found richly in seeds, nuts and green vegetables. Most people are deficient, however, and those with high blood pressure frequently show lower levels of magnesium than those with normal blood pressure. Your health-care practitioner can measure your magnesium status, which is best done by looking at your red blood cell magnesium level.

If you have high blood pressure, it's worth eating the above kinds of magnesium-rich foods as well as supplementing 300mg of magnesium every day.

Although much of the research into magnesium's protective effects has focused on its relaxing role in arteries, there is growing evidence that magnesium can also reduce your cholesterol and triglyceride (blood fat) levels associated with atherosclerosis,[1] and it also has an anti-inflammatory effect.[2] Having a low level of magnesium may be as good an indicator of risk of cardiovascular disease as having a high cholesterol level, yet it is rarely checked.

2. Cut back on sodium (salt) and increase potassium

The other mineral that reduces blood pressure is potassium. It is found mainly in fruits and vegetables, which are also high in magnesium. Unlike magnesium, it's not worth supplementing potassium, as it is so abundant in the fruit and vegetables. You need to aim for seven servings of fruit and vegetables a day to get sufficient. If you fill half a plate with vegetables for each main meal (giving two servings per meal), that will give you four servings per day. Then, having two pieces of fruit as snacks, and a serving of fruit with breakfast on most days, you will have seven servings in total. Vegetables are the more important food to increase, and they also have less sugar – even fruit sugars can increase insulin and cholesterol (see below). These are the best foods, for both potassium and magnesium. Banana is the best fruit for potassium, but it is also high in sugar, so is best generally avoided.

Best fruits and vegetables

The amount in parentheses gives the mg quantity of potassium per 100g (3½oz) of food

Salmon (628mg)	Banana (358mg)
Beans (white) (560mg)	Cauliflower (355mg)
Spinach (558mg)	Pumpkin (or squash) (339mg)
Baked potato (535mg)	Watercress (329mg)
Avocado (485mg)	Broccoli (325mg)
Plums, peaches (398mg)	Celery (285mg)
Mushrooms (371mg)	Courgette (248mg)
Lentils (365mg)	Tomato (207mg)

Sodium (salt) tightens up the blood vessel wall, so cutting back is essential to lower blood pressure.[3] According to one study in the *British Medical Journal*, eating less salt could cut cardiovascular disease risk by a quarter and fatal heart disease by a fifth.[4]

All salt, natural or pure sodium chloride, contains sodium. Adding salt is habit forming, but if you stop adding it to foods you'll soon get used to it. Not adding salt will substantially reduce your intake.

You also need to be aware of reducing foods that are already high in salt. Here are ten foods that have a lot of salt in them. These are important to keep to a minimum:

Ten high-salt foods

Cheese	1,700mg per 100g (3½oz) (about five 2.5cm(1in) cubes)
Olives	1,556mg per 100g (3½oz)
Bouillon (stock) cubes	1,200mg in a 5g (⅛oz) cube
Sun-dried tomatoes	1,040mg per 55g (2oz)
Pretzels	1,357mg per 100g (3½oz)
Crisps (salted)	525mg per 100g (3½oz)
Soy sauce	300mg in 1 teaspoon
Salami	226mg per slice
Yeast extract (Marmite)	216mg in 1 teaspoon
Bacon	194mg per rasher

3. Eat a low-GL diet and reduce insulin

When you eat sugar, and foods containing fast-releasing sugars, such as bread and bananas, your insulin level goes up, because the role of insulin is to take excess sugar out of the blood into storage as fat. Insulin causes the kidneys to retain both water and salt, which leads to high blood pressure. The combination of too much insulin and too much glucose damages the arteries and raises your blood pressure.

The more often your blood sugar levels peak, the more insulin you make and, in time, you become increasingly insensitive to insulin and thus make more, which pushes your blood pressure even higher. It's vital to learn to eat in a way that keeps your blood sugar level even. This is called following a low-GL diet. In essence, this means four things: (1) eating less carbohydrate; (2) eating the right kind of carbohydrate, such as brown rice or wholegrain pasta rather than white; (3) eating protein with carbohydrate (for example, having beans on toast, not jam on toast); and (4) eating little and often, with three main meals and two snacks each day. (See Chapter 1, Part 2 for details on how to follow a low-GL diet.)

Following a strict low-GL diet really can lower not only blood pressure but it can also lower cholesterol and triglycerides substantially.

4. Supplement vitamin C

Supplementing vitamin C daily is an immediate way to lower blood pressure. A meta-analysis of 29 trials confirmed that a mere 500mg of vitamin C a day lowers high blood pressure by 5 points over eight weeks.[5] Higher doses may be even better. In another study, people given 2,000mg of vitamin C a day for 30 days had a 10-point drop in systolic blood pressure. This is comparable to the effect you can get with the best hypertensive drugs, but without the side effects. Taking high-dose vitamin C makes a lot of sense if you have heart disease, because it has been shown to lower LDL cholesterol when given to healthy people, people with diabetes and people on kidney dialysis, and has also been shown to reduce arterial thickening. It is also a natural anti-inflammatory. A study of almost 60,000 people in Japan reported that vitamin C intake is strongly associated with a reduced risk of heart disease, especially in women, cutting the risk by a third.

Unlike the drug alternatives, such as ACE inhibitors and diuretics, which knock out magnesium, there are no adverse effects of taking vitamin C. It is also less expensive.

5. Eat beetroot and drink beetroot juice

Beetroot lowers blood pressure because it promotes levels of nitric oxide in the blood. In a study at the University of Reading, a shot of beetroot juice equivalent to 100g (3½oz) of beetroot (roughly two small beetroots) lowered blood pressure and increased nitric oxide in people with normal blood pressure within 24 hours.[6] This has been confirmed by other studies.[7] The reason for this blood-pressure-lowering effect is that beetroot is exceptionally high in nitrates. These studies have shown that nitrates in beetroot juice have a dose-dependent effect on blood pressure, as well as thinning the blood.

If you don't fancy eating two small beetroots a day, a shot of beetroot concentrate (Beet Active) provides the equivalent of one small beetroot.

6. Reduce stress

Don't underestimate the effect of stress on both raised cholesterol and blood pressure. Stress immediately generates adrenal hormones, which raise blood pressure as part of the 'fight or flight' reaction.

Although there are many other techniques, simple exercises known as HeartMath (which are often taken with a stress-monitoring device, called an Emwave, to give you instant feedback of your reducing stress levels) have been shown to cut stress hormones by a quarter.[8] Blood pressure also drops by 10 points.[9] Meditation also has similar effects.[10]

Reducing your stress level is a very important and highly effective way of reducing your risk of heart disease, lowering your blood pressure and improving recovery from heart disease. Often we look at outside events as the source of stress, but in fact stress is caused by our own emotional reactions to events.

Although there are practical steps that you can take to reduce your stress levels, one of the most important skills to learn is how to master your own stress response the moment it occurs, or in preparation for a potentially stressful situation. (For more information on these stress-reducing techniques, see Part 2, Chapter 6.)

'I used to have ...'

David had spent ten years trying to sort out his hypertension using drugs, with limited benefits, before he discovered that the low-GL diet could do it in six months.

The results were rapid and impressive.

'Within about three weeks I started feeling giddy, and my monitor showed my blood pressure had dropped right down, so I halved my medication. But two weeks later the same thing happened and I had to come off my medication completely! When I showed my cardiologist my blood pressure figures he was astonished and highly delighted. Then I broke the news to him that those figures had been achieved without any medication at all! The initial look of horror on his face changed to total fascination when I explained it was all the result of the low-GL diet and that a further benefit was that my cholesterol had dropped from 5.7 to 4.6.'

Three years later David is still eating low GL and not taking any tablets.

Best foods

- Chia seeds and pumpkin seeds (rich in omega-3)
- Almonds
- Oats
- Beetroot
- Fish
- Beans and lentils (pulses)
- Green vegetables

Worst foods

- Sugar
- Salt
- Cheese
- Bacon and salted meats

Best supplements

- 2 × high-potency multivitamin–minerals providing 100mg of magnesium

- 2 × vitamin C 1,000mg

- 2 × magnesium 100mg (giving a total of 300mg with your multivitamin)

DIG DEEPER

To find out more on this subject, read *Say No to Heart Disease* (Patrick Holford), which includes key referenced studies.

HIGH CHOLESTEROL

Good medicine solutions

1. Follow a low-GL diet

The most important way to lower cholesterol is to eat a low-GL diet. The big myth about high blood cholesterol is that it is caused by eating too much cholesterol in food. This has repeatedly been proven to be untrue. The body makes cholesterol, but when the cholesterol in your blood is damaged, by sugar (glycation) or by oxidation, it accumulates. When your blood sugar level goes high it raises insulin levels, and both high blood sugar and high insulin raise cholesterol. The solution is a low-GL diet, which balances blood sugar levels.

To keep blood sugar levels balanced you need to eat less carbohydrates overall, and choose the right kinds of slow-releasing carbohydrates (for example, oat flakes rather than cornflakes), and always combine protein with carbohydrate, which slows down the release of sugars in food even more. As your blood sugar level stays even by eating this way less insulin is released. This not only lowers cholesterol but it also lowers blood pressure and it is also the easiest way to lose weight or control your weight. (See Chapter 1, Part 2 for details on how to follow a low-GL diet.)

2. Increase your intake of omega-3 fats

A review of ten randomised controlled trials showed that fish oils decrease the triglycerides in the blood, which lead to heart disease by an average of 29 per cent, and they also lower cholesterol by 12 per cent and the so-called 'bad' LDL cholesterol by 32 per cent, as well as increasing the 'good' HDL cholesterol by 10 per cent.[1]

Although eating oily fish generally reduces your level of risk, to lower your cholesterol effectively you need a total daily intake of around 1,000mg of the essential fat eicosapentaenoic acid (EPA). This means supplementing two omega-3-rich fish oil capsules a day. There are three kinds of essential fat found in fish – EPA, docosapentaenoic acid (DPA) and docosahexaenoic acid (DHA). Both EPA and DPA have proven heart benefits. When choosing a fish oil capsule, add up the total EPA and DPA. A good supplement will provide 300–400mg EPA and DPA combined per capsule. Therefore, two provide up to 800mg. A serving of mackerel, herring or salmon will give you about 700mg. If you eat these three times a week and supplement at least 600mg of EPA, plus DPA, and eat omega-3-rich seeds and nuts, such as chia or flax seeds and walnuts, you'll achieve 1,000mg of EPA a day.

Vegetarians please note that, as good as these seeds and nuts are, only about 5 per cent of their type of omega-3 fat (alpha lino-lenic acid – ALA) converts into EPA, so relying on seeds and nuts, or their oils, will not confer the benefit of concentrated fish oil supplements and eating oily fish.

3. Supplement high-dose non-blushing niacin

According to a major review in the *New England Journal of Medicine*, 'the most effective way' to reduce LDL cholesterol is by taking vitamin B$_3$ (niacin).[2] Niacin also comes out top in a review of the drug trials to raise HDL, which is the healthier form of cholesterol associated with less risk.[3] A number of studies confirm that it does both – raising HDL by up to 35 per cent, and reducing LDL by up to 25 per cent. It also reduces levels of another important marker for heart disease: lipoprotein(a).

Niacin is only effective at high doses of 500–2,000mg a day. That's a long way off the recommended daily allowance (RDA) of 18mg.

The most obvious side effect of taking fairly high doses of niacin is a blushing effect, which is diminished by taking the vitamin with food, but non-blush or extended-release niacin is now easily available.

Some people choose to take pure niacin, which gives a very strong blushing effect for up to 30 minutes. Most people find that, within a few days, if they take niacin twice a day with food, the blushing subsides. If you want to try this, you can reduce the blushing by starting with a low dose of 50–100mg per day, then double the dose each week until the minimum effective level, of at least 250mg twice a day, is reached.

Alternatively, there are prescribable forms of niacin, such as Niaspan, that don't cause blushing. These are available on prescription from your doctor.

There is also a non-blushing form of niacin called inositol hexanicotinate, which is available in health-food stores. Clinical trials haven't been carried out on this form, so it's hard to say whether it works as well. Yet another form of niacin, niacinamide, doesn't lower cholesterol.

5. Increase plant sterols and soluble fibres

Plant sterols are present in pulses, including beans and lentils. The most researched in this respect is soya, which is why many soya products rightly claim that they help to lower cholesterol. There are also plant sterol-enriched margarines, such as Benecol, which make similar claims. Studies have shown that the regular consumption of 1–3g of plant sterols per day lowers LDL cholesterol by 5–15 per cent. There's also evidence that the more soya you eat the lower your blood pressure will be.[4]

Taking 2.5g of plant sterols a day is the equivalent of 50g (1¾oz) of soya – roughly a glass of soya milk, a small serving of tofu, or a small soya burger. Other foods, including nuts such as almonds, and most beans and lentils, also provide plant sterols, so you can use these if soya isn't your cup of tea.

Soluble fibres are found in oats, okra and aubergine. They are present in the bran, or rough part, of oats, so you need to eat whole oat flakes or rough oatcakes, or add oat bran to cereals, to obtain them. One of my other favourite sources of soluble fibre is chia seeds, as well as flax seeds, although I think chia tastes much better. These soluble-fibre-rich foods become gel-like when water is added, because they absorb so much of it.

Combining plant sterols with soluble fibres is actually more effective in lowering cholesterol than taking statins. A simple example of putting these principles into action is eating hummus (made from chickpeas) with rough oatcakes, which gives you both plant sterols and soluble fibres.

4. Reduce stress

Don't underestimate the effect of stress on both raised cholesterol and blood pressure. Stress immediately generates adrenal hormones, which raise blood pressure and cardiovascular risk as part of the 'fight or flight' reaction. If you are often in a stressed state, this raises cholesterol. (See High Blood Pressure on page 195 for more on this.)

Although there are practical steps you can take to reduce your stress levels, one of the most important skills to learn is how to master your own stress response the moment it occurs, or in preparation for a potentially stressful situation. (For more information on these stress-reducing techniques see Chapter 6, Part 2.)

'I used to have ...'

Andrew's cholesterol was 8.8mmol/l. He was also gaining weight, feeling tired and stressed, and not sleeping well. His doctor put him on statins and, six months later, his cholesterol level was little changed at 8.7. The lack of response, plus the side effects, led Andrew to stop.

I advised him to follow a low-GL diet and supplement high-dose niacin, vitamin C and omega-3. Three weeks later his cholesterol level had dropped to a healthy 4.9.

He had also lost 4.5kg (10lb), his energy levels were great, he no longer felt stressed and he was sleeping much better.

Best foods

- Chia seeds
- Almonds
- Pumpkin seeds
- Peas
- Oats (oat flakes)
- Beetroot (lowers blood pressure)
- Oily fish (salmon, mackerel, herring, kippers, sardines)
- Beans, chickpeas and lentils (pulses)
- Green vegetables (rich in folic acid, good for heart health)

Worst foods

- Sugar
- Salt (raises blood pressure, narrows arteries)
- Cheese (high in salt)
- Bacon and salted meats (high in salt)

Best supplements

- 2 × high-potency multivitamin–minerals providing 100mg of magnesium

- 2 × vitamin C 1,000mg

- 2 × magnesium 100mg (giving a total of 300mg with your multivitamin)

- 2 × high-potency omega-3-rich fish oil capsules (giving around 800mg of EPA, plus DPA)

- 2 × niacin (extended release or non-blushing. Note: not niacinamide) 500mg

CAUTIONS

There was a hint of a concern in one study that the combination of statins plus niacin might slightly increase stroke risk. It's too early to say if this is really an issue; however, I'd advise caution regarding niacin to someone with a history of stroke, if they are also taking statins, unless advised by a health professional.

If you are taking statins, I advise you to supplement 90mg of co-enzyme Q_{10} (CoQ_{10}), since statins block the function of this critical heart-friendly nutrient. Induced CoQ_{10} deficiency is one of the main reasons for the common side effects, such as muscle aches and fatigue, experienced by some people taking statins.

If you are on blood-thinning medication, or you have a history of stroke, discuss taking omega-3 fish oils with your doctor, as they also reduce blood clotting. Too much blood thinning may increase risk of cerebral haemorrhage.

DIG DEEPER
To find out more on this subject, read *Say No to Heart Disease* (Patrick Holford), which includes key referenced studies.

HIVES (URTICARIA)/RASHES

General information

Hives – medically known as urticaria – are raised white welts on the skin, surrounded by redness. The swelling and redness are caused by the release of one of the body's allergy chemicals, histamine.

Good medicine solutions

1. Look for reactions to chemicals

The most common cause of hives is a reaction to medication – particularly antibiotics (including penicillin). Unfortunately, penicillin is sometimes present in foods and drinks such as milk, meat and poultry, and allergic reactions have been traced back to these 'hidden' antibiotics. People with chronic hives are also often sensitive to aspirin. If you do come up in a rash or hives when you are on medication, contact your doctor to check whether this may be the cause. If it is, you will both have to decide whether the need for drugs outweighs the discomfort of hives.

Salicylates are aspirin-like compounds found naturally in many foods. Hives sufferers who are sensitive to aspirin must look carefully at their salicylate intake. Of all foods, fruits have the highest levels, especially berries, pineapple and dried fruit. I would also avoid all juices, as they can contain concentrated salicylates. High levels have been found in liquorice and mint, including toothpastes, chewing gum and teas. Read the ingredients list of foods and cosmetics to ensure you avoid those containing salicylates.

Our food is increasingly contaminated with chemicals that are used to colour, flavour, sweeten, stabilise and preserve it.

One of the most common food additives that causes reactions is tartrazine, also known as E102, which is used as a dye to colour foods orange and yellow.

Numerous studies have shown that additive-free diets are very helpful to people with hives. Eating fresh food, as close to its natural form as possible, is the main way to avoid the potential hazards of commercially prepared foods. Eating organically grown or produced food is another way of avoiding added chemicals.

2. Test for, and avoid, food allergens

A common cause of hives is a reaction to foods. The foods that are most likely to bring on hives are: milk, fish, meat, eggs, beans and nuts, although any food can do so. Others to consider are chocolate, cured meats, chicken, citrus fruits and shellfish. (See Allergies on page 31 to find out how to test and avoid potential food allergens or intolerances.)

Alcohol aggravates any allergic reaction and is therefore best avoided or minimised. Avoiding suspect foods is only part of the solution. It is also important to make sure the digestive tract is working well. Several studies have shown digestive imbalances in up to 85 per cent of patients who have chronic hives.

The first vital stage of digestion is to chew your food thoroughly. This allows the digestive enzymes a greater surface area to work on and do their job properly. Some people have a lack of, or a reduced amount of, digestive enzymes, which results in food not being properly broken down; this also contributes towards allergies. If you take plant enzyme formulas, the enzymes in the digestive tract can function more efficiently, helping to normalise digestion.

Beneficial bacteria help control allergies by increasing gut immunity. To promote the beneficial bacteria, reduce your intake of sugar and refined foods – these encourage bad bacteria to proliferate. Eat plenty of fibre-rich fruits, vegetables and some live natural yoghurt – these help to encourage the growth of beneficial bacteria. I would also recommend a good-quality probiotic supplement to help restore levels.

The preferred 'fuel' for the cells lining the small intestine is glutamine. A generous supply of glutamine can help repair and maintain a healthy small intestinal lining. You can buy supplements that combine enzymes, glutamine and probiotics. Also, take a supplement programme that includes 10mg of zinc – an important mineral needed to make stomach acid.

3. Supplement vitamin C

Allergic reactions cause a release of histamine that triggers symptoms. Most drugs recommended for hives are anti-histamines; however, vitamin C exerts a number of effects against histamine – specifically, it prevents the secretion of histamine by white blood cells and increases its detoxification. Research shows that 1,000mg of vitamin C reduces blood histamine by approximately 20 per cent, and 2,000mg reduces histamine by over 30 per cent.

Vitamin C is recommended for everyone at an absolute minimum of 1,000mg (1g) a day, although 2,000mg (2g) or more is optimum for most people, whether or not you have allergies. If you are suffering from allergic symptoms, you might want to take twice this amount on a regular basis. Since vitamin C is in and out of the body within six hours, it's best taken in divided doses, either 1,000mg in the morning and 1,000mg at lunch or, if you're taking larger amounts, 1,000mg four times a day. You can increase your vitamin C intake through food by eating plenty of fresh fruit and vegetables, although you would have to eat an enormous amount to get up to 2,000mg; for example, 100g (3½oz) of peppers contains about 100mg of vitamin C, 100g (3½oz) of broccoli contains 110mg and 100g (3½oz) of strawberries contains 60mg, and that's assuming they are fresh. Foods that contain vitamin C typically also contain antioxidant bioflavonoids such as hesperidin, rutin and quercetin, and these bioflavonoids may actually help the body to absorb vitamin C – another good reason to eat vitamin-C-rich foods.

4. Supplement other anti-allergy/anti-inflammatory nutrients

Quercetin is a potent antioxidant that promotes a healthy inflammatory response. One study found that of all the flavonoids, quercetin was the most effective at inhibiting histamine. The best food sources of quercetin are red onions, apples and berries, but you'll be hard pushed to eat more than 20mg a day, so supplementing therapeutic amounts is also necessary if you're suffering from hives. Take 500mg three times a day if your symptoms are severe, then 500mg once a day once your reaction is under control. Best results are achieved by supplementing 250mg twice a day, with some bromelain and vitamin C.

Bromelain is a collection of enzymes found in pineapple stems that have considerable anti-inflammatory and anti-swelling properties. Take up to 300mg daily, if you are having an allergic reaction, or 100mg daily to reduce your allergic potential.

Methylsulfonylmethane (MSM) has so many benefits for allergy sufferers that it's hard to know where to start.

As long as you're still suffering from any allergic symptoms, it's well worth supplementing MSM on a daily basis. Although therapeutic intakes go up to 6,000mg a day, I recommend you start with 1,000mg, or half this if taken in combination with the other anti-allergy nutrients.

Glutamine is an essential part of any regime designed to restore healthy mucous membranes quickly and reduce allergic potential. It is also a powerful nutrient for supporting healthy immune function and gut membranes. As part of a daily anti-allergy regime, take 500mg.

Some supplements contain combinations of these anti-inflammatory nutrients, so you can take them all in one pill. Powerful natural anti-inflammatory foods include oily fish, seeds, ginger and turmeric. I would use these liberally.

5. Deal with stress

Many people find that they react to stressful events with a skin rash or hives. Stress triggers all sorts of changes within our bodies, including a reduction in our immunity, which may well be behind this reaction. Studies have shown that people with chronic hives have more stress in their lives, be it from less family support, negative coping strategies or increased impacts from life events. It seems that people who also suffer from insomnia are even more predisposed to skin rashes.

Dealing with stress by means of relaxation or resolving a stressful situation is important, especially if the hives become chronic. Yoga, meditation and relaxation tapes are recommended or, for a more long-term problem, perhaps counselling would be helpful. (How to manage stress is explained in Chapter 6, Part 2.)

Best foods

- Oily fish (salmon, mackerel, herring, kippers, sardines)
- Vegetables, especially broccoli and peppers
- Red onions
- Ginger

Worst foods

- Alcohol
- Meat and dairy
- Processed foods
- Sugar

Best supplements

- 2 × high-potency multivitamin–minerals providing at least 10mg of zinc
- 2 × vitamin C 1,000mg

- 2 × essential omegas with fish-oil-derived omega-3, plus omega-6 from borage or evening primrose oil (ten times more omega-3 than -6)

- 2 × anti-inflammatory formula containing a combination of quercetin, vitamin C, glutamine, MSM, bromelain

- 1 × digestive formula containing enzymes, glutamine and probiotics

---

CAUTIONS

You should seek the guidance of a nutritionist or other professional when following any elimination diet, especially for children, as it is important to have a full range of essential nutrients.

DIG DEEPER

To find out more on this subject, read *Solve Your Skin Problems* (Patrick Holford and Natalie Savona), which includes key referenced studies.

IMPOTENCE, ERECTILE DYSFUNCTION AND REDUCED SEX DRIVE

General information

Some men suffer from a reduced sex drive but no sexual dysfunction. Others find it increasingly hard to get an erection, which interferes with their enjoyment of sex. This is called impotence. Others have no problem with sexual performance but produce dysfunctional sperm, making conception unlikely for their partners.

Good medicine solutions

1. Check your testosterone levels

Men as well as women can suffer from menopausal symptoms later in life. In men, these are called the andropause. Symptoms include decreased sexual performance, loss of morning erections and decreased potency, as well as fatigue, depression, irritability, rapid ageing, aches and pains, sweating and flushing. The cause of the male menopause is likely to be declining levels of what is known as 'free (unbound)' circulating testosterone. This is the testosterone in the bloodstream that is active and available. It may happen for a number of reasons: stress, too much alcohol, poor diet, and even overheating of the testes. There's a good online test for factors that predict testosterone deficiency (see Resources). If your score says you are at risk, it is worth seeing a health-care practitioner experienced in the andropause and also having your testosterone levels measured. A doctor should measure both your testosterone level and the level of sex hormone-binding globulin (SHBG), which binds to, and hence inactivates, testosterone. By knowing these two figures you can work out the level of 'free' testosterone.

There is an increasing range of testosterone treatments available, including pellets, injections, pills and, more recently, transdermal creams. Try one that suits you for at least three months. It's important to also make the lifestyle changes that reduce risk as well. But if you have lost your enthusiasm for life and love, you can often kick-start these by correcting testosterone deficiency and then you may have more enthusiasm to reduce stress, cut back on alcohol, lose weight and make changes to your diet.

2. Reduce stress and alcohol

Stress is a major factor in testosterone decline, so it makes sense to look at ways to reduce it in your life.

The anti-ageing adrenal hormone, dehydroepiandrosterone

(DHEA), manufactures testosterone, but its efficient functioning is affected by stress. When you are stressed, you produce cortisol, which is needed for a normal response to stress, giving you more energy and alertness when needed, and it has an anti-inflammatory effect. Too much stress means too much cortisol, which then tends to lower testosterone levels and DHEA levels. Continued stress, therefore, lowers your DHEA level, meaning that there is less to manufacture testosterone. (See Chapter 6, Part 2 for more details of how to reduce stress in your life.)

High alcohol consumption is another risk factor for low levels of testosterone. If a man has had a period of heavy drinking in his lifetime, his liver may be able to recover but the testes may be less able to. It is therefore important to reduce your alcohol consumption and look for other ways to switch off and relax. You should also check your testosterone status if you are a heavy drinker, as it is more likely to be low.

3. Reduce your exposure to xenoestrogens

Xenoestrogens are chemicals in the environment with actions similar to the female hormone oestrogen. They have recently been found to be anti-androgenic, blocking the action of testosterone. They are found in pesticides, plastic wrapping and plastic bags, so choose organic vegetables and meat wherever possible to reduce pesticide and hormone exposure, and don't eat fatty foods wrapped in non-PVC clingfilm.

4. Increase protein intake and lose weight

A higher-protein diet tends to increase testosterone, and bring down SHBG, which reduces available testosterone, so it's important to eat enough good-quality protein, such as fish and lean meats. A strict vegetarian or vegan diet with a lot of fibre tends to increase SHBG and so is more likely to be associated with lower testosterone levels. A low-GL diet is good for your sex drive, because it includes healthy levels of protein.

If you are overweight or have insulin resistance or diabetes, this will increase oestrogen dominance, which inhibits testosterone. Following the low-GL diet will help you to lose weight and therefore correct this problem. The basic principles of a low-GL diet are: (a) eat foods that release their sugar content slowly, such as whole grains, oats, lentils, beans, apples, berries and raw or lightly cooked vegetables; (b) eat protein with every meal or snack; for example, chicken or fish with brown rice, fruit with nuts or seeds, oatcakes with hummus; and (c) limit refined or processed carbohydrates found in cakes, white bread and biscuits. (See Chapter 1, Part 2 for details on how to follow a low-GL diet.)

5. Think zinc

A high degree of impotence and infertility is found in men who suffer from zinc deficiency. Zinc is found in high concentrations in the male sex glands and in the sperm itself, where it is needed to make the outer layer and the tail. The average dietary intake of zinc is half the recommended daily allowance (RDA), so include more high-zinc foods in your diet, including oysters, lamb, nuts, egg yolks, rye and oats, and take a zinc supplement.

6. Protect your cholesterol

Testosterone is made in the body from cholesterol. Very low-cholesterol diets, as well as cholesterol-lowering medication, can therefore lower testosterone levels, but antioxidant nutrients such as vitamin E help to protect valuable cholesterol from being damaged. Seeds and nuts are rich sources of vitamin E.

'I used to have . . .'

Reg was in his mid-forties when he first started feeling irritable much of the time. Over the next few years things got worse – he began having night sweats, his memory became poorer, he had outbursts of irrational anger and his libido plummeted.

'I no longer felt like myself. I went right off sex, I had no energy whatsoever and my memory was so bad I had to write simple instructions on my hand, such as "lock office door".'

Dr Malcolm Carruthers, at the Centre for Men's Health clinic in Harley Street, tested Reg's hormone levels, and they showed that Reg's testosterone level was less than 10pg/ml of 'free', or available, testosterone – the normal range for men is 14–40pg/ml.

'I had half the normal level for a seventy-year-old man – and I was still in my forties,' Reg said.

Dr Carruthers prescribed testosterone capsules, and the results were extraordinary.

'Within two days my memory returned, my depression had lifted and my libido had returned. I felt sharp, bright and full of energy.'

Reg's other symptoms took several months longer to respond, but eventually they all disappeared.

Best foods

- Oysters
- Lamb
- Nuts
- Egg yolks
- Rye and oats
- Organic vegetables and fruit
- Seeds and nuts
- Fish, prawns

Worst foods

- Refined foods (anything made with white flour or sugar)
- Alcohol
- Bran

Also, limit exposure to, or use of, industrial chemicals and pharmaceutical drugs.

Best supplements

- 2 × high-potency multivitamin–minerals providing at least 10mg of zinc
- 1 × zinc 10–15mg (giving a total of 20mg with the multivitamin)
- 1 × vitamin E 400mg
- 1 × high-potency omega-3-rich fish oil capsule (choose products with the most EPA)

DIG DEEPER
To find out more on this subject, read *The Testosterone Revolution* (Malcolm Carruthers).

INDIGESTION AND HEARTBURN

General information

If you don't fully digest your food, bacteria in the gut feast on it, and this can result in bloating. Other symptoms of poor digestion are digestive discomfort and sleepiness. If the stomach either overproduces stomach acid or the top valve, called the oesophageal sphincter, doesn't shut fully, stomach acid can move up into the oesophagus giving a feeling of burning in the chest, or throat, perhaps accompanied with an acidic taste, a desire to cough and some difficulty swallowing. These are the symptoms of heartburn.

Good medicine solutions

1. Improve digestion

Gas and bloating are indications that you are not digesting your food adequately. The first vital stage of healthy digestion is to chew your food thoroughly. Aim to have reduced your mouthful to a liquid mush before you swallow. This allows the digestive enzymes in your stomach and intestines to have a greater surface area to work on and do their job properly. Also, it is important to eat when not stressed, as the adrenal hormones shut down digestion.

Some people have a lack of digestive enzymes in the small intestine, resulting in food not being properly broken down. Inefficient digestion of food in the intestines can result in malabsorption, bacterial imbalance, diarrhoea and indigestion.

Although the body should make enough of all the necessary enzymes if you are well nourished, some of us don't produce sufficient levels of certain enzymes; for example, some people underproduce lactase – the enzyme that digests milk. Other critical enzymes that can be lacking are amyloglucosidase, which digests leafy greens, and alpha-galactosidase, which digests beans.

The simplest way to find out if your digestion isn't up to scratch is to supplement a comprehensive digestive enzyme formula which contains all the above, plus the enzymes lipase, amylase and protease, which digest fat, carbohydrate and protein, respectively. If your symptoms immediately improve, you will then know that at least part of your problem is that you are not able to digest foods properly. If this is the case you can persist with taking digestive enzymes, especially with main meals or with foods you find hard to digest or are associated with your main symptoms.

2. Find the cause of acid indigestion and heartburn

The other critical digestive substance, made in the stomach, is betaine hydrochloride, known as stomach acid. Its production is dependent on zinc, but if you have insufficient zinc you won't be producing enough stomach acid and your body cannot break proteins down properly. Some people lack stomach acid and benefit from supplementing betaine hydrochloride (called betaine-HCl – betaine is also known as tri-methyl-glycine or TMG, so it might be called TMG-HCl).

Other people appear to produce too much acid or have 'leaking' of stomach acid from the circular muscular valve at the top of the stomach into the oesophagus. This may be diagnosed as gastro-oesophageal reflux disease (GERD). In an extreme form, this is called hiatus hernia. Although unproven, there is a simple home test that you can do to find out if you are producing enough stomach acid. It is based on the fact that baking soda (sodium bicarbonate) reacts with stomach acid to produce gas, which you'll experience as a need to burp. Here's what you do:

1 Mix ¼ teaspoon of bicarbonate of soda in 125–175ml (4–6fl oz) cold water first thing in the morning before eating or drinking anything.

2 Drink the solution.

3 Time how long it takes you to burp. Time for up to five minutes.

If you are burping within two to three minutes, it is likely that you are producing enough stomach acid. If you really burp a lot, it may be that you are producing too much.

You might want to do this test two or three times to check, but always do it first thing in the morning before food.

The most accurate test is called the Heidelberg Stomach Acid Test, but this has to be performed by a laboratory and is quite expensive. It is best to seek the guidance of a nutritional therapist if you want to explore this area further.

One common reason for heartburn is eating a food you are allergic to. Babies, when given cow's milk too early, regurgitate it; also, some dairy-based formula milks do the same. This normal reflux is what the body does to expel something that doesn't suit it. If you continue to eat foods that disagree with you, this can weaken the circular muscle at the top of the stomach until some stomach acid enters the oesophagus, producing symptoms of heartburn.

Other things that aggravate the digestive tract include alcohol, coffee and non-steroidal anti-inflammatory drugs (NSAIDs) – painkillers, such as aspirin and ibuprofen. These should be avoided if you suffer with indigestion. Most important is to test for food allergies or intolerances.

High-protein foods, such as meat, require a greater release of stomach acid, so it's sensible to have smaller portions such as a palm-sized piece of meat. High-protein diets, for this reason, can be aggravating for some people's digestive systems.

Another possible cause of digestive pain is the presence of stomach ulcers, often caused by infection with *Helicobacter pylori* (see Stomach Ulcers and *Helicobacter pylori* Infection, page 356, for more details on this). Other gut infections from bacteria, yeasts (see *Candida*/Thrush on page 82) or parasites can cause digestive symptoms. If you have followed the advice given here and still not found relief, this is an avenue worth exploring, especially if your problems started after a trip abroad in a 'high-risk' region that has unsafe drinking water and lacks good food-hygiene practices.

3. Restore your gut bacteria

Quite a significant amount of research has pointed to an overgrowth of 'bad' bacteria in the gut as a possible cause of digestive problems, including irritable bowel syndrome (IBS) (see Irritable Bowel Syndrome on page 247).

Taking probiotics, which are good bacteria, helps to maintain a healthy balance of bacteria in the gut. This also helps to keep the digestive tract healthy and reduce a predisposition to developing food allergies.

To promote the good bacteria in your gut, reduce your intake of sugar and refined foods – these encourage bad bacteria to proliferate. Eat plenty of fibre-rich fruits, vegetables and some live natural yoghurt to help encourage the growth of beneficial bacteria. I would also recommend a good-quality probiotic supplement to help restore levels. Probiotics are certainly worth taking for a month to re-inoculate the gut and restore gut health. Choose supplements that provide both *Lactobacillus acidophilus* and bifidobacteria, as these are the two main strains of bacteria that colonise a healthy gut.

4. Heal and repair the gut

The gut is a very sensitive organ, and if you're not digesting food adequately, or you have an imbalance of bacteria, or if you are eating too many foods that irritate it, the gut lining will be prone to becoming inflamed and 'leaky'. It is essential to restore balance before healing and repair can take place. There are a number of substances that will aggravate a leaky gut by causing irritation to the delicate lining. The most important ones to avoid are alcohol, caffeine, NSAIDs, such as aspirin and ibuprofen, antacids and, for some people, very spicy foods.

The preferred 'fuel' for the cells lining the small intestine is an amino acid called glutamine. You can obtain glutamine powder, 1 heaped teaspoon of which provides about 5g, which is best taken on an empty stomach; for example, last thing at night in a glass of cold water, as heat destroys glutamine. A generous supply of glutamine can help repair and maintain a healthy small intestinal lining. Taking this for ten days can help to restore gut health.

Some digestive enzyme formulas contain both probiotics and glutamine, although usually not sufficient glutamine if you need to heal 'leaky gut' syndrome, which needs to be tested for. A nutritional therapist can do this for you. The test involves drinking a liquid that contains molecules of different sizes. If certain-sized molecules are detected in a urine sample taken afterwards, this denotes a leaky gut, in which case you'll need to take larger amounts of glutamine.

Another key to gut healing and repair are omega-3 fats from oily fish, nuts and seeds. These have been shown to help calm an inflamed gut.

5. Test for, and eliminate, hidden food allergies

Allergies are the most common cause of digestive problems. Studies have found that IBS sufferers have significantly raised levels of IgG antibodies to specific foods, and eliminating these foods greatly improves digestion. The most common foods that cause food intolerances are dairy products, wheat and yeast. If you have indigestion or heartburn, checking for hidden food allergies through proper testing should be the first place to start. (For more on this see Allergies on page 31.)

Best foods

- Whole foods
- Fruit
- Vegetables
- Yoghurt (unless you are dairy intolerant)
- Oily fish (salmon, mackerel, herring, kippers, sardines in small portions)

Worst foods

- Alcohol
- Coffee
- Spicy foods
- Dairy products
- Wheat and other gliadin grains (rye, barley, but not oats)
- Yeast
- Meat (in large portions)

Best supplements

- 2 × high-potency multivitamin–minerals providing at least 5mcg of B_{12} and 10mg of zinc

- 1–2 × vitamin C 1,000mg

- 1–2 × essential omegas with fish-oil-derived omega-3, plus omega-6 from borage or evening primrose oil

- 1 × digestive enzyme supplement with each main meal

- 1 × probiotic supplement, giving 5–10 billion viable organisms

- 1 teaspoon glutamine powder in water last thing at night

Or

- 3 × combined digestive enzyme, probiotic and glutamine formula

CAUTIONS

Proton pump inhibitor drugs (PPIs) – whose names end in -azole – inhibit the production of stomach acid and may provide relief from indigestion or heartburn; however, the long-term use of these drugs is dangerous, because stomach acid is needed for the absorption of vitamin B_{12} and minerals.

Vitamin C, although good for general health, can further aggravate a stomach ulcer. If you feel worse after taking vitamin C, or if you have a burning sensation, see a doctor to investigate the possibility of stomach ulcer.

DIG DEEPER

To find out more on this subject, read *Improve Your Digestion* (Patrick Holford), which includes key referenced studies.

INFECTIONS

General information

Infections can be caused by bacteria, viruses and sometimes other parasitical organisms. Not infrequently, infections, such as of the lung (pneumonia), can be caused by a combination, in this case of both bacteria and viruses. Colds and flu are viral infections (see Colds and Flu on page 101). The standard treatment for bacterial infections is the appropriate antibiotic; however, there are other ways to boost the body's natural defences against pathogenic bacteria, viruses and pathogens.

Good medicine solutions

1. Take vitamins C and D, and other immune-boosting nutrients

There is virtually no infectious disease that hasn't been shown to respond to high-dose vitamin C. Although vitamin C is often thought of as primarily a strong anti-viral agent, it also does many things to strengthen the immune system against other infections. It makes immune cells stronger, helps the immune system identify and attack invaders, helps make interferon – which is part of the body's own natural defence system, enabling you to fight off infection – and is antibacterial. The trick is to maximise intake at the start of infection by taking 2,000mg of vitamin C immediately, followed by 1,000mg an hour, or whatever level can be tolerated without having diarrhoea, known as 'bowel tolerance'. This level of tolerance will be much higher during an infection, because the body uses up more vitamin C to fight infection. It is important to take vitamin C at least every three hours to keep blood levels consistently high.

Vitamin D is also of vital importance to immunity and is made principally when the skin is exposed to sunlight. Vitamin D inhibits cold viruses, but the lack of sunlight across the winter months leads to a weaker immune system that is less able to identify and attack viral invaders. Although it might not have an immediate effect in the same way as vitamin C, it is wise to supplement 50mcg (2,000iu), or two drops, of vitamin D a day while you have an infection.

Many other nutrients are also vital for immune system functioning, and it is best to take a high-strength multivitamin–mineral during times of infection. Choose one that is relatively high in the two key infection fighters: zinc (at least 10mg) and vitamin A (3,000mcg). Vitamin A strengthens the mucous membranes in the lungs and the digestive tract. It can be taken in relatively high amounts (25,000iu or 8,000mcg) for short-term use to boost immunity.

2. Take probiotics during infections and after a course of antibiotics

Beneficial bacteria, known as probiotics, are not only essential to supplement in order to re-inoculate the gut after a course of antibiotics but they also speed up recovery from a wide variety of infections, ranging from diarrhoea to colds. If you are taking a course of antibiotics and want to benefit from probiotics, take the probiotics at a completely different time of day from when you take the antibiotics.

If you know the antibiotic is going to work, you can choose to wait until the course is over and then supplement the probiotics for at least two weeks to re-establish your healthy gut bacteria. Choose probiotic supplements that provide both *Lactobacillus acidophilus* and bifidobacteria, giving a total of at least 10 billion viable organisms a day. You can easily double this amount in the first few days after taking antibiotics to speed up your recovery.

3. Consider niacin – a potential antibiotic?

One of the problems with the widespread use of antibiotics is the development of drug-resistant strains. This is not a theory but a reality, and antibiotic over-use has already resulted in antibiotic-resistant staphylococci infections killing thousands of people worldwide. A recent study found that high-dose vitamin B$_3$ (niacinamide) increased by 1,000 times the ability of immune cells to kill *Staph.* bacteria. The work was done both in laboratory animals and with human blood. The vitamin, given in the form of niacinamide, boosted natural immunity, dramatically increasing the numbers and efficacy of 'neutrophils', a specialised type of white blood cell that can kill and eat harmful bacteria. In human blood, clinical doses of vitamin B$_3$ appeared to wipe out the *Staph.* infection in only a few hours.[1] Supplement 1,000–3,000mg of niacinamide (the non-blushing form of vitamin B$_3$). There is no known harm from taking this dose of niacinamide, especially for short-term use and, judging by these results, it could potentially make a large difference to fighting bacterial infections. It is certainly worth a try if you're suffering from a bacterial infection, and especially if you are antibiotic resistant. The recommended daily allowance (RDA) for vitamin B$_3$ is 18mg, so this is way beyond any amount that could be achieved through diet.

4. Try herbal and other natural remedies

There are many other natural immune-boosting herbs, remedies and foods, some more applicable than others depending on the nature of the infection.

Artemisia is a natural anti-fungal, anti-parasitical and anti-bacterial agent. A form of artemisia (*Artemisia annia*), also known as Chinese wormwood, inhibits the development of malaria.

Cat's claw, officially called *Uncaria tomentosa*, is a powerful anti-viral, antioxidant and immune-boosting agent. The plant grows in the Peruvian rainforest. Cat's claw is available as a tea or supplement.

Colloidal silver is a natural antibacterial agent, which can either be consumed or sprayed onto an infected wound.

Aloe vera is also good for wound healing.

Echinacea is a useful all-round immune-booster, containing anti-viral and antibacterial properties. It's the original 'snake-root' used by Native American Indians as a natural immune booster. The active ingredients are thought to be specific mucopolysaccharides.

Garlic contains allicin, which is anti-viral, anti-fungal and anti-bacterial. Rich in sulphur-containing amino acids, it also acts as an antioxidant. It is a great all-rounder and can either be eaten (raw or cooked) or taken as a capsule.

Grapefruit seed extract, also called citricidal, is a powerful antibiotic, anti-fungal and anti-viral agent. Unlike antibiotics, it doesn't adversely affect beneficial gut bacteria. It is available as drops and can be swallowed or gargled with, or used as nose drops or ear drops, depending on the site of infection. For internal use, take 20 drops twice a day during an infection.

Honey, bee pollen and propolis all have infection-fighting properties. This is especially true for manuka honey-derived products.

Tea tree oil is an Australian remedy with antiseptic and anti-fungal properties. It is great for rubbing on the chest or gargling (diluted), adding to bathwater, or for steam inhalation, it also helps keep mosquitoes away. Go easy on how much you use, because it is strong. Add two or three drops if inhaling, and five to ten drops in a bath.

White thyme oil is also good for chest infections, as is **Olbas oil**.

General advice

If your body is in a state of fever, and you have no desire to eat, it is probably best not to do so temporarily. A high body temperature – above the normal body temperature of 37°C (98.6°F) – enhances immune function, which is why the body produces a fever, and for this reason it is important to keep warm. You can, for example, take hot baths. If the infection continues, however, your immune system needs protein, so perhaps eat a meat consommé, or fish, or a bean soup. Ginger is anti-inflammatory, so drinking strong ginger teas is a good idea, perhaps with some lemon or lime (for vitamin C) and a little manuka honey added.

Alcohol, caffeine, sugar and refined foods weaken immunity, as does fried food, which is high in oxidants. (Oxidants are formed whenever our cells turn food into energy. They are also created when something is burned. The damage they cause in the body, oxidation, is harmful.) Dairy products can be mucus forming and are also best avoided during an infection.

Best foods

- Fruits, vegetables and fresh juices (such as carrot and ginger)
- Fish
- Beans (pulses)
- Garlic
- Ginger and ginger tea with lemon and manuka honey
- Cat's claw tea

Worst foods

- Alcohol
- Sugar
- Caffeinated drinks
- Refined food
- Fried food
- Dairy products

Best supplements

- 2 × high-potency multivitamin–minerals providing at least 10mg of zinc and 3,000mcg of vitamin A and beta-carotene
- 2 × vitamin D 25mcg (1,000iu) drops
- Vitamin C 1,000mg up to 'bowel tolerance'
- 20 drops of echinacea tincture, or herbal concentrate, as directed

Optional

- 2 × niacinamide 1,000mg (for resistant bacterial infections) (Note: not 'niacin' – a form of B$_3$ that makes you blush when taken in high doses)
- 2 × *Lactobacillus acidophilus* and bifidobacteria capsules, giving 10 billion active organisms, ideally on an empty stomach or before meals, if you suspect a bacterial infection or have digestive symptoms
- 20 drops of either grapefruit seed extract or artemisia tincture, depending on the nature of the infection
- Plus other herbs for inhalations or topical application as listed previously

CAUTIONS

Bacteria need iron to survive. If you are fighting a bacterial infection, be careful not to supplement too much iron. Certainly limit it to a maximum of 10mg a day.

Vitamin A should not be taken in high doses if you are pregnant or could become so.

DIG DEEPER

To find out more on this subject, read *How to Boost Your Immune System* (Patrick Holford), which includes key referenced studies.

INFERTILITY

General information

This section relates to female infertility. For male infertility see the section on Impotence, Erectile Dysfunction and Reduced Sex Drive on page 213.

Good medicine solutions

1. Tune up your sex hormones with vitamins and essential fats

Zinc is absolutely vital for reproductive health. Together with vitamin B_6, zinc affects every part of the female sexual cycle. Working in partnership, these two nutrients ensure that adequate levels of sex hormones are produced. A deficiency in either zinc or B_6, for example, affects the luteinising hormone-releasing hormone (LHRH), whose role is to cause your pituitary gland to stimulate the development of an egg (or ovum) that causes ovulation. Such a deficiency results in decreased fertility.

Adequate levels of zinc and B_6 also increase your desire for sex. After conception, zinc and B_6 ease pregnancy sickness and post-natal depression, as well as increasing the chances of having a healthy baby.

Oysters, lamb, nuts, egg yolks, rye and oats are all rich in zinc, while B_6 is found in cauliflower, watercress, bananas and broccoli.

Like zinc and B_6, omega-3 and -6 fats (found in oily fish, raw nuts and seeds, respectively) are needed for healthy hormone functioning, so a deficiency is likely to affect your menstrual cycle and therefore your fertility. (See Chapter 3, Part 2 for more on essential fats.)

2. Increase antioxidants

Although oxygen is essential to life, it also causes damage – and reproductive organs are particularly sensitive. When oxygen is broken down in our bodies, highly reactive molecules, called free radicals, are formed, and these harm, or oxidise, other molecules, which can start a chain reaction of damage. Antioxidant nutrients are essential to minimise this damage. If these are lacking, we age faster and can become less fertile.

To keep your body young, you need a good intake of antioxidants and phytonutrients. The main antioxidant nutrients are vitamins A (both the animal form, retinol, and the plant form, beta-carotene), C and E, plus the minerals zinc and selenium. Phytonutrients enhance our absorption and utilisation of other antioxidant nutrients, as well as having protective qualities themselves. They are often responsible for giving a plant its colour, and this is why eating a 'rainbow' selection of fruit and vegetables ensures that you get a good variety. (See Chapter 2, Part 2 for more about antioxidants.)

3. Protect yourself from 'anti-nutrients'

Anti-nutrients are substances that deplete your body of vital resources while contributing nothing nutritionally themselves. Refined sugar can be classed as such, because it contains no nutrients of its own yet it uses up stores of vitamins and minerals as your body processes it. But anti-nutrients that have a greater impact on your fertility are those that actually damage your body: alcohol, cigarettes, drugs (including pharmaceutical and over-the-counter drugs) and environmental toxins.

Women who drink fewer than five units of alcohol (that is, fewer than five small glasses of wine or 1.4 litres/2½ pints of beer) a week are twice as likely to conceive within six months compared with those who drink more.[1] Also, just one cup of coffee a day can halve your chances of conceiving, as can smoking.[2] (Note: In the US, the Food and Drug Administration (FDA) advises pregnant women to avoid caffeine-containing foods and drugs (and this includes colas) completely.)

Weight matters, because fertility decreases in both obese and skinny women.[3] Slimmers and underweight women run the risk of becoming infertile if they don't eat enough to maintain a regular menstrual cycle.

Likewise, if you are overweight, your fertility can be reduced. Even being moderately overweight – classified as a body mass index (BMI) of 25–30 – reduces your chances of conception and increases the risk of miscarriage.

4. Lower your homocysteine

Homocysteine is a protein-like substance found naturally in our blood. A diet lacking in sufficient nutrients, or a genetic impairment, can mean increased levels, which can contribute to all kinds of health problems, including infertility.

I suggest you test yourself before you get pregnant and, if necessary, reduce a high level (below 6 is optimum) with the right supplements and dietary measures *before* you attempt to conceive. Not only can it boost your fertility but it will also help you to avoid many of the problems that can occur during pregnancy. (See Chapter 4, Part 2 for more information on lowering your homocysteine level.)

Getting your partner tested for homocysteine may also be helpful. In men, high homocysteine is strongly associated with low sperm motility. In one study, high homocysteine was associated with 57 per cent less motility![4] As for women, high levels can be reduced by taking supplements, as explained in Chapter 4, Part 2.

5. Relax and know when to try

Stress is an everyday fact of life in the 21st century, but when you're trying to conceive, too much can reduce your fertility and play havoc with your health. So it's important to find a relaxation technique that works for you. T'ai chi and yoga, having a regular massage or simply creating 'me time' are useful ways to help you relax. (See Chapter 6, Part 2 for more on how to reduce stress levels.)

During your cycle there is only one day in which an egg is available for fertilisation. Sperm, by comparison, usually live for three days, and under excellent conditions they can survive for five. Therefore, if you know when you ovulate, having frequent sex in this five-day window will dramatically increase your chances of conception. How, then, do you find out when ovulation occurs?

Look out for fertile mucus, which is sticky and thread-like – a bit like egg white – and unlike the vaginal mucus you produce during the rest of the month. It's designed to nourish and protect the sperm, providing it with channels to move along, thereby greatly increasing its chances of reaching the egg. You can also monitor your resting temperature (as soon as you wake up in the morning). This will drop and then rise very slightly as you ovulate. There are also ovulation-predicator kits that you can buy without prescription from chemists and large supermarkets.

Once you're ready to get pregnant, being in good health at the expected time and shortly after conception is especially important. Catching flu or a virus in the early stages of pregnancy might harm your baby or increase your risk of miscarriage. For that reason it is probably best to stop trying to conceive, if you become unwell, until you have fully recovered. You can reduce the risk of getting ill in the first place by supporting your immune system (see Colds and Flu on page 101).

Best foods

- Oysters
- Lamb
- Nuts
- Eggs
- Rye and oats
- Cauliflower
- Watercress
- Bananas
- Broccoli
- Oily fish (salmon, mackerel, herring, kippers, sardines)
- Flax, chia and pumpkin seeds
- Vegetables and fruits in a variety of colours

Worst foods

- Refined foods (anything made with white flour or sugar)
- Alcohol
- Tobacco
- Caffeine

Also, limit your exposure to, or use of, industrial chemicals and pharmaceutical drugs.

Best supplements

- 2 × multivitamin–minerals providing at least 20mg of B_6, 10mg of zinc, 100mg of magnesium
- 2 × antioxidant formula (together with the multivitamin, aim to supplement 15mg of zinc, 100mcg of selenium and 400iu of vitamin E)
- 2 × vitamin C 1,000mg
- 2 × essential omegas with fish-oil-derived omega-3, plus omega-6 from borage or evening primrose oil

DIG DEEPER

To find out more about how to increase your fertility, read *Optimum Nutrition Before, During and After Pregnancy* (Patrick Holford and Susannah Lawson), which includes key referenced studies.

INSOMNIA

Good medicine solutions

1. Increase melatonin – the sleep hormone

Melatonin's main role in the brain is to regulate the sleep–wake cycle. Without melatonin it's difficult to get to sleep and stay asleep. It's an almost identical molecule to serotonin, from which it is made. One way to increase melatonin is to provide more of the building blocks used to make serotonin: 5-hydroxytryptophan (5-HTP), which is made from various nutrients, including folic acid, vitamins B_3 (niacin), B_6 and C and zinc, plus tryptophan. There is a biochemical chain that stretches from foods that are particularly high in tryptophan (chicken and turkey, seafood, tofu, eggs, nuts, seeds and milk) to melatonin.

You could also supplement melatonin directly. Taking between 3mg and 6mg is proven to help you get to sleep. In Britain, melatonin is classified as a medicine and is available only on prescription. Another option is to take 5-HTP or tryptophan. They've been consistently proven to be effective in promoting sleep. Ideally, both need to be taken one hour before you go to bed and with a small amount of carbohydrate (such as an oatcake), because this causes a release of insulin which carries tryptophan into the brain.

The best natural source of melatonin is a supplement called asphalia, which comes from a grass called *Festuca arundinacea*, also available as a supplement. Other good sources include oats and sour cherries. A concentrate of the Montmorency cherry has been shown to aid sleep.

2. Stay away from stimulants

Avoid well-known stimulants such as caffeine, but also be aware that sugar can raise the activity of the two adrenal hormones: adrenalin and cortisol. When your blood sugar dips too low, the adrenal hormones start rising. Raised cortisol levels at night will stop you sleeping.

A sensible starting place for a good night's sleep is to eat a low-GL diet. The diet focuses on (a) cutting back on sugar; (b) choosing low-GL foods (the foods that keep blood sugar levels even, such as wholegrain pasta or brown rice, instead of white); and (c) eating protein with carbohydrates to slow the release of sugars in those carbohydrates further. These are immediate ways to lower the GL of your diet. (See Chapter 1, Part 2 for details on how to follow a low-GL diet.)

Caffeine keeps you awake because not only is it a stimulant but it also depresses melatonin for up to ten hours. Coffee drinkers take twice as long to drop off to sleep than those who don't drink coffee and they sleep on average one to two hours fewer than those given decaf coffee, so it is wise to avoid caffeinated drinks in the afternoon.

Although tea contains caffeine, it also contains L-theanine. This amino acid seems to encourage a relaxed state, inducing calming alpha waves in the brain. You can supplement L-theanine, thus avoiding the caffeine in tea, and some sleep formulas contain it.

The main neurotransmitter that switches off adrenalin is called gamma-aminobutyric acid (GABA). When your levels of GABA are low, you feel anxious and have trouble sleeping. Almost all sleeping pills work to promote a GABA-like effect. In many parts of the world you can buy GABA over the counter or on the internet, but in the UK it's only available on prescription. That's a shame because GABA is a natural antidote to anxiety.

Although alcohol is classified as a relaxant precisely because it promotes GABA, it actually also promotes anxiety. The net consequence of regular alcohol consumption is GABA *depletion*, which leads to more adrenalin and that causes less good-quality sleep. To bring your brain chemistry back into balance, it's better to avoid alcohol.

3. Consider behavioural techniques

Therapy, such as cognitive behavioural therapy (CBT), can help insomnia by encouraging patients to acknowledge the stress that is preventing them from sleeping and helping them to develop ways of dealing with it.

One method is to identify negative or unhelpful thoughts, such as 'I just can't sleep without my pills', and changing them. Research shows that various forms of counselling and psychological help are not only the most effective but also the safest way to tackle insomnia. Ask your doctor about getting psychological help, or contact the Sleep Assessment Advisory Service (see Resources).

'Sleep hygiene' forms part of most sleep regimes. The idea is to create regular sleep-promoting habits, such as keeping the bedroom quiet, dark and at a temperature that's good for you. Don't have a large meal in the evening and avoid coffee and alcohol from at least three hours before bedtime. Exercise regularly, but not within three hours of bedtime.

A similar but more systematic approach is known as 'stimulus control therapy' (SCT). This involves ensuring that the bed is associated only with sleeping and sex. People are advised against having naps during the day, and to go to bed when feeling sleepy, but to get up again after 20 minutes if they haven't fallen asleep. They are then advised to do something relaxing until they feel drowsy again and to try – but to get up again if it fails. This breaks the cycle of 'trying' to get to sleep.

You could also try specialist sleep-music recordings, which

have a calming effect similar to that generated by yoga or meditation. Music can induce a shift in brain-wave patterns to alpha waves, which are associated with the deep relaxation you experience before you go to sleep, and this induces less anxiety. My favourite CD is called *Silence of Peace* by John Levine (see Resources), composed especially to induce a relaxation response. Put it on quietly in the background when you go to bed.

4. Take minerals that calm

If you're not getting sufficient calcium and, more particularly, magnesium, this can trigger or exacerbate sleep difficulties. The reason for this is that these two minerals work together to calm the body and help the nerves and muscles to relax, thus reducing cramps and twitches.

If you're very stressed, or you consume too much sugar, your magnesium levels may well be low. Your diet is more likely to be low in magnesium than calcium – so make sure you're eating plenty of magnesium-rich foods such as seeds, nuts, green vegetables, whole grains and seafood. Milk products, green vegetables, nuts and seeds are particularly good sources of calcium. Some people also find it helpful to supplement up to 500mg of calcium and 300mg of magnesium at bedtime. Magnesium is the more important of the two for a relaxing effect.

5. Try help from herbs

Many herbs are said to have sleep-inducing properties. The best known of these is valerian, which is sometimes referred to as 'nature's Valium'. It seems to work in two ways: by promoting the body's release of GABA, and by providing the amino acid glutamine, from which the brain can make GABA. Valerian is a good alternative to GABA, if you just can't get to sleep and you live in a country that prohibits GABA.

Other useful herbs include chamomile, passion flower, lavender, hops, Californian poppy, lemon balm and bitter orange. These can also be used as essential oils in a relaxing bath before going to bed. For more detailed advice about herbal remedies, find a medical herbalist in your area (see Resources).

'*I used to have . . .* '

Pauline from Ireland says:

'After a very bad viral infection, my doctor put me on Zimovane [a non-benzodiazepine tranquilliser] because I needed to sleep. I remained on it years. I tried so many times to come off it and failed. Once I didn't have any for three days, but I couldn't sleep, and one day I drove into the back of a car! I decided I wanted to come off the tablets and followed your advice. I took a supplement containing 5-HTP, B vitamins and magnesium, plus some valerian and, after a week, I was off Zimovane. To this day I still take these nutrients and I feel great.'

Best foods

- Sour or Montmorency cherries, or cherry-concentrate drinks, such as Cherry Active
- Chicken or turkey
- Seafood
- Green vegetables
- Raw nuts and seeds
- Milk products
- Eggs

Worst foods

- Sugar
- Refined 'white' foods
- Caffeinated drinks
- Alcohol

Best supplements

- 2 × high-potency multivitamin–minerals providing at least 50mg of niacin (B$_3$), 20mg of vitamin B$_6$, 200mcg of folic acid, plus 100mg of vitamin C and 10mg of zinc

- 1 × 5-HTP 100mg or 3–6mg of melatonin or 2g of tryptophan an hour before bed

- 2 × GABA 500mg. If you can't get GABA, find a combination formula providing L-theanine as well as taurine and glutamine, which are precursors of GABA

- 1 × magnesium 300mg, possibly with calcium

- 1 × valerian 150–300mg

CAUTIONS

If you are on SSRI antidepressants and also take large amounts of 5-HTP, this could theoretically make too much serotonin. I don't recommend combining the two.

Valerian can promote drowsiness, so it's best to take it in the evening. It can interact with sedative drugs and should therefore be taken in combination only under medical supervision.

Don't combine GABA with drugs that target GABA, such as most sleeping pills.

Too much melatonin can have undesirable effects, such as diarrhoea, constipation, nausea, dizziness, reduced libido, headaches, depression and nightmares.

INSULIN RESISTANCE

General information

When we eat sugary foods and carbohydrates, the level of sugar (glucose) in the blood rises. The hormone insulin is then released into the bloodstream to help escort glucose out of the blood into cells for energy, and the excess goes to the liver which turns sugar into fat for storage; however, our bodies have not evolved to deal with large quantities of sugars, and constantly producing insulin to process them causes a number of serious health problems. Insulin resistance is when your insulin receptors become less efficient and, consequently, the body tends to produce more insulin, which works less well at processing the sugars.

Good medicine solutions

1. Eat a low-GL diet

Diets high in sugar and foods that have a high glycemic load (GL) – that is, carbohydrate-rich foods, particularly those made with refined carbohydrates – are strongly linked to insulin resistance, because they demand that the body makes more insulin. To prevent blood sugar spikes, it's vital to avoid too much sugar or fast-releasing carbohydrates, found in white bread, cereals, white rice, pastries, sweets and sugared drinks, as well as too much fruit juice. Even raisins, bananas, dates and grapes contain fast-releasing sugars, whereas berries, cherries and plums have a low GL, meaning that they release their sugars into the blood more slowly, thereby avoiding spikes.

Becoming aware of the GL of what you eat, and knowing how to lower the GL of a meal, is one of the fastest routes to controlling insulin levels. Hundreds of studies now prove that a low-GL diet makes you less insulin resistant. The basics of a low-GL diet

are: (a) eating little and often; (b) eating foods that are low-GL –
these are foods that release their sugar content slowly, such as
brown rice or wholegrain pasta instead of white rice or pasta;
and (c) combining carbohydrate foods with protein to further
slow down their release of sugars and help keep your blood sugar
levels even. Examples of protein and carb combinations are fish
with brown rice, or an apple with some almonds. (See Chapter 1,
Part 2 for details on how to follow a low-GL diet.)

2. Eat the right fats

Insulin resistance can cause unpleasant symptoms and knock-on
diseases, because it switches your whole system towards inflammation. Inflammation in turn promotes insulin insensitivity.
A diet high in omega-3 fats lowers inflammation and improves
insulin resistance. On the other hand, a diet high in saturated
fat, found in meat and dairy, promotes inflammation. The best
sources of omega-3 fats are oily fish such as salmon, mackerel,
tuna, herring and sardines. Good plant sources include flax,
chia, pumpkin seeds and walnuts. Although you can, and should,
obtain omega-3 fats from your diet, I also recommend you supplement omega-3 fish oils every day. To give you a rough idea,
I recommend you take the equivalent of 1,000mg of combined
EPA and DHA (these are the two most powerful omega-3 fats)
a day, or 7,000mg a week. A 100g (3½oz) serving of mackerel
might give you 2,000mg, whereas a serving of salmon might give
you 1,000mg. If you eat fish three times a week, you'll probably
achieve 3,500mg. To make up the remaining 3,500mg, I recommend you take an omega-3 fish oil supplement providing 500mg
of combined EPA and DHA a day.

3. Increase levels of soluble fibres

Soluble fibres slow the release of sugars in food and lower the
amount of insulin required. To increase the soluble fibre in your
diet, eat whole grains (such as oats and barley), lentils, beans

and chickpeas. Chia seeds are also a rich source of soluble fibre. I recommend eating a small handful of chia or flax seeds every day. Also include raw or lightly steamed vegetables in your daily diet and eat whole, unpeeled fresh fruit to benefit from the fibre contained in their skins. There are also 'super-fibres', such as glucomannan, that you can buy as powders or capsules. Taking capsules before a meal, or a spoonful of glucomannan dissolved in water, makes a massive difference to the GL of the meal you are about to eat. Pure glucomannan is not allowed to be sold in the UK; however, konjac root (which contains about 60 per cent glucomannan extract) is. A daily intake of 5g konjac root would be equivalent to 3g of glucomannan, hence you'll need five capsules or 1 heaped teaspoon before meals.

Another super-fibre is PGX, created by reacting glucomannan with other plant fibres. I recommend taking 1 heaped teaspoonful (5g) in a glass of water before meals. Ideally, take your super-fibre drink up to 15 minutes before a meal to help bulk up the food you are about to eat with much more water and fibre, thus lowering the GL of the meal.

4. Take daily exercise

Exercise does so much more than burn calories. When you exercise, your muscles need glucose, so they stimulate the insulin receptors to become more sensitive. This means that regular exercise helps your blood sugar to become more balanced, because insulin starts to work properly. Resistance exercise – exercise that uses weights, for example, to help build muscle – makes your body more sensitive to insulin. Also, simply moving around after a meal, such as taking a brisk, ten-minute walk, helps to move the glucose out of the blood into the cells that need it. Even if you are not significantly overweight, exercise is critical in the process of reversing insulin resistance. Aim for about 20–30 minutes a day, even if it is just walking.

Exercise not only directly improves insulin resistance but also its effect on stress levels and improved sleep helps to regulate blood sugar levels. People with insulin resistance need to be especially careful not to lead a stressful lifestyle or get insufficient sleep, because the stress greatly exacerbates their symptoms.

When the effect of insulin is continually blocked by stress hormones, the body simply produces more insulin – and the more it produces, the more insulin-resistant you become. So, over the long term, stress can actually lead to insulin resistance and weight gain. Exercise is a biochemical, physiological and psychological antidote to stress. (Learn other techniques to reduce your stress level in Chapter 6, Part 2.)

5. Take 'insulin helpers'

Chromium The mineral, chromium, is essential for insulin receptors to work properly, thereby improving sensitivity to insulin and reversing insulin resistance. In some trial participants, it normalises sugar levels completely. Although chromium is naturally present in foods such as beer, whole grains, cheese, liver and meat, the typical intake – thought to be in the region of 28–35mcg – is much lower than the recommended daily requirement of 50–200mcg per day. One reason for this low consumption is that white flour, which is the most frequently type eaten, has 98 per cent of its chromium removed. Furthermore, typical Western diets, which are high in sweetened and refined foods, such as white bread, cakes, sweets and biscuits, increase chromium losses, because it is used up by the body to process the sugar. Every time you binge on something sweet, you are depleting your body's stores of chromium. The critical issue is the amount of chromium you take, ranging from the minimal effective dose of 200mcg up to 600mcg for diabetics. The ideal dose for someone with insulin resistance is 400mcg split between breakfast and lunch.

Cinnamon, which mimics insulin, is also a valuable addition to your diet. In trials the amount of this spice needed to help stabilise blood sugar is around 6g. That's 1 heaped teaspoon.

Cinnamon extracts, such as Cinnulin, are high in the active ingredient methylhydroxychalcone polymer (MCHP), and are 20 times more potent than taking the spice, so 300mg equals 6g of cinnamon. Having ½ teaspoon daily and 150mg of a cinnamon extract gives you the equivalent of 6g of cinnamon. Some supplements combine chromium with cinnamon extract high in MCHP.

Zinc, **magnesium**, **B vitamins** and **vitamin C** are also needed for insulin production and blood sugar control. A dose of 2,000mg of vitamin C a day helps to stabilise blood sugar and improve insulin sensitivity.

Best foods

- Whole foods
- Oily fish (salmon, mackerel, herring, kippers, sardines)
- Raw nuts and seeds
- Oats and barley
- Vegetables – raw or lightly steamed
- Beans and lentils (pulses)
- Berries, cherries and plums
- Cinnamon

Worst foods

- High-sugar foods
- Refined 'white' foods
- Sweetened drinks, including fruit juice
- Bananas, dates, grapes and raisins

Best supplements

- 2 × high-potency multivitamin–minerals providing 10mg of zinc and 150mg of magnesium, plus B vitamins including at least 10mcg of B_{12}

- 2 × high-potency omega-3-rich fish oil capsules (choose products with the most EPA)
- 2 × chromium 200mcg, plus cinnamon extract (such as Cinnulin) 75mg
- 1 heaped teaspoon of PGX in water before each main meal, or 3g of glucomannan fibre before meals
- 2 × vitamin C 1,000mg

CAUTIONS

Chromium and cinnamon can have a dramatic impact on blood sugar levels. If you are taking diabetes medication, it's best to start on a low dose and build up, because it's important not to drop too low too quickly. Talk to your doctor about adjusting your medication accordingly.

If you are taking metformin, this knocks out vitamin B_{12}, so it is important to supplement at least 10mcg of B_{12} a day.

DIG DEEPER

To find out more on this subject, read *Say No to Diabetes* (Patrick Holford), which includes key referenced studies.

IRRITABLE BOWEL SYNDROME (IBS)

Good medicine solutions

1. Watch out for allergies, intolerances and lectins

People who have IBS are often found to have a food allergy, and clinical studies have found that the most commonly offending foods are grains (especially wheat), dairy products, coffee, tea and citrus fruits. Many IBS sufferers find relief by avoiding all gluten grains, but it is usually those who have diarrhoea that find they do better without dairy products. It is also worth taking an IgG food intolerance test, which you can do as a home test kit (see Resources), but don't cut out any foods prior to the test.

Alternatively, contact a nutritional therapist to arrange an allergy test. (See Allergies on page 31.)

The next possibility to explore is whether you are eating something you are intolerant, but not allergic, to. The most common intolerance is to the lactose in milk. Many people – in fact, most of the world's adult population – do not have the digestive enzyme, lactase, in their bodies that is necessary to digest the lactose in milk. Others are unable to digest beans and foods that contain a type of sugar called oligosaccharides, such as cruciferous vegetables. The solution here is to take a digestive enzyme containing alpha-galactosidase (for beans) and amylo-glucosidase (for cruciferous vegetables). You can also try eating fermented soya, such as tempeh or miso, as this may be easier to digest. The most common sign that you need digestive enzymes is bloating after eating a particular food.

All beans and grains also contain lectins. Lectins can be damaging to the digestive tract and initiate immunological reactions. Therefore, it's best to consume less of these foods if you're suffering from IBS, or possibly avoid them completely for a couple of weeks and see if that makes a difference.

2. Eat the right kind of fibre and drink up!

To ensure good bowel movement it's important to eat plenty of the right kind of fibre. Contrary to the popular image of fibre as mere 'roughage', it can actually absorb water and, as it does so, it makes faecal matter bulkier, less dense and easier to pass along the digestive tract. This decreases the amount of time food waste spends inside the body and reduces the risk of infection or cell changes due to carcinogens that are produced when some foods, particularly meat, degrade. The bulkier faecal matter also means less chance of a blockage or constipation.

The soluble fibres in oats, chia and flax seeds are particularly beneficial. Brown rice is also a reasonably good source of soluble fibre, as are all pulses. You can help 'bulk up' these fibres by either soaking 1 tablespoon of flax seeds in water overnight, then drinking it, or putting 1 tablespoon of ground flax or chia seeds in a bowl of oats and soaking for 30 minutes before eating for breakfast. These soaked seeds can help you become more regular. The other critical ingredient is drinking the equivalent of eight glasses of water or herb tea a day.

3. Test your ileocaecal valve

It's worth considering whether the muscular 'rhythm' of your intestines is working properly. Basically, if everything is working well you should feel the urge after a main meal, or perhaps once or twice in the morning. As the valve at the bottom of the stomach opens up to pass food along, this should trigger the opening of the ileocaecal valve (ICV), which separates the small from the large intestine. You can find the location of your ICV by putting your thumb in your belly button and your little finger on the protrusion of your right hip. Your ICV is roughly halfway between. If this area is tender, you might have a slightly inflamed ICV.

Your ICV can often become inflamed and aggravated by intestinal irritants – either something you're allergic to or an irritant like coffee or spicy foods. Ileocaecal valve function can be restored by two methods. One is a physical technique, or manipulation, practised by naturopaths, some nutritionists and kinesiologists. The other is by eating a diet that is very low in digestive irritants, such as grains, spicy food and stimulants, especially coffee, for a couple of weeks (see below for foods to avoid).

4. Check for a leaky gut that's full of unfriendly bacteria

If IBS is persistent, it may well be linked to a 'leaky gut' (increased intestinal permeability), in which case you can take steps to heal it by: (a) removing irritating or allergenic foods from your diet; (b) following the dietary tips below; and (c) supplementing gut-friendly nutrients such as zinc, vitamin A, essential fats and glutamine. A nutritional therapist can arrange a simple test for increased intestinal permeability.

Problems can also arise when you have more unfriendly bacteria in your gut than the beneficial ones. This can happen if you've repeatedly taken antibiotics and antacids. Altering your diet using the dietary tips below, and taking probiotic supplements, will help to repopulate your gut with these essential friends.

Some digestive enzyme supplements also provide probiotics and glutamine.

5. Recognise the stress connection

When you are stressed, your body automatically diverts its energies to essential systems in your body necessary to activate it for the 'fight or flight' mechanism. Systems such as digestion are not immediately required and therefore shut down, which can result in constipation and a build-up of toxins. Reducing stress really helps; for example, a study training IBS sufferers in 'mindfulness' – an approach to becoming more in the present and less stressed – cut symptoms by a quarter.[1]

To help reduce stress you can try to find a relaxation technique that works for you, such as meditation, t'ai chi, yoga, having a regular massage or simply creating 'me time' – whatever helps you to relax. (See Chapter 6, Part 2 for more on how to reduce stress levels.)

Best foods

- Fresh fruit and vegetables (especially apples and bananas, if you have diarrhoea)
- Water, herbal teas and diluted juices
- Brown rice and oats
- Flax seeds

Worst foods

- Foods rich in sulphur such as bread, eggs, onions and most dried fruits
- Beans (pulses) and cruciferous vegetables
- Sugar and wheat
- Refined/processed foods
- Animal fats and dairy products (especially in cases of diarrhoea)
- Alcohol, coffee, tea and cigarettes
- Spicy foods

Best supplements

- 2 × high-potency multivitamin–minerals providing B vitamins, plus at least 10mg of zinc and 150mg of magnesium, which has a calming effect on the mind, muscles and digestive tract

- 1 × *Lactobacillus acidophilus* and *bifidobacteria*, giving 5 billion active organisms, ideally away from food or before meals

- 1 × digestive enzymes with each meal (some also provide probiotics)

- 1–2 teaspoons (5–10mg) of glutamine powder in a glass of cold water last thing at night or first thing in the morning on an empty stomach

Optional

1 tablespoon fructo-oligosaccharides (FOS) taken daily. Sprinkle it on cereal or fresh fruit, or blend into yoghurt or fruit juice

CAUTIONS

It is better to avoid the temptation to use laxatives, except as an emergency measure. Even natural laxatives containing the herbs senna or cascara are gastrointestinal irritants and, although they work, they don't really solve the underlying issue. As you increase the fibre in your diet they should not be necessary anyway, but if you are 'blocked up' you could try a new kind of laxative, fructo-oligosaccharides (FOS), which comes as a powder and works in a more beneficial way than conventional ones. FOS is a type of complex carbohydrate that helps keep moisture in the gut and also stimulates the production of healthy gut bacteria. This keeps faecal matter softer and easier to pass along. Although results are not quite so rapid, this is a highly preferable way of reducing constipation.

DIG DEEPER

To find out more, read *Improve Your Digestion* (Patrick Holford), which includes key referenced studies.

LIVER DISEASE, HEPATITIS AND CIRRHOSIS

General information

The liver is the hardest-working organ of the body, converting sugar into fat, detoxifying the blood and storing some nutrients such as vitamins A, D and B$_{12}$. The most common liver disease is 'fatty liver disease' when too much sugar (or alcohol) is being converted into fat and the liver becomes unhealthily loaded with fat. This can lead to hepatitis (inflammation of the liver) and cirrhosis (the scarring and dying off of liver cells). Hepatitis can be caused by excess alcohol or a viral or other kind of infection. One of the most common causes is infection with the hepatitis A or C virus, the latter being prevalent among heroin addicts due to sharing dirty needles.

Good medicine solutions

1. Follow a low-GL 'detox' diet

The liver is the main detoxifying organ of the body, and therefore reducing toxic foods, drinks and substances will help to reduce the load the liver has to deal with. Toxic substances include alcohol, caffeine, burned and crispy fats, and refined foods, especially sugar – this is because the liver converts sugar into fat. The second most-common cause of a fatty liver, the precursor to cirrhosis (or liver damage), is excess sugar, the first being alcohol. Infection causing hepatitis (an inflamed liver) also leads to cirrhosis.

The best diet for repairing the liver is a low-GL diet that excludes any nutrient-depleted, refined foods while focusing on whole foods, vegetables and fresh fruits instead. (See Chapter 1, Part 2 for details on how to follow a low-GL diet.)

2. Increase glutathione by supplementing NAC

Glutathione is the body's most powerful detoxifying antioxidant, which helps the body to repair damage caused by alcohol and other drugs including pharmaceutical and over-the-counter drugs. People with reasonably healthy diets, who are not abusing alcohol, have an adequate supply of glutathione, which is constantly being used up by the body and then replenished.

Alcoholics and heavy drinkers, on the other hand, invariably suffer with glutathione depletion.

Liver disease and dysfunction are strongly associated with long-term glutathione deficiency. People with chronic hepatitis C also tend to have lower glutathione levels and, as a consequence, they are at greater risk of developing liver cirrhosis and cancer of the liver.

Glutathione is made in the body from three amino acids (specifically, cysteine, glutamate and glycine). Supplementing with these amino acids, including glutamate's precursor amino acid, glutamine, helps to increase your glutathione levels. Glutathione itself is less effective if supplemented directly, unless it is also supplemented with anthocyanidins – for example, present in blueberries – which help to preserve it. Glutathione is made from N-acetyl-cysteine (NAC), and the body can absorb NAC better. Milk thistle and turmeric help to promote glutathione levels. (Read on for specific instructions for supplementing these nutrients and herbs.)

NAC is one of the most powerful naturally occurring antioxidants, which, when supplemented, dramatically increases glutathione levels in the body. Animal studies have shown that treating a damaged liver with NAC not only works directly as an antioxidant to decrease dangerous lipid oxidation but it also increases the levels of beneficial glutathione. Similarly, many studies in humans have shown that treatment with NAC improves liver function following liver damage and may even offer protection against cancerous liver cells. The effective dose of NAC used in the studies ranged from 1,100 to 1,700mg per day. Take 500–1,000mg NAC mid morning and again in the mid afternoon.

3. Try help from herbs

Milk thistle is a plant native to the Mediterranean region and has been used for thousands of years as a remedy for a variety of illnesses, especially liver problems. Milk thistle contains a flavonoid-lignan called silymarin, which possesses a number of unique liver-protective functions and is a particularly powerful antioxidant. Silymarin also increases glutathione levels. Another way the liver can be damaged is through the action of substances known as leukotrienes. Silymarin prevents these leukotrienes from attacking the liver.

Recently, milk thistle has been shown to have anti-cancer effects. Specifically, researchers found that a compound in milk thistle called silibinin can significantly reduce the growth of several human liver cancer cells.

Other studies have indicated that milk thistle is beneficial for the treatment of hepatitis C; for example, researchers found that milk thistle extract normalises the levels of damaging liver enzymes that are raised in hepatitis C.

A meta-analysis of six studies of milk thistle and chronic alcoholic liver disease found that four studies reported significant improvement in at least one measurement of liver function with milk thistle compared with a placebo. One study that specifically looked at acute viral hepatitis showed significant improvement in liver enzyme levels after 28 days of milk thistle supplementation.

Milk thistle is generally well tolerated and has been shown to have few side effects in clinical trials. It may, however, cause a laxative effect, and occasionally nausea, diarrhoea, abdominal bloating, fullness and pain. Milk thistle can produce allergic reactions, which tend to be more common among people who are allergic to plants in the same family (such as ragweed, chrysanthemum, marigold and daisy). This is not common but worth bearing in mind.

Take 600mg milk thistle twice a day (ideally taken in the high-absorption formula combining standard milk thistle with phospholipids to enhance its absorption).

Turmeric The Indian spice, turmeric, has been used for years in traditional medicines. It contains an ingredient called curcumin, a powerful anti-inflammatory and antioxidant, which increases glutathione levels (the body's most powerful antioxidant), and a detoxifying and liver-protective enzyme. Curcumin also has the ability to reduce homocysteine levels, high levels of which lead to a number of health problems, including increased risk of heart disease, age-related memory loss and osteoporosis.

A recent scientific review of all the research on turmeric concludes that curcumin not only regulates immune cells but can also reduce harmful pro-inflammatory substances, which contribute to the formation of cancer cells. Specific studies on the liver have demonstrated that curcumin can decrease the levels of liver enzymes and markers of fat oxidation that are usually increased in alcoholic liver disease. In addition, levels of beneficial antioxidants, such as glutathione, vitamin C and vitamin E, are increased when curcumin is given. I recommend taking 900mg of curcumin twice daily.

Sho-saiko-to (SST) is a Japanese herbal formula that has been used to reduce the symptoms and severity of liver cirrhosis. This mixture of seven herbs helps to prevent liver fibrosis, or 'scarring', by preventing oxidative stress in the liver's cells. The formula has also been shown to have anti-cancer properties in animals, decreasing the growth of cancer cells. The active components of SST appear to be flavonoids, which have a similar structure to the silibinin found in milk thistle.

A key ingredient in the formula is the herb bupleurum. This has been found to reduce symptoms and blood liver enzyme levels in children and adults with chronic active viral hepatitis. Most of these studies focused on people with hepatitis B infection, although one preliminary human trial has also shown a benefit in people with hepatitis C. SST was also found to decrease the risk of people with chronic viral hepatitis developing liver cancer. Another trial found that SST could reduce the rate of liver cancer in people with liver cirrhosis.

I recommend 500–2,000mg of bupleurum dry root, taken three times a day in capsules, or making a tea using 4g per day (or about 1,300mg per cup of tea), and drinking this three times a day. Ideally, take the whole SST formula as a capsule (1.8–2.5g) three times a day.

Side effects of SST and bupleurum include stomach upset, but this is lessened by taking it with food or in capsule form.

4. Supplement glutamine

This amino acid has many functions in our body, including: increasing brain levels of the key neurotransmitters GABA and glutamate; healing the 'leaky' lining of the gut (found commonly in alcoholics and substance abusers); reducing cravings for alcohol; increasing the release of human growth hormone; and increasing the production of the detoxifying enzyme glutathione.

Glutamine is found in large amounts in all animal protein, but when you cook it, at least 95 per cent of this is destroyed, and when you are stressed, either physically or emotionally, your body needs much more glutamine than can be provided by the diet. In these cases, supplement 8–24g daily. One heaped teaspoon is approximately 5g.

One study of alcoholics found that 10–15g of glutamine daily helped 75 per cent of them to control their drinking. In addition to this, glutamine supplementation has been shown to improve liver healing and can be used as a treatment in early stage liver cirrhosis.

However, those with advanced liver cirrhosis or a history of or a risk of liver failure must not take large amounts of glutamine, unless under the supervision of a medical practitioner. This is because glutamine is the only amino acid that contains an additional nitrogen molecule, which the liver has to process. Taking large amounts of amino acids, especially glutamine, can further tax the liver in advanced cases of liver cirrhosis, as does eating a high-protein diet.

5. Increase essential fats

Fish oil, which is high in the omega-3 fatty acids eicosapentaenoic acid (EPA) and docosahexaenoic acid (DHA), may also protect your liver. In an animal study, sections of damaged liver were treated with fish oil or vitamin E (a known potent anti-oxidant). The livers treated with fish oil and vitamin E showed more regeneration than the control group, and this was most significant in the fish oil group. When examined for glutathione levels, these were increased in the fish oil group and the vitamin E group, indicating that they both improve the antioxidant system of the liver. Supplementing 1–3g of EPA- and DHA-rich fish oil may therefore be beneficial.

'I used to have . . . '

'A blood test revealed poor liver function. I did your 9-day Liver Detox, lost 7lb [3.2kg], and my re-test results are perfect! It's really good – I'd highly recommend it to anybody.' Angie

Best foods

- Green vegetables, especially cabbage, Brussels sprouts, broccoli, cauliflower and kale
- Berries, apples and plums
- Good-quality water (such as filtered or mineral water, which has fewer potential toxic substances)
- Unfried fish, particularly oily fish (salmon, mackerel, herring including kippers, sardines)
- Quinoa, beans, lentils (pulses) (for protein)
- Chia seeds

Worst foods

- Alcohol
- Caffeinated drinks
- Sugar
- Refined foods
- Deep-fried foods

Best supplements

- 2 × high-potency multivitamin–minerals providing 10mcg of B$_{12}$, 200mcg of folic acid, 20mg of B$_6$, 10mg of zinc and other antioxidants

- 2 × high-potency omega-3-rich fish oil capsules (choose products with the most EPA)

- 2 × antioxidant formula providing NAC or glutathione, ALA, beta-carotene, vitamins E and C

- 2 × vitamin C 1,000mg

- 2 × NAC 500mg (away from food, morning and afternoon)

- 1 teaspoon glutamine powder in a glass of cold water last thing at night on an empty stomach

Optional

- 2 × milk thistle (silymarin) 600mg

- 2 × turmeric 900mg

Or

- SST herbal formula, as directed by a health-care practitioner

---

CAUTIONS

Do not supplement glutamine or follow a high-protein diet if you have advanced liver damage, unless under the guidance of your health-care practitioner.

Bupleurum and SST are not recommended during pregnancy or while breastfeeding.

Although there are few known side effects at the dosage given for NAC above, a recent research study questioned the safety of high doses of NAC, suggesting that it may raise blood pressure. Although this is not my experience, you might also want to monitor your blood pressure.

DIG DEEPER
To find out more on this subject, read *The 9-Day Liver Detox Diet* (Patrick Holford and Fiona McDonald Joyce), which includes key referenced studies.

MACULAR DEGENERATION

see **EYESIGHT DETERIORATION**

MEMORY LOSS

General information

Memory decline is a problem many people fear as they get older but it is not always easy to recognise whether you have the problem or not. Many people who think their memory is getting worse are actually fine, for example, whereas others who think there is no problem are not. It is worth taking a screening test every few years from the age of 50, since memory decline is preventable, although there is no good evidence that Alzheimer's disease is reversible. The charitable organisation Food for the Brain has a free online cognitive function test that takes about 15 minutes to complete. Although the test is not diagnostic, it gives a very good indication of whether or not your memory may be becoming an issue. If it is, the site gives you a letter you can take to your doctor recommending homocysteine testing. Homocysteine is a toxic amino acid, high levels of which are linked to a number of health problems, including Alzheimer's and dementia, as well as heart disease and osteoporosis.

The first degree of significant memory loss is called 'mild cognitive impairment' (MCI). Beyond that the classification is dementia. Most dementia (75 per cent) is Alzheimer's disease, which can only be diagnosed with a specific kind of brain scan. The second most common type of dementia is vascular dementia, which is linked to narrowed arteries and a poor supply of nutrients to the brain (see Angina on page 38).

See Dementia and Alzheimer's Disease on page 126 for details of how to prevent memory loss.

MENOPAUSAL SYMPTOMS

Good medicine solutions

1. Reduce hot flushes

Most menopausal women, particularly those who are thin, experience some hot flushes. Although not a direct sign of oestrogen deficiency, it's possible to reduce their frequency and severity by supplementing phytoestrogens, which are plant-derived compounds that are structurally and functionally similar to the body's own oestrogen. Both red clover and soy have high concentrations of isoflavones, one type of phytoestrogen.

Eating fermented soy products, such as miso, tempeh, natto and tamari, will increase the amount of isoflavones in your diet. Although levels are lower in tofu, soya milk and soya yoghurt, they will also provide some isoflavones, while highly processed forms of soy, such as burgers, often have very little. Other foods that contain phytoestrogens are alfalfa, linseeds, lentils, beans, rye and chickpeas.

Natural progesterone cream (see below), from which the body can make oestrogen, has also proven effective in reducing hot flushes.

A low-GL diet also helps because hot flushes can be triggered by dips in blood sugar levels. The best foods are indicated in Chapter 1, Part 2, which also explains how to follow a low-GL eating plan.

Regular exercise is also important, because women who take

more vigorous physical exercise are less likely to suffer with hot flushes. Several trials have shown that breathing from the diaphragm – a practice followed in many health systems, such as yoga and t'ai chi – can reduce the frequency by half, and it tends to work best when practised at the start of a flush.

Single herbs or combinations of black cohosh, dong quai, sage and agnus castus can be effective, and can also minimise other symptoms like sweating, anxiety, depression and insomnia.

2. Enhance vaginal lubrication

Oestrogen stimulates secretions and also helps to maintain the elasticity and acidity of vaginal tissue, which together promote health and defend against infections. With less oestrogen, the vaginal lining becomes thinner and more fragile, and women become more prone to dryness as well as vaginal and urinary tract infections.

Supplementing vitamins A, C, E and zinc can keep vaginal membranes healthy and encourage normal mucus production. These nutrients are available in good high-potency multivitamin–mineral supplements which should be taken on a daily basis. The omega-7 fatty acid, found in macadamia nuts and in high concentrations in the plant sea buckthorn, also supports mucous-membrane health, reducing dryness in intimate areas, as well as the eyes, mouth and nasal passages. So does ensuring adequate progesterone levels (see below).

3. Consider natural or bio-identical progesterone

Often overlooked is the decline in progesterone, oestrogen's counterpart, which typically prepares the body for pregnancy but also protects breast tissue and blood vessels and increases bone strength in later years. Using natural progesterone cream, available on prescription, can reduce many of the symptoms of the menopause, especially hot flushes.

Confusingly, it's possible to be oestrogen deficient and

oestrogen dominant at the same time – where oestrogen is low but there is also very little progesterone, resulting in more oestrogen signals than progesterone. Symptoms of oestrogen dominance and progesterone deficiency overlap, and they include mood swings, weight gain around the hips and thighs, loss of libido, breast tenderness, depression and insomnia. Many of these can show up during the menopause along with the more common hot flushes, vaginal dryness, fatigue and headaches. If you're experiencing many symptoms, I strongly recommend taking a salivary hormone test (see Resources) to shed light on whether you need to address a progesterone deficiency, oestrogen excess or a combination of the two. A nutritional therapist can arrange such a test and interpret the results for you.

The usual solution is to supplement natural progesterone, provided as a skin cream, which can be prescribed by your doctor. Oestrogen can be made from progesterone, as can testosterone (important for sex drive) and stress hormones, so progesterone is the most versatile of hormones. Natural progesterone is not associated with any increase in cancer, unlike synthetic progestins used in conventional HRT. For more information contact the Natural Progesterone Information Service (see Resources).

4. Manage stress and maintain your sex drive

Although vaginal dryness is an obvious cause for loss of sex drive, you should also consider a hormonal involvement, such as a deficiency in testosterone, which determines sex drive in both men and women. Testosterone and the stress hormone cortisol are both made from progesterone. If you're constantly stressed, the adrenal glands produce more cortisol at the expense of testosterone. In addition, producing lots of cortisol will rapidly deplete your progesterone levels, which has the knock-on effect of reducing thyroid gland function, a common symptom of which is low sex drive.

Regular physical exercise is a great stress buster and can increase sex drive. Short-duration, intense exercise for about 20 minutes is especially beneficial; however, you'll most likely find that managing stress is key to minimising many menopausal symptoms. (See Chapter 6, Part 2 for how to reduce your stress levels.)

5. Follow a low-GL diet, plus exercise, to avoid weight gain

Many menopausal women find they're more prone to weight gain. Once again, stress doesn't help. One consequence of raised cortisol is that triglycerides are removed from storage and deposited in visceral fat stores in the abdomen – that's why stress causes weight gain around your middle. Another effect is that cortisol increases your blood glucose levels but at the same time it makes your cells less sensitive to insulin. This prevents glucose from entering the body's cells, leaving them under-fuelled – a state that can lead to hunger signals, overeating and weight gain. There's also a greater tendency to store fat around the middle, because adipose tissue is metabolically active and becomes one of the major sources of oestrogen following the menopause; the other source is your adrenal glands.

To correct this, first, follow a low-GL diet to balance your blood glucose. (See Chapter 1, Part 2 for details.) By eating beans (pulses) and whole grains, you'll get more chromium from your diet – a mineral that is essential for promoting insulin sensitivity. You'll also be reducing stimulants, such as sugar and caffeine, which will reduce cortisol. Raised cortisol levels at night stop you sleeping, so the diet will help if you're prone to insomnia. (For more on managing insomnia see page 236.)

Whether you need to lose weight or not, take regular exercise. It will encourage weight maintenance if you are a healthy weight. Ideally, include both aerobic and resistance exercises (such as skipping, dancing and walking, and using weights), because weight-bearing exercises drive the movement of calcium into the bones. This will reduce the rate of bone thinning and the risk of osteoporosis, which increases following the menopause.

Take antioxidants, essential fats and St John's wort, which also helps to improve mood.

There's a strong link between oestrogen, which declines at the menopause, and mood and mind. Oestrogen helps to: raise levels of the neurotransmitter acetylcholine; stimulate the receptors for serotonin and noradrenalin in the brain, which improve your mood and motivation; slow the processes which break down these neurotransmitters so that you feel better for longer; and improve blood flow and nutrient supply to the brain. Serotonin, noradrenalin and acetylcholine are important neurotransmitters involved in memory, so it's no surprise that memory lapses can increase as oestrogen declines.

Eating fish, organ meats and, especially, whole eggs will supply choline, a vital nutrient used in acetylcholine synthesis. Dietary antioxidants can also support neural function. Compounds with memory-boosting potential include turmeric, green tea, blueberries and resveratrol – an antioxidant found in red grapes.

The foods we eat also play a part in mood, because nutrient deficiencies can cause depression. The essential omega-3 fats are particularly important for hormone balance, so include oily fish, nuts and seeds (such as walnuts, pecan nuts, pumpkin and chia seeds), and their cold-pressed oils, in your diet at least three times a week.

St John's wort, a herb renowned for its antidepressant effects, has been effective for women experiencing menopause-related depression, irritability and fatigue. When taken in combination with black cohosh, it may also relieve other menopausal symptoms, including decreased libido, palpitations, headaches and lack of concentration.

Best foods

- Miso, tempeh, tofu, natto
- Alfalfa
- Chia and flax seeds
- Beans, lentils and chickpeas (pulses)
- Eggs

- Oily fish (salmon, mackerel, herring including kippers, sardines)
- Turmeric
- Blueberries

Worst foods

- Sugar
- Refined foods
- Caffeinated drinks

Best supplements

- 2 × high-potency multivitamin–minerals providing B vitamins, at least 20mg of B_6, at least 10mg of zinc and 150mg of magnesium

- 1–2 × essential omegas with fish-oil-derived omega-3, plus omega-6 from borage or evening primrose oil

- 1 × red clover or fermented soy isoflavones

Optional, if required

- Black cohosh 50mg twice a day

Or

- Agnus castus 4mg a day of a standardised extract (containing 6 per cent agnusides – one of the active ingredients)

Or

- Dong quai 600mg a day

- St John's wort 300mg a day (also helps low mood)

- 2 × omega-7 fat capsules giving 500mg (best for vaginal dryness)

DIG DEEPER

To find out more on this subject, read *Balance Your Hormones* (Patrick Holford), which includes key referenced studies.

MOUTH ULCERS

Good medicine solutions

1. Check for, and avoid, allergies

Food sensitivities can be an underlying factor, particularly in cases of recurring mouth ulcers. Wheat is often a culprit, but fruit such as tomatoes, melons, pineapples and strawberries can also trigger occurrences.

For some people, the response is almost instantaneous, making it easier to identify and avoid these poorly tolerated foods. In other cases, however, the effects are slower to appear.

Allergies promote the release of inflammatory chemicals, such as histamine and prostaglandins. If these are frequently released it can lead to inflaming and weakening of the mucosal membranes in the mouth and gut, thereby increasing the likelihood of ulceration. Indeed, people with Crohn's disease, a disorder where areas of the intestine become chronically inflamed, often develop mouth ulcers.

Dairy products, grains, nuts and eggs are the most common allergens and should be excluded from your diet, especially if you notice other symptoms such as itching, sneezing, watery eyes, headache, muscle pain or excessive tiredness after eating any of them. It's best to avoid eating such foods permanently if you find your ulcers or other symptoms come back when they're reintroduced. (For more on identifying and managing food intolerances and allergies see Allergies on page 31.)

To encourage faster healing, limit citrus fruits such as lemon, lime, oranges and pineapple. Although they may not be causing intolerances, their high acidity can aggravate existing ulcers.

2. Take vitamin A and omega-7 to heal the mucous membrane

Ulcers are most commonly caused by irritation or rubbing; splayed-out toothbrush bristles or brushing teeth too hard can cause ulceration in the mouth. Vitamin A and omega-7 help to regenerate mucosal cells, which form the moist membrane lining the mouth. An essential building block for all mucous membranes, omega-7 is found richly in macadamia nuts and the plant, sea buckthorn, which also contains other ulcer-repairing antioxidant and anti-inflammatory substances, including carotenoids, vitamin E and omegas-3, -6 and -9. A sea buckthorn supplement can be taken long term and will support mucous membrane health throughout the body; for example, reducing dryness in the eyes, nasal passages and intimate areas.

Carotenoids provide the plant form of vitamin A, which is converted to retinol in the body. Taking high doses of vitamin A for a month can help speed up the healing of mucous membranes; however, this is not advisable if you are pregnant or likely to become pregnant because of the potential risks of toxicity.

3. Correct nutritional deficiencies

A lack of B vitamins can cause recurrent ulcers. Significant, long-term, clinical improvements have been achieved by giving B-complex vitamins to people with an identified lack of one or more of vitamins B_1, B_2 and B_6. These are also provided in a high-strength multivitamin. In other cases, there have been clear links to a deficiency in B_{12}. If you are also extremely tired, it is worth exploring if you are B_{12} deficient, which is most often caused by chronic poor absorption leading to pernicious anaemia (see page 301). If so, you'll either need to supplement high doses (500–1,000mcg) or have B_{12} injections. Meat, fish, eggs and dairy products are rich in B_{12}.

A dry mouth and throat, cracked lips and ulcers can all result from a lack of iron. There are two simple tests that you can do at home to check your iron status. Look in the area under your lower eyelids. This should be a rich pink/red colour, not washed out and pale. Or press on the end of your fingernail, turning the bed white. The colour should return quickly when you release it, not remain pale. For more accuracy, ask your doctor to test your iron levels. Female menstruating vegans who do not take supplements are more likely to be iron deficient.

Eating liver, lean red meat and shellfish will provide iron, as well as B_{12}. Beetroot, eggs, spinach, beans, lentils, pumpkin seeds and dried apricots are also good vegetable sources of iron, although in a form that is less well absorbed, so eat plenty of these as well. Eating two eggs for breakfast, a large handful of roasted pumpkin seeds as a snack and a serving of red meat, beans or lentils, with a beetroot (either roasted or in salad), would more than meet your daily 14–18mg iron requirement.

Vitamin C deficiency is also a factor in ulcers – and vitamin C also assists the absorption of iron – so include foods that have high levels, perhaps focusing on vegetables such as Brussels sprouts, cabbage and broccoli rather than fruit, which tends to be more acidic.

4. Handle stress and fight infection

Your need for vitamin C, along with magnesium and B$_6$, will increase if you're under stress, since they are both required for the healthy functioning of your adrenal glands, which are responsible for producing cortisol, the stress-coping hormone. If you are under stress, the adrenals are likely to be getting the lion's share of your vitamin C supplies, leaving other areas low. There's a direct link between higher stress levels, depleted vitamin C and an increased occurrence of ulcers, so take 1,000mg of vitamin C three times a day, especially during periods of greater pressure.

Along with a supplement, it's also a good idea to tackle the way you deal with stress so that it is not so much of a burden. (See Chapter 6, Part 2 for ways to manage stress.)

There's a further consequence of depleted levels of vitamin C in the body. The adrenal hormone cortisol rises when vitamin C is low. High cortisol can depress your immune system, leaving you less able to mount a strong response against bacteria and viruses, and an infection can prolong the occurrence of ulcers. To help with this, you can suck zinc lozenges – try one every 3 hours for two days – to provide 15mg of zinc. Along with encouraging wound healing, the zinc also stimulates the production and activity of immune cells that attack, destroy and remove invaders.

Best foods

- Red meat, especially liver
- Eggs
- Beetroot
- Pumpkin seeds
- Beans (pulses), lentils
- Broccoli, cabbage and Brussels sprouts

Worst foods

- Lemons, limes and oranges
- Pineapple
- Alcohol

Best supplements

- 2 × omega-7 (sea buckthorn oil) 500mg

- 2 × vitamin A 2,250mcg (15,000iu)

- 2 × B complex giving 50mg of most of the B vitamins, and at least 10mcg of B_{12}

Or

- 2 × high-potency multivitamin–minerals providing the same levels

- 1 × zinc 15mg lozenge every three hours

- 1 × vitamin C 1,000mg three times a day

CAUTIONS

Don't take more than 7,500iu (2,250mcg) of vitamin A if you are pregnant.

MULTIPLE SCLEROSIS

General information

Multiple sclerosis is an autoimmune disease that leads to degeneration of the myelin sheath around the nerves. Any autoimmune disease requires investigating for the possibility of a cross-reaction between food proteins and proteins in the body. The development of food allergies is also often associated, and should be suspected, particularly if you have digestive problems.

Good medicine solutions

1. Explore food intolerances

Food intolerances can involve different kinds of antibody reactions, the most common being IgG, IgE and IgA antibodies, which are produced by the body to protect you from undesirable substances, a bit like the role of a bouncer at a nightclub. IgG antibodies are responsible for most food intolerances. Generally, it is worth testing for both IgE and IgG antibody reactions with a reliable laboratory using the ELISA immuno-assay method (see Resources). (See Allergies on page 31 for more details on testing and food elimination.)

Foods particularly associated with MS are wheat and legumes (pulses), both of which contain lectins, and also dairy products. One stream of investigation is the possibility of a cross-reaction between lectins and proteins within the myelin sheath. Lectins are found richly in lentils and beans such as soya, although not all lectins in food are bad, because few bind to the gut wall, which is what is needed to initiate a reaction. If you test intolerant to beans, nuts or seeds, however, a low-lectin diet might be worth trying for a trial period.

One common contributor to developing food intolerances is

increased gastro-intestinal permeability where the lining of the digestive tract is compromised. Excessive alcohol, or frequent antibiotic and painkiller, use is a common cause of this. (This is easily investigated with a urine test available through nutritional therapists.) The gut wall, consisting of rapidly multiplying epithelial cells, can be restored to full integrity by a combination of probiotics and glutamine powder (taken in a glass of cold water last thing at night on an empty stomach).

2. Increase vitamin D

Vitamin D is made in the skin in the presence of sunlight. The further from the equator you live, the less is your exposure to the sun. The fact that multiple sclerosis incidence increases with decreasing sunlight exposure has led to investigation of the role of vitamin D. Research to date tends to show that: (a) sufficient vitamin D in pregnancy reduces risk; (b) children with MS tend to have low levels; and (c) supplementing high levels of vitamin D reduces the frequency of relapses. On this basis, I think it is worth supplementing as much as is necessary to get your blood level up to 75–100nmol/l. Vitamin D levels are easily tested (see Resources). You will probably need 2,000iu (50mcg) a day to achieve this, and possibly more. Some research groups have used much higher levels short term.

3. Ensure you are getting enough essential fats and phospholipids

The formation of nerves is very dependent on omega-3 and -6 fats and phospholipids – vital nutrients found in eggs and fish that are essential for building nerve cells – so there is a good reason to optimise your intake of these. There is growing evidence that omega-3 fats may improve the body's immune response and thereby lessen the symptoms of MS. The most critical fats for the nervous system are arachidonic acid (omega-6), eicosapentaenoic acid (EPA), docosapentaenoic acid (DPA) and docosahexaenoic acid (DHA; omega-3). I would recommend supplementing a combination of these as well as eating oily fish three times a week and seeds every day, emphasising flax and chia seeds, then also eat pumpkin seeds for their omega-3 content; however, omega-3s from oily fish are much more potent.

The principal phospholipid in the brain is phosphatidylcholine (PC), followed by phosphatidylserine and then dimethylaminoethanol (DMAE). The best food source of PC is eggs, and also lecithin granules. A spoonful a day of lecithin granules is a good way to ensure you have an optimal supply.

General advice for MS sufferers is to avoid saturated fat; however, I would keep an open mind about organic virgin-pressed coconut butter, which is high in medium chain triglycerides (MCTs). These are easily converted into ketones, which serve as an alternative energy source for neurons and, in a number of neuronal diseases, have been linked with improvement.

4. Check your homocysteine level and for efficient methylation

Homocysteine is a toxic amino acid, high levels of which are linked to a number of health problems, ranging from cardiovascular disease through to Alzheimer's and cancer. Reducing your homocysteine levels can therefore reduce your risk of developing many different diseases. (See Chapter 4, Part 2 to find out more about homocysteine.) Evidence is growing of an association between an increased risk of MS and associated depression and cognitive decline in those with high homocysteine levels. High homocysteine also increases inflammation and damage to neurons.

Homocysteine is produced from the amino acid methionine, which is found mainly in animal protein. Optimal levels of B vitamins and other nutrients in the diet convert methionine into one of two things: either glutathione (a potent antioxidant) or S-adenosyl methionine (SAMe), which is known to alleviate depression and aid liver detoxification. If the body cannot turn methionine into these helpful factors, its route becomes stuck at the damaging homocysteine. People with MS may have an extra need for B vitamins, which could lead to a build-up of homocysteine and its detrimental effects.

The key nutrients needed for healthy methylation and low homocysteine levels are vitamins B_6 and B_{12} and folic acid. Methylation is vital for building nerve cells, so it is very important to have an optimal daily supply of these methylation nutrients. Vitamin B_{12} is necessary for the formation and repair of myelin; it is also needed for immune function and is a component of neurotransmitters, such as serotonin (needed for good mood) and adrenalin (needed for motivation). Vitamin B_{12}, as well as folic acid, is needed for a healthy digestive tract, and also for the prevention of depression. Vitamin B_6 is needed for protein digestion, also helping to prevent depression and PMS in women. Together, these three nutrients have been shown to greatly reduce homocysteine levels in a more powerful way than when supplemented alone. In addition, the co-factor vitamins and minerals, zinc and vitamin B_2, have been shown to assist in the process.

Some people absorb vitamin B_{12} very poorly because they have pernicious anaemia (see Pernicious Anaemia on page 301) and therefore need very high supplemental levels of B_{12}. For some people, high oral doses of supplemental B_{12} are not sufficient to work and they need to have B_{12} by injection, which bypasses the gut. There is no harm in having a few B_{12} shots (usually 1,000mcg). If these greatly improve your symptoms, it is worth investigating if you have pernicious anaemia and poor B_{12} absorption.

Best foods

- Vegetables
- Berries, apples and pears
- Oily fish (salmon, mackerel, herring including kippers, sardines)
- Raw nuts and seeds
- Oats (they are gliadin-free – the main offending type of gluten in wheat)
- Eggs

Worst foods

These all act as 'anti-nutrients', robbing the body of vital nutrients:

- Alcohol
- Sugar
- Caffeinated drinks
- Refined foods
- High saturated fat from meat and dairy

Best supplements

- 2 × high-potency multivitamin–minerals providing at least 20mg of B_6, 10mcg of B_{12}, 200mcg of folic acid, 15mcg of vitamin D, 10mg of zinc and 150mg of magnesium

- 2 × vitamin C 1,000mg

- 2 × essential omegas with fish-oil-derived omega-3, plus omega-6 from borage or evening primrose oil (supplying EPA, DPA, DHA and GLA)

- 3 teaspoons of lecithin granules or 2 × phospholipid complex

- 2 × vitamin D 1,000iu (25mcg) drops

Optional

- X* × homocysteine-modulating nutrients (*dose and need dependent on your homocysteine score – must provide 500mcg of B_{12})

> **CAUTIONS**
>
> Vitamin D toxicity has been observed in doses in excess of 50mcg (2,000iu) a day for several months. If you do supplement this amount, it is wise to check your vitamin D status after a couple of months.

DIG DEEPER
To find out more on this subject, visit the website of the charitable Multiple Sclerosis Resource Centre (see Resources).

MUSCLE CRAMPS, TREMORS AND SPASMS

General information

Muscle cramps, tremors and spasms can occur either when a muscle is over-stressed or when it runs out of nutrients to fire properly; for example, after an extensive period of exercise, or through insufficient diet.

Good medicine solutions

1. Look into calcium/magnesium imbalance

Muscle spasms are caused by the inability of the muscles to relax. This is likely to be caused by low magnesium and potassium in the diet, which work with the sodium (in salt) and with calcium to control muscle contraction and relaxation. A diet rich in foods that have a lot of magnesium – such as green vegetables, nuts and seeds – is important. Most fruits and vegetables are rich in potassium (bananas are a great source, for example), so eat at least five portions of fruit and vegetables a day. To be absolutely sure you are achieving the correct calcium–magnesium balance you can supplement 500mg of calcium and 300mg of magnesium.

2. Cut down on salt and increase fluids

Although cramps are popularly believed to be the result of a salt deficiency, this is actually very rare. In fact, it is best to avoid added salt and to keep your fluid intake high. Fruit is naturally rich in potassium and water, and contains sufficient sodium for the body's needs. If you do like to add salt to your food for flavour, you could switch to Solo Salt, which has 60 per cent less sodium content than sea salt and significantly more potassium and magnesium.

3. Warm up, cool down and breathe properly

It's important to warm up and cool down properly before and after you exercise. Also, if you habitually breathe shallowly, this can make your muscles go into spasm, because they are not getting enough oxygen. Practise daily breathing exercises, such as taking ten deep breaths, holding them in and slowly exhaling.

4. Reduce stress and stimulants, sleep well and eat well

Muscle tremors can be induced by stress, so it is important to reduce the stress in your life as much as possible and to find ways of coping with it when you do have it. (See Chapter 6, Part 2 on reducing your stress level.) Stimulants, such as caffeine (found in coffee, tea and many fizzy drinks) and nicotine, can trigger tremors, so cut these out of your diet and find something to replace them, such as herbal teas. Reducing stress and cutting out stimulants may also help to improve your sleep, a lack of which can contribute to tremors. (If you do have trouble sleeping, see page 238 in the section on Insomnia for more help on how to get a good night's sleep.)

Tremors can also be induced by low blood sugar, but following a low-GL diet might help to prevent them. The basic principles of a low-GL diet are: (a) to eat foods that release their sugar content slowly, such as whole grains, oats, lentils, beans, apples, berries and raw or lightly cooked vegetables; (b) to eat protein with every meal or snack; for example, chicken or fish with brown rice, fruit with nuts or seeds, and oatcakes with hummus; and (c) to limit refined or processed carbohydrates found in cakes, white bread and biscuits. (See Chapter 1, Part 2 for details on how to follow a low-GL diet.)

5. Ensure adequate B vitamins and vitamin D

Muscle aches can also occur when cells are not able to make energy efficiently from glucose. Magnesium, particularly in the form of magnesium malate, helps here, as do the B vitamins, and it's important to eat green leafy vegetables, and nuts and seeds, which are rich in both magnesium and B vitamins. Also, think about taking a good B complex providing 100mg of vitamin B_5 and 75mg of vitamin B_6, as a deficiency of these two B vitamins is particularly associated with muscle cramps and tremors.

As vitamin D is vital for proper muscle function, it may be worth supplementing it as well as eating oily fish, such as mackerel, herring and salmon. Also, expose your skin to sunlight when possible as this is how your body makes vitamin D.

6. Have a structural check-up, stretch and check your posture

Muscle spasms and cramping can also be linked to structural problems. An examination by an osteopath can ascertain whether you have any nerves that are trapped, which could be cutting off circulation or somehow interfering with the muscles involved.

If you sit for long periods, you may find it useful to get up regularly during the day to have a good stretch and walk around. Also, look into the way you are sitting, and your chair itself, to make sure that you are maintaining good posture. An ergonomic chair, designed to align the body properly, could be a good investment if your chair is broken or poorly designed.

Best foods

- Nuts and seeds
- Green leafy vegetables
- Whole grains
- Bananas
- Fruit and vegetables (five portions a day)
- Water

- Oily fish (salmon, mackerel, herring, kippers, sardines)

Worst foods

- Caffeine (coffee, tea and fizzy drinks)
- Nicotine
- Sugary and refined foods
- Salt and salty foods

Best supplements

- Bone mineral complex (to provide 500mg calcium and 300mg magnesium) or magnesium malate, plus calcium

- B complex (to provide 100mg B_5 and 75mg B_6)

- Vitamin D (to provide 15–25mcg) – a good multivitamin might provide this – or have 1 × vitamin D 25mcg (1,000iu) drop

> ### CAUTIONS
>
> Muscle tremors can be a sign of a neurological disorder. It is therefore important to be checked by your health-care practitioner.

NICOTINE DEPENDENCE

General information

Smoking and nicotine addiction contribute to so many health problems and risks that it is therefore a health essential to stop. If you've become addicted, however, that is easier to say than do.

Here are some behavioural and nutritional changes that make stopping much easier.

Good medicine solutions

1. Quit other stimulants and follow a low-GL diet

Most withdrawal symptoms and cravings kick in when your blood sugar level dips. By following a low-GL diet, with frequent smaller meals, and an emphasis on foods containing slow-releasing carbohydrates combined with foods rich in proteins, your cravings will decline significantly. As you do this it will also become easier to reduce any other stimulants (such as tea, coffee and chocolate) or sugar, and so make it much easier to stop smoking. (See below, and Chapter 1, Part 2 for details on how to follow a low-GL diet.)

2. Break all the associated habits

The average smoker is addicted not only to nicotine, but also to smoking when tired, hungry or upset, on waking, after a meal with a drink, and so on. So before you give up smoking altogether, it's best to break these mental associations.

At first, don't attempt to change your smoking habits. Just keep a diary for a week, writing down every situation in which you smoked, how you felt before, and how you felt after.

When the week is up, add up how many cigarettes you smoked in each situation. Your list might look something like this:

With a hot drink: 16

After a meal: 6

With alcohol: 4

In a difficult situation: 4

After sex: 3

Now set yourself weekly targets. For the first week, smoke as much as you like whenever you like but not when you drink a hot drink. For the next week, smoke as much as you like whenever you like but not when you drink a hot drink or within 30 minutes of finishing a meal. Continue like this until, when you smoke, all you do is smoke, without the associated habits. Set yourself a maximum of six weeks to complete this phase. This will be tremendously helpful for you when you finally quit. Most people start again because the phone rings with a problem, or someone brings in a coffee, offers you a cigarette . . . and before you know it you're smoking.

To help you kick the habit, put your cigarette butts in a big glass jar with a sealing lid. Fill it half with water. Keep this in clear view in your living room. You will begin to associate cigarettes with the nasty stuff in your jar.

3. Lower your nicotine load

Once you have recognised, and hopefully broken, your smoking habits it's time gradually to reduce your nicotine load. Week by week, switch to a cigarette brand that contains less nicotine, until what you smoke contains no more than 2mg per cigarette. Now reduce the number of cigarettes you are smoking until you smoke no more than five cigarettes a day, each with a nicotine content of 2mg or less. If you wish, stop smoking and replace cigarettes with nicotine gum or a 'smokeless cigarette' as an intermediate step. (Nicotine gum comes in two strengths: 4mg and 2mg.)

You want to be down to a maximum of 10mg of nicotine a day before quitting – that is, five pieces of 2mg nicotine gum, or five 2mg smokeless cigarettes.

4. Look into supplements that can help

During the first week or two of quitting, if you are craving cigarettes and not feeling great, also take an extra 10g of vitamin C a day. Buy some ascorbate powder containing calcium and magnesium ascorbate. Put 8g of the ascorbate powder in a bottle containing half water and half juice and drink it throughout the day. It is likely that you will get slightly looser bowels. Vitamin C helps to speed up the body's detoxification of nicotine, helping you to get on an even keel more quickly.

Also take 2 × 200mcg chromium: one tablet with breakfast and one with lunch. This helps to stabilise your blood sugar level.

Take 50mg of niacin (nicotinic acid) twice a day. (You'll probably need to buy a 100mg niacin tablet and break it in half.) You will experience a blushing sensation when first taking niacin. This is harmless and usually occurs 15–30 minutes after taking it, and lasts for about 15 minutes (so don't take it at work). The blushing is less likely to occur if you take niacin with a meal. It should diminish and, in most cases, stop completely after a week, if you keep taking it. The reason for taking this is that both nicotine and niacin occupy the same receptors in the brain – so giving yourself more niacin is likely to reduce your craving. If you are craving a cigarette, and take some niacin, it will be virtually impossible to smoke during the blush and your desire will reduce thereafter.

5. Eat an alkaline-forming diet

An alkaline-forming diet means eating a lot of fruit, vegetables and seeds. (It's better to have a more alkaline-forming diet than one that is acid forming.) Also, make sure you are supplementing a total of 850mg of magnesium and calcium combined. A good multivitamin–mineral will provide 300mg of calcium and 150g of magnesium, and there will be at least 500mg in the ascorbate powder noted above (this is an alkaline form of vitamin C). These alkaline minerals will have an alkalising effect on your body.

Whenever you feel the need for nicotine, first drink a glass of water and then eat an apple or a pear. This will raise a low blood sugar level, which is often the factor that triggers such a craving.

6. Improve your breathing and sleeping

Your lungs will have been damaged by smoking, and it's really important to do something that stimulates breathing and their recovery. At the least, go for a brisk walk every day, ideally in clean air or in the park. Any exercise that focuses on the breath, such as some forms of yoga and Psychocalisthenics® (see Resources), is ideal. This is a great time to sign up at your local gym or to start jogging, cycling or swimming.

If you have difficulty sleeping, or are irritable or depressed, supplement 200mg of 5-hydroxytryptophan (5-HTP). This is an amino acid that the body converts into serotonin, an important brain chemical that controls mood. Nicotine withdrawal tends to lower serotonin levels. The supplement 5-HTP is better absorbed if you don't take it with protein foods, so take it either on an empty stomach or with a piece of fruit or an oatcake. Because serotonin levels rise at night, promoting a good night's sleep, the best time to take your 5-HTP is one hour before bed. (Also see Insomnia on page 236.)

Best foods

- Fruits
- Vegetables
- Raw seeds and nuts
- Herb teas
- Whole foods
- Fish, especially oily fish (salmon, mackerel, herring, kippers, sardines – high in omega-3 fats, which help to stabilise mood)
- Quinoa, beans and lentils (pulses), whole grains (good sources of amino acids for reducing cravings)
- Oats (help keep blood sugar level even)

Worst foods

- Caffeinated drinks
- Sugar
- Refined foods
- Alcohol (which robs the body of nutrients)

Best supplements

- 2 × high-potency multivitamin–minerals
- 2 × vitamin C 1,000mg
- 1 × essential omegas with fish-oil-derived omega-3, plus omega-6 from borage or evening primrose oil

During the first week or two

- 8g of calcium/magnesium/sodium ascorbate powder in water and juice
- 2 × chromium 200mcg
- 2 × niacin (nicotinic acid) 50mg (note: not niacinamide)

CAUTIONS

Niacin makes you blush, and get hot and itchy for about 20 minutes. You then feel a little cold afterwards. For this reason, it is best to take it at home for the first couple of times.

DIG DEEPER

To find out more on this subject, read *How to Quit without Feeling S**t* (Patrick Holford, David Miller and Dr James Braly), which includes key referenced studies.

OSTEOPOROSIS

Good medicine solutions

1. Include essential bone-building minerals

Building and maintaining strong bones is like building a wall. Although the bricks provide the bulk of the material, you also need cement; without it you'll never have a strong, resilient structure. It's the same with bones. A calcium-studded, collagen frame is the starting point, but you also need other vitamins and minerals to hold the calcium in place and to build a strong bone matrix.

A common misconception is that bones become thinner due to a lack of calcium; however, many osteoporosis sufferers have adequate calcium but a deficiency in other minerals, such as zinc and magnesium. You also need vitamins D, C and K, along with the minerals boron, selenium, copper and phosphorus. Together these enhance the way that calcium is absorbed by the body and enable it to be effectively incorporated into your bones. A good bone complex and high-strength multivitamin–mineral will provide you with all of the above.

If you already eat dark green leafy vegetables and seeds, along with some milk and cheese, you'll be getting a good amount of calcium in your diet. Dried herbs also contain relatively high levels, so cook with these too. To ensure calcium is well absorbed, include nuts, whole grains and seafood. These will provide you with magnesium, which is often low in the diet. Eating brightly coloured vegetables and fruit (berries, squash, tomatoes), shellfish – especially oysters – and a handful of brazil nuts will provide you with vitamin C, vitamin K and the trace minerals, which are typically only needed in small amounts.

The following are the best foods to include to get the maximum calcium from your diet:

Almonds	Oysters
Beans (pulses)	Prawns
Broccoli	Sardines (with their bones)
Chestnuts	Sea vegetables
Chickpeas	Sesame seeds and tahini
Kale	Soya milk (fortified)
Kelp	Tofu
Nuts	Wheatgerm
Oats	

Collagen, the matrix of bone, is made from vitamin C. When targeting bone health, I recommend a daily intake of 1,000–2,000mg a day.

2. Supplement vitamin D, the sunshine vitamin

The combination of vitamin D and calcium is more effective than calcium alone at improving bone mass density (BMD) and reducing the risk of fractures, especially if your level of calcium is low. A simple blood test, available from your doctor or privately, will determine your vitamin D level (see Resources), which should be above 75nmol/l. If low, you'll need to take a high-dose daily supplement of 2,500–5,000iu (50–100mcg) for 6–8 weeks and, if possible, test again.

The greatest gains are made with a daily intake of between 800 and 1,200iu (25mcg) of vitamin D, along with at least 1,000mg of calcium.

Vitamin D is commonly known as the 'sunshine' vitamin; you need to be exposed to natural sunlight to start making vitamin D in your skin. If you sit in the sun for 30 minutes each day and you also eat foods rich in vitamin D – say oily fish at least three times a week, plus six eggs – you might make the equivalent of 600iu a day (15mcg). This, however, leaves you short by 200–600iu. If you do none of the above, your vitamin D shortfall will be greater.

There will be some vitamin D in your bone mineral complex and high-strength multivitamin–mineral but you should also take a separate vitamin D supplement to get the extra 1,000iu (25mcg) each day.

3. Check your homocysteine level and supplement accordingly

Homocysteine is a toxic amino acid, high levels of which are linked to a number of health issues. It accumulates if you have an insufficient intake of B vitamins. More and more studies are showing the relationship between high homocysteine, low B_{12} levels and decreased BMD, osteoporosis and an increased risk of fractures, particularly in women. It appears that homocysteine actually damages bone by encouraging its breakdown and interfering with the collagen matrix, which holds the bone together.

If you have decreasing bone mass, or you wish to prevent it, it is important to test your homocysteine levels. If they are high, you can lower your homocysteine with a combination of vitamins B_{12} and B_6, folic acid and tri-methyl-glycine (TMG). (See Chapter 4, Part 2 for more on lowering homocysteine.)

4. Cut out the calcium robbers

Carbonated drinks, such as cola and lemonade, are high in phosphates, but contain no calcium. Although we need phosphorus – it's the second major mineral component of bone – it really needs to be balanced by calcium. If not, blood phosphate becomes relatively high, which leads to calcium being drawn out of the bones.

The same is true with sugar and caffeine, which both encourage calcium loss through your urine; in the case of caffeine, this can be for up to three hours. To avoid constantly dipping into your calcium stores, exclude all sugary or caffeinated drinks, and drink water and herbal teas, which are naturally caffeine-free.

Eating a diet that is very high in animal protein can also pull calcium out of the bone matrix. Once in the body, protein is acid forming, and extra calcium is needed to act as a neutralising 'buffer'. So the more protein you eat, the more calcium you need. In fact, countries with high protein intakes actually have a higher incidence of osteoporosis.

Ideally, you should aim to eat 20–40g (¾–1½oz) of protein each day, mainly from vegetable sources. Vegetarians show significantly less bone loss when compared to meat eaters. Eating two servings a day of lentils, beans or tofu would provide adequate amounts. As for meat, have no more than one serving a day, and ideally a maximum of three each week. There is about 30g (1oz) of protein in an average chicken breast, and 35g (1¼oz) in a salmon fillet. High-protein diets, although effective for weight loss, are not good for bone mass.

Introduce a low-GL diet. You'll get lots of vegetable protein and will also radically reduce your sugar intake. This means that you'll be less likely to experience the blood sugar lows that fuel the need for stimulants like caffeine. Blood sugar and insulin imbalances affect bone health too. (See Chapter 1, Part 2 for details on how to follow a low-GL diet.)

5. Check your progesterone levels and supplement as necessary

Bones have two kinds of cell: osteoblasts, which build new cells; and osteoclasts, which get rid of old bone material, such as calcium. Oestrogen, which influences osteoclast cells, doesn't actually help to build new bone. It only stops the loss of old bone. Progesterone, on the other hand, stimulates osteoblasts, which actually build new bone.[1] In the time leading up to the menopause, most women start to have cycles in which ovulation doesn't occur (known as anovulatory cycles). After the menopause ovulation never occurs. If no egg is released, no progesterone is produced (because progesterone is made in the ovary sac only once the egg is released).

You can test your progesterone level using blood and saliva tests available through your health-care practitioner. If you are low, taking natural progesterone increases bone density more than taking oestrogen, but without the risks. Natural progesterone, which is prescribable as Projuven, is applied as a cream to the skin. It doesn't increase breast cancer risk and may even help to prevent it.

6. Minimise negative habits and increase your exercise

Together with nutrient deficiencies, there are a number of factors that contribute to low bone mass density: being stressed, smoking, being underweight, using prescription medication (particularly steroids), regularly using antacids, especially PPI drugs, and being sedentary. Stopping smoking is essential (see Nicotine Dependence on page 280, and for ideas on managing stress, see Chapter 6, Part 2).

Incorporate exercise, especially weight-bearing exercise, to increase your muscle strength and to give additional support to your skeletal frame and help increase bone density. Any activity that involves your feet hitting the floor – be it walking, dancing, jogging or skipping – drives the movement of calcium from your bloodstream back into the bones. Exercise every other day, choosing activities that use both your upper- and lower-body muscles. If you're new to exercise, start with a 15-minute walk, gradually increasing the pace and incline, and using arm movements.

Best foods

- Beans and chickpeas (pulses)
- Vegetables, particularly broccoli
- Chia seeds
- Dairy products
- Sesame seeds and tahini
- Oats

- Oily fish (salmon, mackerel, herring including kippers, sardines) and shrimps and prawns (eat the shells or tails as a rich source of calcium and glucosamine)
- Soya and oat milk (fortified)
- Brazil nuts

Worst foods

- Caffeinated drinks
- Meat
- Sugar and carbonated, sugary drinks

Best supplements

- 1 × bone mineral complex, containing at least 400mg of calcium, 200mg of magnesium, 1mg of boron, plus 40mcg of vitamin K and 10mcg of vitamin D. The most absorbable forms of calcium and magnesium are citrate, ascorbate and malate

- 2 × multivitamin-minerals – check the calcium, magnesium and vitamin D (ideally 15mcg)

- 1 × vitamin D 1,000iu (25mcg), if your multivitamin and bone support supplement don't provide enough

- 2 × vitamin C 1,000mg

Optional

- X* × homocysteine-modulating formula with 500mcg of B_{12}, plus folic acid, B_6 and other homocysteine-lowering nutrients (*dose and need dependent on your homocysteine score, as explained in Chapter 4, Part 2)

Note Oestrogen HRT is typically prescribed to menopausal women as a safeguard against changes in bone mass density; however, when taken for over a decade, it doubles a woman's risk of breast cancer. Consequently, drugs called bisphos-phonates are often prescribed to help get calcium into the bone. They are remarkably ineffective unless your vitamin D level is good. They also become ineffective if taken with antacid (PPI) drugs. The combination of the two is not recommended.

DIG DEEPER

To find out more on this subject, read *Say No to Arthritis* (Patrick Holford), which includes key referenced studies.

PARKINSON'S DISEASE

General information

Parkinson's disease is a progressive neurological disorder that is caused by a degeneration of cells in the part of the brain that produces the neurotransmitter dopamine (a chemical messenger). It is characterised by the loss of motor control, such as slowness of movement, rigidity, tremor and balance problems, as well as other symptoms, including constipation, low mood, fatigue, sleep and memory problems.

Conventional treatment can involve medication that is primarily aimed at increasing dopamine activity. As dopamine is made in the body from amino acids – the building blocks of protein – diet can play a key part in ensuring that the correct nutrients are available to support the body's production of dopamine.

Good medicine solutions

1. Check and lower your homocysteine level

Homocysteine is an amino acid that is toxic if elevated, and some studies have found that it is elevated in people with Parkinson's. At this stage it isn't known whether higher levels of homocysteine contribute to the development of Parkinson's disease or whether the Parkinson's (or the medications to treat it) contributes to higher levels of homocysteine, or both. Either way, reducing homocysteine to a healthy level is a good idea. The nutrients needed to reduce homocysteine include folic acid, vitamins B_{12} and B_6, zinc and tri-methyl-glycine (TMG). Some of these are required for dopamine production too, so increasing your intake of B vitamins, especially B_6, is important. (See Chapter 4, Part 2 for more details on how to test and lower your homocysteine level.)

2. Increase your intake of omega-3s and vitamin D

The omega-3 essential fats are anti-inflammatory, and may be beneficial because neuro-inflammation is a feature of Parkinson's. Mood problems are also a common feature, and there has been a lot of research into the mood-boosting properties of the omega-3 essential fats. Parkinson's patients treated with omega-3 fat supplements have shown mood improvements. The richest dietary source is from fish such as salmon, mackerel, herring, sardines, trout, pilchards and anchovies.

Vitamin D has been a hot topic for research since it was discovered that we have receptors for this vitamin in the brain. This nutrient is mainly produced by the action of sunlight on the skin. In a small pilot study, bright light therapy was found to be superior to placebo (less bright light) in Parkinson's patients. Vitamin D deficiency is increasingly likely as we get older (and it has a number of implications for health), so it makes sense to ensure that you have a good level.

3. Increase your magnesium

Magnesium is a mineral that acts as a natural relaxant. Some indications of deficiency are: muscle tremors or spasm, muscle weakness, insomnia or nervousness, high blood pressure, irregular heartbeat, constipation, hyperactivity, depression. Magnesium's role in supporting good sleep may also be quite important here, since many people with Parkinson's experience poor sleep patterns. It is also a relaxant and is certainly worthy of consideration to reduce spasms and anxiety, and to improve sleep.

4. Reduce your toxic load

Higher levels of pesticides and herbicides than usual have been found in the brains of Parkinson's sufferers, and the incidence of Parkinson's is higher in areas where there is greater use of these chemicals. It makes sense to avoid any environmental toxins that you can. Also, consider your intake of dietary toxins such as sugar, refined foods, alcohol and caffeine – avoiding or reducing these may reduce the load on your body's detoxification pathways.

Many people with Parkinson's have poor digestion and liver function. Ensuring that you take in plenty of antioxidants from fresh fruits and vegetables is therefore recommended. (Antioxidants are substances that remove or disarm potentially damaging oxidising agents in the body, which are created like 'exhaust fumes' when our cells turn food into energy.) These nutrients may help to combat inflammation (a feature of Parkinson's) and support your body's detoxification pathways as well.

A number of studies have shown benefit from high-dose co-enzyme Q_{10} (CoQ_{10}), a key antioxidant that protects the energy factories within cells.

5. Eat a 'dopamine-friendly' diet

Eating the correct diet is essential when following a strategy that aims to tackle every piece of the jigsaw of Parkinson's. The drug

L-dopa is the most frequently prescribed medication given to Parkinson's sufferers to increase dopamine activity; however, movement problems can become worse if protein foods containing certain amino acids in high proportions are eaten too close to the times that the L-dopa medication is taken. This is because L-dopa competes with the amino acids for absorption at the receptor sites in the intestine and at the blood–brain barrier, so less of it gets through. Therefore, to make the best use of the L-dopa, protein-rich foods should not be eaten at the same time as taking L-dopa medication, as explained in the following guidelines*:

- L-dopa is affected by protein-containing foods, which contain significant amounts of the amino acids tyrosine, phenylalanine, valine, leucine, isoleucine, tryptophan, methionine and histidine. Foods that contain these amino acids include eggs, fish, meat, poultry, dairy produce (not butter), pulses, green peas, spinach, sago, soy, couscous, bulgar wheat, coconut, avocado, asparagus and gluten-containing grains (oats, rye, wheat, barley, spelt).

- Take the L-dopa medication, then **wait one hour**, or until the drug takes effect, before eating any of the foods listed above.

- After eating any of the foods listed above, **wait two hours**, if possible, before taking L-dopa medication again, if it is needed.

*This dietary protocol has been developed and proven helpful by Dr Geoffrey and Lucille Leader and is reproduced with their kind permission.

Best foods

- Vegetables
- Berries, apples and pears
- Raw nuts and seeds (good protein sources)
- Oats
- Oily fish (salmon, mackerel, herring including kippers, sardines)

- Eggs
- High-protein foods (but not with medication)

Worst foods

- Alcohol
- Sugar
- Caffeinated drinks
- Refined foods

Best supplements

- 2 × high-potency multivitamin–minerals providing at least 20mg of B_6, 10mcg of B_{12}, 200mcg of folic acid, 15mcg of vitamin D, 10mg of zinc and 100mg of magnesium

- 2 × vitamin C 1,000mg

- 2 × magnesium 100mg (giving a total of 300mg with your multivitamin)

- 2 × high-potency omega-3-rich fish oil capsules (giving around 600mg of EPA, or EPA, plus DPA)

- X* × homocysteine-modulating nutrients (*dose and need dependent on your homocysteine score, as explained in Chapter 4, Part 2)

- 3 × CoQ_{10} 100mg

- 1–2 × vitamin D 1,000iu (25mcg) drops

CAUTIONS

Parkinson's disease is a complex condition and the exact dietary strategy in relation to medication needs careful management. It is therefore best to follow the guidance of an experienced health practitioner. The Brain Bio Centre, near London, offers support (see Resources).

DIG DEEPER

To find out more on this subject, read *Parkinson's Disease: Reducing Symptoms with Nutrition and Drugs* (Dr Geoffrey and Lucille Leader), which includes key referenced studies.

PERIODONTAL DISEASE

see **TOOTH DECAY AND PERIODONTAL (GUM) DISEASE**

PERIODS – IRREGULAR, HEAVY OR PAINFUL

Good medicine solutions

1. Balance your hormones

Heavy periods are one of the warning signs of oestrogen dominance. This can be due to excess exposure to oestrogenic substances or a lack of progesterone, or a combination of both. Oestrogen can be found in meat, but particularly in dairy products, in many pesticides and potentially in soft plastics, some of which leach into food (although these are being phased out in the EU). Oestrogen is also contained in most birth-control pills and HRT.

Aim to reduce the amount of animal fats and dairy produce in your diet, choose organic vegetables and meat wherever possible to cut down on your exposure to pesticides and hormones, and don't eat fatty foods that have been wrapped in non-PVC cling-film or microwaved in plastic containers.

2. Reduce stress

Stress is an everyday fact of life in the 21st century and it can play havoc with your hormones. Stress raises levels of the adrenal hormone cortisol, which has the effect of lowering progesterone. Extreme stress can, therefore, lead to missed periods. It's important to find a way to reduce stress using methods such as meditation, t'ai chi or yoga, or by having a regular massage or simply creating 'me time' – whatever helps you to relax. (See Chapter 6, Part 2 for more on how to reduce stress levels.)

3. Take vitamins

Zinc is absolutely vital for reproductive health. Together with vitamin B_6, zinc affects every part of the female sexual cycle. Working in partnership, these two nutrients ensure that adequate levels of sex hormones are produced. Oysters, lamb, nuts, egg yolks, rye and oats are all rich in zinc, while vitamin B_6 is found in cauliflower, watercress, bananas and broccoli.

Studies have shown that vitamin A may be deficient in women with heavy periods. This may be because vitamin A is lacking in their diet or because of a lack of zinc and Vitamin E, which are needed to release vitamin A from the liver. Vitamin E can also help to reduce cramps. Foods rich in vitamin E include seeds and nuts, while the best food source of vitamin A is liver.

Vitamin C and bioflavonoids (found mainly just beneath the surface skin of fruit) have been shown to help control heavy periods. Low levels of iron are common with heavy periods, which may be causal or an effect of the blood loss, but either way it's important to correct these levels. Vitamin C is found plentifully in berries, citrus fruits and leafy green vegetables, while iron, which is best absorbed if taken with vitamin C, is found in seeds and nuts. Meat is also a good source.

For those with very painful periods, eating foods rich in calcium and magnesium, plus taking supplements, should help. These minerals help to control the muscles of the womb, which are working extra hard during menstruation. Calcium helps the womb muscle to contract, and magnesium helps it to relax. Many diets that rely heavily on dairy produce are rich in calcium but relatively low in magnesium. Including nuts, seeds and dark green leafy vegetables in your diet often helps, as these foods are rich in both calcium and magnesium.

4. Have enough essential fats

Prostaglandins are needed for healthy hormone functioning, as they sensitise your cells to hormones. They are made from the essential fats omega-3 and -6 (found in oily fish, as well as nuts and seeds, respectively). A deficiency is likely to create hormone imbalances and contribute to painful, heavy periods, especially if the blood has a tendency to clot, so it's important to eat oily fish such as salmon or mackerel, and nuts and seeds, such as almonds, brazil nuts and pumpkin seeds, every day. You could also take supplements of evening primrose or borage oil (omega-6) or flax oil (omega-3). (See Chapter 3, Part 2 for more on essential fats.)

5. Fill up on fibre

Including adequate soluble fibre in your diet is an essential part of helping to balance your hormones and reduce problems with painful and heavy periods. Fibre helps to eliminate hormones from the body after they have been used. If there is too little fibre they will be reabsorbed, creating a hormone imbalance. It is therefore important to include plenty of oats, lentils, beans, fruit, vegetables and flax seeds in your diet.

6. Check whether you are too thin or do too much exercise

Absent or irregular periods are associated with low weight, strenuous exercise and anorexia nervosa. They can also be a sign of impending menopause (see Menopausal Symptoms on page 261).

Best foods

- Organic fruit and vegetables
- Nuts and seeds
- Oily fish (salmon, mackerel, herring including kippers, sardines)
- Oats
- Beans and lentils (pulses)
- Eggs
- Green leafy vegetables such as broccoli and spinach
- Liver
- Berries

Worst foods

- Animal fats
- Dairy
- Refined foods made with white flour and sugar, as these rob your body of nutrients
- Caffeine and cigarettes (which promote stress hormones)
- Alcohol (which depletes B vitamins and zinc)

Best supplements

- 2 × high-potency multivitamin–minerals providing at least 150mg of magnesium, 10mg of zinc, 20mg of vitamin B_6 and 100mg of vitamin E

- 2 × vitamin B_6 50mg and zinc 10mg (enough to achieve *at least* 20mg of zinc and 100mg of B_6 with your multivitamin)

- 1 × magnesium 150mg (enough to achieve 300mg in total)

- 1 × vitamin C 1,000mg

- 2 × essential omegas with fish-oil-derived omega-3, plus omega-6 from borage or evening primrose oil

> **CAUTIONS**
>
> Heavy, irregular or painful periods can be caused by fibroids, ovarian cysts, endometriosis, pelvic inflammatory disease, cervical erosions or dysplasia. Relief and/or prevention of these can be helped by following the advice above, but you should also check with your health-care practitioner for any unexplained pain or bleeding.

DIG DEEPER

To find out more about how to relieve heavy, painful or irregular periods, read *Balance Your Hormones* (Patrick Holford).

PERNICIOUS ANAEMIA

General information

Pernicious anaemia (PA) is caused by a deficiency in vitamin B_{12} due to a lack of production of a protein in the stomach known as intrinsic factor, which is needed for B_{12} absorption. Some PA sufferers produce antibodies that destroy intrinsic factor. PA is responsible for a variety of symptoms including:

- Shortness of breath

- Extreme fatigue

- Brain fog

- Poor concentration

- Short-term memory loss

- Confusion (putting familiar objects in the wrong places, such as putting a handbag in the fridge)

- Nominal aphasia (forgetting the names of objects)

- Clumsiness/lack of coordination

- Brittle, flaky nails; dry skin anywhere on the body

- Mood swings, heightened emotions

If untreated, PA can result in neurological symptoms and damage, leading to symptoms that include:

- Imbalance

- Dizziness, fainting

- Frequently bumping into, or falling against, walls

- General unsteadiness, especially when showering and dressing

- An inability to stand up with eyes closed, or in the dark

- Numbness/tingling – especially in the hands, arms, legs or feet

- Tinnitus (caused by nerve damage in the brain)

The average sufferer takes over two years to be diagnosed, because PA is often not considered and therefore is not properly tested for. A delay in diagnoses can lead to permanent neurological damage, hence the need for the possibility of PA to be taken seriously in those with extreme fatigue and other related symptoms. The website of the Pernicious Anaemia Society (see Resources) has a checklist that gives you a score indicating your likelihood of suffering from PA.

Good medicine solutions

1. Get properly tested and diagnosed

The first step is to get properly tested and diagnosed. The first test usually given is a standard B_{12} test, but the problem with this is twofold. Firstly, there is no consistent 'reference' range. In the UK, the cut-off point for indicating PA is often 150ng/l – which is a measurement of B_{12} in the blood – whereas, in Japan PA sufferers are treated at a level below 500ng/l, which is a much higher level of B_{12} than in the UK. A healthy level is above 500ng/l. Secondly, the test is not completely reliable, because not all B_{12} in circulation is in the active form, known as holo-transcobalamin (holo-TC). Measuring holo-TC is therefore a much more accurate determinant of need, but this test is not readily available.

Another test, called methylmalonic acid (MMA), is a more reliable marker for B_{12} deficiency than simple B_{12} levels, because MMA accumulates only if you are deficient in B_{12} or if you are not using B_{12} efficiently. If you want to be sure of your B_{12} status, it is best to have your MMA level tested. This should be below 0.37mol/l. If your homocysteine level is also high it is wise to assume you are not getting sufficient vitamin B_{12}. (Homocysteine is a toxic amino acid that is linked to a number of health issues. High levels of homocysteine are connected to low levels of vitamin B_{12}.)

2. Take high-dose B_{12} supplements or injections

Vitamin B_{12} is found only in foods of animal origin – meat, fish, eggs and dairy products. The B_{12} in fish is more bio-available than that found in meat. Although blue-green algae, such as spirulina or chlorella, are said to contain B_{12}, it is not the same as animal-derived B_{12}, and will not correct a deficiency. The recommended daily allowance (RDA) for vitamin B_{12} is only 1mcg and is seriously inadequate. I recommend that everyone achieves 10mcg, but people with PA need much higher levels so that the stomach is able to absorb a little more than normal.

If you are diagnosed with PA, or if you have a number of the symptoms listed above, it is worth supplementing 500–1,000mcg of B_{12}. Some PA sufferers find this works, and some report that supplementing methylcobalamine (methylB_{12}) works best. There is no risk of overdose with either.

Some PA sufferers respond only to injections of B_{12}, however. These are available from your doctor. If a B_{12} injection gives immediate relief it is one of the clearest indicators of PA and not a bad option to explore the cause of your symptoms, given the unreliability of B_{12} tests. Vitamin B_{12} is stored in the liver, and it is not needed every day, so the frequency of injections to relieve symptoms will vary from person to person. For many, monthly injections will suffice, but this is not the case for everybody.

Best foods

- Fish
- Meat
- Eggs
- Dairy products

Worst foods

- Alcohol
- Coffee and caffeinated drinks
- Sugar and refined foods (which deplete B vitamins)

Best supplements

- 2 × high-potency multivitamin–minerals providing 10mcg of B_{12}, 20mg of B_6, 2,300mcg of folic acid
- 1–2 × methylB_{12} (methylcobalamine) 500mcg

Or

- Injectable B_{12} at a frequency of one every two weeks to two months, depending on response to treatment.

DIG DEEPER

To find out more on this subject, read *Pernicious Anaemia* (Martyn Hooper), which includes key referenced studies. Also visit the website of the Pernicious Anaemia Society (see Resources).

PNEUMONIA

see **INFECTIONS**

POLYCYSTIC OVARIES

General information

As many as one in ten women suffers from small cysts that form in the ovary. The presence of these cysts, plus the associated symptoms, is known as polycystic ovarian syndrome (PCOS). The symptoms are abdominal pain, but usually only on one side, and often especially painful at certain times of the month. The primary cause is often insulin resistance, or insensitivity, which leads to more insulin being produced by the body, stimulating the growth of cysts. PCOS is therefore especially common in women with diabetes or pre-diabetes.

Good medicine solutions

1. Follow a low-GL diet

High levels of insulin appear to stimulate and increase blood levels of androgens (the male hormones) in PCOS and suppress a protein called sex hormone-binding globulin (SHBG), which makes sex hormones less biologically active. Eating a low-GL diet can improve insulin sensitivity and help to lessen the symptoms of PCOS. A low-GL diet will also help you to lose weight, if applicable, or maintain a healthy weight. As well as reducing the amount of insulin the body produces, weight loss can reduce androgens, and may restore ovulation.

Becoming aware of the GL of what you eat and knowing how to lower the GL of a meal is one of the fastest routes to controlling insulin levels. Insulin is released whenever your blood sugar spikes, for example when you eat sugar or fast-releasing carbohydrates from white bread, cereals, white rice, pastries, sweets and sugared drinks as well as too much fruit juice. To prevent blood sugar spikes, it's important to restrict these foods. Essentially, a low-GL diet focuses on: (a) eating little and often; (b) eating foods that are low-GL – those that release their sugar content slowly, such as brown rice or wholegrain pasta instead of white; and (c) combining carbohydrate foods with protein; for example, eating fish with brown rice, or an apple with almonds, to help keep blood sugar levels even. (See Chapter 1, Part 2 for details on how to follow a low-GL diet.)

2. Take chromium supplements

Controlling your blood sugar levels and weight is key to managing PCOS. For this reason insulin-sensitising drugs, such as metformin, may be recommended. Metformin has been shown to decrease blood levels of insulin in women with PCOS, reducing circulating androgens and improving ovulation. Metformin is, however, also associated with some unpleasant side effects. It interferes with the action of vitamin B_{12} and may raise your homocysteine level. Homocysteine is a toxic amino acid, high levels of which are connected to a number of health issues. Make sure you are supplementing vitamin B_{12} to keep your homocysteine level healthily low if you are on this drug.

There is a mineral that has the same action as metformin, but with no significant downsides. It's called chromium, and insulin can't work properly without it. In some trial participants, chromium has normalised sugar levels completely. Although chromium is naturally present in foods, such as beer, whole grains, cheese, liver and meat, the typical intake is much lower than the recommended daily requirement of 50–200mcg. One reason for this low consumption is that white flour, which is the most frequently eaten type, has 98 per cent of the chromium removed. Also, diets that are high in sweetened and refined foods, such as white bread, cakes, sweets and biscuits, increase chromium depletion, because it is used up by the body to process the sugar. The critical issue is the amount of chromium you take, ranging from the minimal effective dose of 200mcg up to 600mcg for diabetics. The ideal dose for someone with PCOS is 400–600mcg split between breakfast and lunch.

3. Reduce your stress

Stress, depression or mood swings are common in women with PCOS. Too much stress may aggravate many aspects of the syndrome, including insulin resistance. Whenever you take in a stimulant, such as coffee or a cigarette, or if you react stressfully to an event, your body produces the adrenal hormone cortisol. Cortisol, to deliver its stress message, has to lock onto receptors, or docking ports, on cells, but it uses the same receptors as the hormone progesterone, thereby making it harder for progesterone to deliver its message. In prolonged stress, with continued high cortisol, the net result is progesterone deficiency, because progesterone is effectively inactivated. Stress also upsets the balance of the 'male' hormone, testosterone, which is also present in women in lesser quantities. It is still vital, though – for example, for libido. A disturbance in the balance of male and female hormones in women can lead to a lack of ovulation, a decreased desire for sex and the development of excessive facial hair and other male characteristics. The vast majority of women with PCOS show this kind of hormone imbalance. When the blood sugar level is too low this stimulates the adrenal glands to make more cortisol. It's because of the link between stress hormones and your blood sugar that the right diet can make a big difference to the way you handle stress. Comforting cakes and sugary snacks are a particularly bad idea when you are stressed. To manage stress, keep your blood sugar balanced and avoid stimulants, such as alcohol, caffeine and cigarettes.

Another key way to beat stress and depression is exercise, which is a biochemical, physiological and psychological anti- dote to stress. It helps PCOS by reducing stress, improving your insulin sensitivity, increasing your metabolism and helping to shed any excess weight. Regular exercise helps your blood sugar become more balanced, because insulin starts to work properly. Even if you are not significantly overweight, exercise is critical in the process of reversing PCOS. You should be aiming for about 20–30 minutes a day, even if it is just walking. (How to manage stress is explained in Chapter 6, Part 2.)

4. Get your fats right

Apart from helping to control your weight, eating the right fats can lower inflammation, which is strongly associated with PCOS. Insulin resistance switches your whole system towards inflam- mation. Inflammation, in turn, promotes insulin insensitivity. Eating and supplementing essential fats, both omega-3 and -6, are also vital for keeping your hormones in balance, because they turn into hormone-like molecules, called prostaglandins. From a dietary point of view, I recommend cutting back on saturated and hydrogenated fats (found in meat, dairy products and processed foods such as cakes, biscuits and junk food), as these increase inflammation and oestrogen. Replace these fats with the essential fats found in oily fish (salmon, mackerel, herring, tuna, sardines), nuts (walnuts) and seeds (chia, flax, sunflower and hemp).

Although you can, and should, obtain omega-3 fats from your diet, I also recommend you supplement omega-3 fish oils every day. To give you a rough idea, I recommend you have the equivalent of 1,000mg of combined EPA and DHA a day, or 7,000mg a week.

A 100g (3½oz) serving of mackerel might give you 2,000mg, whereas a serving of salmon might give you 1,000mg. If you eat fish three times a week you'll probably achieve 3,500mg. To make up the remaining 3,500mg, I recommend you take an omega-3 fish oil supplement providing 500mg of combined EPA and DHA a day.

5. Consider natural progesterone

Progesterone plays a pivotal role in the balance of other hormones: the body makes oestrogen as well as testosterone and the stress hormone cortisol from progesterone. The competition from synthetic hormones, which are messed-up oestrogen- or progesterone-like molecules, plus environmental hormone-disrupting chemicals, called xenoestrogens, is often too much of a challenge for the body to deal with and can lead to oestrogen dominance and/or the underproduction of progesterone. In addition to this, women make more oestrogen relative to progesterone from their mid thirties onwards. The effect of this is that the body is exposed to a relative excess of oestrogen throughout the month. It is xenoestrogen exposure that is considered to be the most potent factor involved in this. (See 'Increase your intake of phytoestrogens' in Breast Cancer, page 71, for more on this.)

Addressing the problem of oestrogen dominance through an optimum diet and lifestyle alone may not be enough for some women. In certain instances, it is appropriate to correct a hormone deficiency by supplementing a bio-identical one – derived from a natural source, such as soya or wild yam. Such a hormone is called a natural, or bio-identical, hormone. The late Dr John Lee found that supplementing natural progesterone from day 10 to day 26 of the cycle for a few months is often enough to shrink ovarian cysts and no further treatment is required. Taking progesterone from day 10 effectively suppresses ovulation and gives the ovaries time to rest and repair. A nutritional therapist can test your progesterone levels and advise you accordingly.

Best foods

- Oily fish (salmon, mackerel, herring, kippers, sardines)
- Raw nuts and seeds
- Cruciferous vegetables (broccoli, cauliflower, kale, cabbage, Brussels sprouts – these help to detoxify excess oestrogen)
- Phytoestrogens (fermented soya, chickpeas, lentils)

Worst foods

- Sugar
- Refined 'white' foods
- Meat and dairy

Best supplements

- 2 × high-potency multivitamin–minerals providing 10mg of zinc and 150mg of magnesium, plus B vitamins, including at least 10mcg of B_{12}

- 2 × high-potency omega-3-rich fish oil capsules (choose products with the most EPA)

- 1–3 × chromium 200mcg. Start with 1 for two weeks then double the dose. A dose of 3 may be required for diabetics (see page 137)

> ### CAUTIONS
>
> Chromium can have a dramatic impact on blood sugar levels. If you are taking metformin, it's best to start on a low dose of chromium and build up to avoid dropping too low too quickly. Too much chromium can lead to too low blood sugar, so higher doses are not needed once you are feeling better and have good blood sugar control without dips in energy or cravings and a stable weight. Talk to your doctor about adjusting your medication accordingly. If you are taking metformin, this knocks out vitamin B_{12}, so it is important to supplement at least 10mcg of B_{12} a day.

DIG DEEPER

To find out more on this subject, read *Balance Your Hormones* (Patrick Holford), which includes key referenced studies.

PREMENSTRUAL SYNDROME (PMS)

General information

PMS is experienced by seven out of ten women, and one in ten women will suffer with it badly. The most common symptoms of PMS are acne, anxiety, fatigue, irritability, fluid retention, forgetfulness, mood swings, bloating, breast tenderness, sweet cravings and weight gain. In the Holford 100% Health Survey of over 45,000 women, 63 per cent reported often having PMS, 60 per cent menstrual cramps, 51 per cent breast tenderness, 51 per cent cyclical water retention and 42 per cent irregular/heavy periods.

Good medicine solutions

1. Eat a low-GL diet

There's an intricate relationship between the body's hormones, including those required for balancing blood sugar, responding to stress, and maintaining thyroid function and menstrual cycles. One of the most important dietary factors for balancing hormones is to keep your blood sugar level even, because many of the symptoms of PMS are blood sugar-related. You can do this easily by following a low-GL diet. The essentials of this are to: (a) eat plenty of complex, unrefined carbohydrates, such as whole grains (oats, brown rice, barley, wholegrain bread and pasta, millet), pulses (lentils, soya beans, kidney beans, and so on) and plenty of vegetables; (b) always combine carbohydrates with protein; for example, eat fish with brown rice, or an apple with some almonds; and (c) cut out all refined carbohydrates, such as white bread, white pasta and rice, cakes, biscuits and sweets, and any foods or drinks containing added sugar. A low-GL diet also provides lots of soluble fibre, which plays a key role in balancing the female hormones. The fibre found in vegetables, fruit and whole grains can absorb excess oestrogen in the gut and prevent it from re-entering the blood, thus lowering the level of circulating oestrogen and relieving PMS symptoms. Oat fibre, or whole oats or rough oatcakes, is particularly good. (See Chapter 1, Part 2 for details on how to follow a low-GL diet.)

2. Increase phytoestrogens

Phytoestrogens are oestrogen-like, plant-derived substances found in high amounts in soya products and various vegetables, such as peas and beans (pulses). Despite being similar to oestrogen, they can protect against the negative effects of too much oestrogen. There is a growing body of evidence that eating foods rich in phytoestrogens, called isoflavones, helps to keep the hormones in balance. Studies show that the higher a woman's isoflavone intake, the lower her PMS symptoms. Much of the attention has focused on soya due to its high isoflavone levels; however, other pulses, for example chickpeas, have high levels too. Other food sources are lentils, seeds, rye, oats and alfalfa.

Before you go overboard on soya, a word of caution: non-fermented soya products can have very high levels of phytates and genistein – natural substances that block the uptake of nutrients. Fermented soya products, such as miso, tempeh and natto, are much better for you, with occasional tofu or soya milk. Fermentation of soya also substantially increases the active isoflavone concentration. Even so, I recommend you have only about 30g (1oz) a day. This provides a daily dose of about 20–30mg of isoflavones. Supplements of isoflavones from fermented soya are another option. Research has found that soya supplementation can help with many premenstrual symptoms, including headache, breast tenderness and cramps. Phytoestrogens are also found in several herbs, such as Mexican yam, black cohosh, dong quai and agnus castus. These can be bought in combination formulas and can help with hormonal balance.

3. Increase liver-friendly foods

The liver is one of the key organs for controlling and balancing hormones, as this is where excess hormones can be removed. If the liver is over-taxed by a poor diet and/or alcohol, this elimination will not occur. The better your diet and intake of antioxidant nutrients and fibre, the more efficient your liver will be. I recommend drinking no more than six units of alcohol a week (that's four small glasses of wine, three half-pints of light beer, cider or lager, or six single shots of spirits a week) and eating at least five servings of fresh fruit and vegetables a day. Especially important are the liver-friendly foods such as onions, garlic, artichokes, watercress and rocket. Cruciferous vegetables both support the liver and contain di-indolylmethane (DIM) and indole-3-carbinol (I3C), which are a vital part of the process of eliminating excess oestrogen. Cruciferous vegetables include cabbage, Brussels sprouts, broccoli, cauliflower, kale, turnip, swede, radish, horseradish, mustard and cress. I suggest eating some cruciferous vegetables every day if you suffer from PMS. Some supplements also provide I3C.

4. Eat the right fats

Essential fats, both omega-3 and -6, are vital for keeping hormones in balance, because they turn into hormone-like molecules called prostaglandins. The most beneficial fat for PMS is called gamma-linolenic acid (GLA), found richly in evening primrose oil and borage oil. From a dietary point of view, I recommend cutting back on 'bad' saturated and hydrogenated fats (found in meat, dairy products and processed foods such as cakes, biscuits and junk food) as these increase both inflammation and oestrogen. Replace these fats with the essential fats found in oily fish (salmon, mackerel, herring, tuna, sardines), nuts (walnuts) and seeds (chia, flax, sunflower and hemp). These good fats are especially important for menstruating women as they help to prevent inflammation and reduce abnormal blood clotting. I would also suggest supplementing on a daily basis an omega-3 and -6 supplement, ideally containing ten times more omega-3, from fish oil, than omega-6, from borage oil; for example, if you took two capsules providing 750mg of fish oil (giving you about 650mg of active omega-3), plus 250mg of borage oil (giving you about 50mg of GLA) would be a good insurance policy. Most studies show the best results from supplementing the equivalent of up to 300mg of GLA a day, however. This is the equivalent of six 500mg evening primrose oil capsules. You can buy concentrated GLA capsules using borage oil, containing 150mg or 300mg in one capsule.

If a basic change in diet plus taking a daily omega-3 and -6 combination supplement doesn't alleviate your PMS, try taking 150mg or 300mg of GLA in the week before your period.

5. Get help from B vitamins and magnesium

There are extensive interactions between vitamin B_6 and magnesium in the body, as they work together in many enzyme systems. Vitamin B_6 is needed for clearing oestrogen from the liver. If oestrogens are not cleared efficiently, this can lead to symptoms such as PMS. Interestingly, women taking the contraceptive pill are often deficient in vitamin B_6. Some women have the inability to covert B_6 to its active form (pyridoxal-5-phosphate, or P5P) due to a deficiency in another nutrient, such as other B vitamins or magnesium, so it is a good idea to take a B complex that includes magnesium.

The best evidence for relieving PMS symptoms comes from studies giving vitamin B_6 (usually 100mg a day) and magnesium (200–300mg a day). Trials on B_6 have consistently shown that this vitamin reduces symptoms, but there is also evidence that magnesium does the same – especially with respect to water retention and mood swings.

Magnesium deficiency and PMS share many features. If you suffer from PMS, and you are very stressed or consume too much sugar, your magnesium levels may well be low, so make sure you're eating plenty of magnesium-rich foods such as seeds, nuts, green vegetables, whole grains and seafood, as well as supplementing.

I used to have ... '

Elaine told me:

> 'My PMS starts a week before a period. For the first two days I can handle it, but then my stomach starts churning, I get worse and worse, and I won't listen to anyone; I go nuts, get breast tenderness and have heavy, painful periods.'

The children would flee, and her husband cower, but two cycles later Elaine told me a very different story:

> 'I haven't had any PMT   it should be really bad right now. I've had none of my outbursts. No breast tenderness. I've stuck to the diet completely. My energy has gone through the roof. I just feel like a completely different person. I can't believe it's happened so quickly. My husband can't believe the change . . . I'm really enjoying the diet. I'm trying new foods and the taste is great.'

Best foods

- Oily fish (salmon, mackerel, herring, kippers, sardines)
- Raw nuts and seeds
- Cruciferous vegetables (broccoli, cauliflower, kale, cabbage, Brussels sprouts)
- Phytoestrogens (fermented soya, chickpeas, lentils)

Worst foods

- High-sugar foods
- Refined 'white' foods
- Alcohol
- Meat and dairy

Best supplements

- 2 × high-potency multivitamin–minerals

- 2 × essential omegas with fish-oil-derived omega-3, plus omega-6 from borage or evening primrose oil (with up to 300mg of GLA)

- 1 × female-balance formula containing at least 30mg B_3, 50mg of B_6, 10mcg of B_{12}, 300mcg of folic acid, 300mg of magnesium,150mg I3C and 200mg isoflavones

- 2 × vitamin C 1,000mg

DIG DEEPER

To find out more on this subject, read *Balance Your Hormones* (Patrick Holford), which includes key referenced studies.

PROSTATE CANCER

General information

Prostate cancer can vary from a relatively harmless condition to a potentially fatal illness, and its frequency increases with age. It is increasing at an alarming rate. The World Cancer Research Fund estimates that by 2018 one in four men will have a diagnosis of prostate cancer during their lives.

A small amount of prostate cancer is commonly found in older men who have died from other causes. For instance, it is present in up to 80 per cent of 80-year-olds. According to Professor Jonathan Waxman of Imperial College, London, little spots of cancer occur in 70 per cent of 70-year-olds, 60 per cent of 60-year-olds and 50 per cent of 50-year-olds, but their relationship with the development of aggressive cancer is unknown. A non-aggressive type of prostate cancer is known as prostatic intra-epithelial neoplasia or PIN. Some doctors regard PIN as being a precursor of cancer, however not all agree.

The main screening test involves measuring prostate-specific antigen (PSA) and a digital rectal examination. The symptoms are similar to prostate enlargement and the unreliability of PSA screening leads to over-diagnosis. A study in the *New England Journal of Medicine* followed 76,000 men, aged 55 to 74, who were randomly assigned to have annual PSA tests, plus digital rectal exams or 'usual care' which did not involve regular PSA screening.[1] After seven years, there was a 22 per cent increase in prostate cancer diagnosis in the screening group compared to the control, but no difference in the death rate from this disease. PSA testing clearly did not save lives. A second study involving 182,000 men of similar ages, emphasised the risks of over-diagnosis, and reported that it may be as high as 50 per cent.[2] Thus, some men have their prostate glands removed unnecessarily.

Prostate tissue, like breast tissue, is hormonally sensitive and the causes and nutritional approaches for the two are very similar. Follow the advice for Cancer (page 74) and see below. You should be especially wary of dairy products, which are the second most predictive risk factor – age being the first.

Good medicine solutions

1. Control the factors that stimulate growth

Cancer cell growth is influenced by hormones and growth factors. Eating too much sugar and refined carbohydrates promotes high insulin levels, which stimulate the growth of prostate cells. High-sugar diets also lead to weight gain – another risk factor for prostate cancer. Both healthy and cancerous prostate cells have receptors for insulin. Once insulin has attached to the receptor, it encourages the cell to divide and multiply, encouraging the tumour to grow.

Losing weight and eating less sugar can make a big difference to prostate cancer survival, as does taking regular exercise and staying relaxed. The best way to lose weight is to follow a low-GL diet. Essentially, that means: (a) eating plenty of complex, unrefined carbohydrates, such as whole grains (oats, brown rice, barley, wholegrain bread and pasta, millet), pulses (lentils, soya beans, kidney beans, and so on) and lots of vegetables; (b) you should always combine carbohydrates with protein; for example, eat fish with brown rice, or an apple with some almonds; and (c) cut out all refined carbohydrates, such as white bread, white pasta and rice, cakes, biscuits, sweets and any foods containing added sugar. (See Chapter 1, Part 2 for details on how to follow a low-GL diet.)

Another major promoter of insulin, which is strongly linked to prostate cancer, is milk (see Section 5 below).

Other growth promoters can come from excess hormone disruptors, which are carcinogens found in some pesticides, cosmetics and cleaning products. Follow the guidelines given in the general cancer advice (page 74) to see how to switch to alternatives.

2. Increase your intake of phytoestrogens

Phytoestrogens in beans, especially soya beans, but also in chickpeas, lentils, nuts, seeds and rye, help to block oestrogen receptors from powerful hormone-disrupting chemicals that mimic oestrogen, such as PCBs, dioxins and some pesticides. Much attention has focused on soya due to its high levels of phytoestrogens; however, other pulses (for example, chickpeas) have high levels too. Eat at least some beans, lentils, rye, alfalfa, raw nuts or seeds every day. When you do have soya, try fermented soya products such as miso, natto or tempeh. Fermenting breaks down digestion inhibitors, making the protective components (isoflavones) more available. Of the seeds, flax and pumpkin seeds are the best anti-cancer types.

I recommend you aim for about 15,000mcg (15mg) of phytoestrogens a day. This is easily achieved by having a small portion of
tofu. A 100g (3½oz) serving provides 78,000mcg, while a 100ml
(3½fl oz) glass of soya milk or soya yoghurt provides 11,000mcg
and a portion of chickpeas, perhaps prepared as hummus, contains 2,000mcg. Supplements of isoflavones made from fermented soya are another option.

The liver is the main organ responsible for removing excess
hormones from the body. Eating cruciferous vegetables (including
broccoli, kale, cabbage, cauliflower and Brussels sprouts), which are
rich in di-indolylmethane (DIM), helps the liver to do this. Growth
hormones stop cancer cells from committing suicide; DIM switches
this suicide signal back on. Making cruciferous vegetables part of
your daily diet, therefore, is essential. You might also think about
boosting your levels of DIM by taking supplements.

3. Increase your intake of vitamin D

Numerous studies show an association between higher levels of
vitamin D and a lower risk of developing and/or surviving cancer.
Interestingly, a high-meat-protein diet and high-calcium diet, which
is what you get from dairy products, blocks the body's ability
to create active vitamin D. Testing for vitamin D levels is the only
way we can really know how much we have in our bodies. Family
doctors will often test for this, and there are home test kits available, or you could visit a nutritional therapist who can do it
for you.

There are three ways to increase your blood level of vitamin
D: eat it, supplement it or expose yourself to more sunlight.
The best dietary sources are oily fish and eggs, but to reach
optimum levels you'll need to supplement, especially if you are
not exposed to much sunlight. Better-quality high-potency
multivitamin–minerals should give you 600iu (15mcg). During
the winter months this is certainly not enough, so it's worth
supplementing an additional 1,000iu (25mcg), and possibly more.

4. Increase key antioxidants, including zinc

Antioxidants are substances that remove or disarm potentially damaging oxidising agents in the body, which are created like 'exhaust fumes' when our cells turn food into energy. (See 'Increase Your Intake of Antioxidants' in Cancer, page 76, for the background information relating to cancers.) As well as following the recommendations for improving antioxidant status, certain nutrients are especially vital for a healthy prostate:

Zinc is often found to be deficient in prostate cancer patients, and low levels are a good predictor of risk. Zinc protects against harmful oxidants created in anything burned, including cigarettes and crispy meat. The body also generates oxidants from 'burning' sugar for energy. Zinc is also anti-inflammatory, and helps to repair damaged DNA. Most of us don't get enough zinc. I recommend supplementing 10–20mg a day as well as eating zinc-rich foods (seafood, nuts and seeds and nut/seed butters, such as tahini).

Selenium Low selenium levels are also a good predictor of prostate cancer. Foods rich in selenium include garlic and onions, sunflower seeds, mushrooms, whole grains (brown rice, oats, wheatgerm), brazil nuts and fish (tuna, halibut, sardines, salmon); however, this mineral is often deficient in the soil where foods are grown today, so I recommend people also supplement about 100mcg of it each day. The recommended amounts of both zinc and selenium can be found in a good-quality multivitamin–mineral.

Lycopene in tomatoes, **quercetin** in red onions, and *vitamins C* and *E* are all important antioxidants with good evidence suggesting an anti-prostate cancer effect both from foods and isolated nutrients.

Spices are amazing antioxidants, especially turmeric, cinnamon, chilli and ginger. I recommend you maximise your use of all these foods in your diet.

5. Avoid dairy products and limit meat

The foods most strongly linked to a higher risk of prostate cancer are dairy products and, to a lesser extent, meat, particularly processed meat, as well as alcohol. According to the National Cancer Institute (NCI), 19 out of 23 studies have shown a positive association between dairy intake and prostate cancer: 'This is one of the most consistent dietary predictors for prostate cancer in the published literature . . . In these studies, men with the highest dairy intakes had approximately double the risk of total prostate cancer, and up to a fourfold increase in risk of metastatic or fatal prostate cancer relative to low consumers.'[3] Vegetarians have a lower prostate cancer risk and countries with the lowest dairy intake have the lowest rate of prostate cancer fatalities.

Dairy products promote high levels of an insulin-like growth factor (IGF-1), which has been found to directly stimulate the growth of cancer cells. Both high IGF-1 levels and high insulin levels are predictive of prostate cancer risk. You can keep your insulin levels down by following a low-GL diet. (See Chapter 1, Part 2 for details on how to follow a low-GL diet.)

If you have prostate cancer, I recommend the complete avoidance of dairy products. If you don't have cancer, keep your intake of dairy products low; that is, below 300ml (10fl oz/½ pint) a day and ideally less than 1.2 litres (2 pints) a week. Try rice milk, oat milk or soya milk instead. I would also recommend avoiding red meat.

6. Choose helpful herbs

The most consistently helpful herbs for prostate cancer are saw palmetto and pygeum. Saw palmetto has been proven to help inhibit cancer growth and to reduce inflammation. It also inhibits an enzyme, called 5-alpha reductase, which turns testosterone into dihydrotestosterone (DHT) – the form of testosterone that promotes prostate cancer. It has been shown to inhibit the growth-promoting effects of IGF in milk. The fatty acids in saw palmetto seem to be the most biologically active, so choose a supplement that is standardised to 45 per cent fatty acids. This means it is high quality. I recommend 120mg a day for prevention and 360mg a day if you have prostate cancer.

The other prostate-friendly herb that shows many similar beneficial properties is the African bark pygeum. It also lessens the harmful effect of too much IGF and, in animal studies, is profoundly anti-cancer. When supplementing pygeum, it's worth getting a high-quality standardised extract with up to 5 per cent B-sitosterol. I recommend 40mg a day for prevention and 120mg a day if you have prostate cancer.

7. Consider salvestrols, and high mega-doses of vitamin C

The holy grail of chemotherapy has been to find a way of targeting only cancer cells while leaving healthy cells untouched. More than a decade ago now it was discovered that cancer cells have an active enzyme, called CYP1B1 (pronounced sip-one-B-one), which differentiates them from healthy cells. A major conceptual breakthrough for cancer treatment is the discovery that many plants contain compounds, called salvestrols, that are converted by the CYP1B1 enzyme into a compound that kills cancer cells. By flooding the body with harmless salvestrols, theoretically the cancer cells should self-destruct.

This is exactly what happens in the laboratory when you expose cancer cells to salvestrols. Although we lack human clinical trials, more and more cases of successful cancer treatment are being reported using high-dose salvestrols. Taking high-dose salvestrol supplements is a sensible precaution (see Resources). The dose required for general protection is 350 salvestrol points, while the dose for cancer treatment is 4,000 points. (Salvestrols are measured in relation to their comparative effect against cancer cells, in points, rather than in milligrams.)

The other 'natural' chemotherapy that has no harmful effects on healthy cells but effectively destroys cancer cells is the use of high-dose vitamin C. Both high-dose oral and intravenous vitamin C therapy have been used in the successful treatment of cancer for over 40 years. The aim, in this kind of cancer treatment, is to raise blood levels of vitamin C as high as possible. This means taking as much orally as you can before it induces diarrhoea (known as the 'bowel tolerance' level). This varies from individual to individual, but is usually between 5g and 20g a day. Vitamin C is most easily taken as ascorbic acid powder, dissolved in water with some juice, and sipped throughout the day. An alternative way of achieving very high levels is through intravenous vitamin C therapy. A number of cancer specialists are providing this. (For doctors in the UK, see Resources.)

Taking high-dose salvestrols and vitamin C for three months would give cancer cells a very hard environment in which to survive.

8. Look at HIFU – a breakthrough in prostate cancer treatment

If you are diagnosed with prostate cancer one of the least invasive and most effective treatments is high-intensity focused ultrasound (HIFU). The treatment uses a special form of ultrasound to heat the tumour. The treatment thus involves hyperthermia, one of the few effects known to kill cancer cells totally while leaving healthy cells relatively unscathed.

The procedure usually involves a hospital stay of three days at most, with minimal side effects, namely a burning sensation in a few cases. The original claims for the treatment were that it had over 87 per cent five-year survival rates, compared with a UK norm at the time of about 54 per cent. The beauty of the treatment is that it melts the cancer away, liquefying the tumour. It is not effective for all prostate tumours, however, so please discuss this with your oncologist. It can be repeated at a later stage, if required, unlike radiotherapy, for example. Moreover, side effects such as impotence or incontinence are greatly reduced compared to surgery and radiotherapy.

Best foods

- Cruciferous vegetables (broccoli, Brussels sprouts, cabbage, cauliflower, kale)
- Fish
- Garlic
- Raw nuts and seeds
- Tomatoes
- Beans (lentils, soya beans, kidney beans, chickpeas)

Worst foods

- Alcohol
- Meat
- Dairy
- Sugar

Best supplements

- 2 × high-potency multivitamin–minerals providing at least 10mg of zinc and 15mcg of vitamin D

- 1 × antioxidant complex (containing beta-carotene, vitamin E and selenium, plus other antioxidant nutrients such as glutathione, alpha lipoic acid, co-enzyme Q_{10} (CoQ_{10}) and resveratrol)

- 1 × 1,000iu (25mcg) vitamin D drops

- 1 × 360mg saw palmetto, plus 120mg pygeum

- 5,000mg or more vitamin C

- 2 × salvestrols 2,000 points for recovery; 350 points for prevention

---

CAUTIONS

Many chemotherapeutic drugs are oxidants. It may therefore not be a good idea to take lots of antioxidants while undergoing certain types of chemotherapy. (Vitamin C in high doses acts as a pro-oxidant so should not interfere.) Please check with your oncologist if you are undergoing chemotherapy.

You must not undertake an extensive nutritional strategy on your own. It is important to ensure that you get the correct guidance from a nutritional therapist.

Calcium supplements above 400mg should be avoided by prostate cancer patients, as they may reduce the amount of vitamin D activated by the kidneys.

PROSTATE ENLARGEMENT AND HYPERPLASIA

General information

The prostate is a small gland, about the size of a walnut, that sits under the bladder by the urethra (the urine duct) and makes fluid that passes into the seminal duct to help sperm swim along.

If the prostate becomes swollen it can act like a clamp, making it harder to urinate. This is very common in men later in life. It's caused by either inflammation of the prostate (prostates) or, more commonly, benign prostatic hyperplasia (BPH), which affects one in three men over the age of 60. Although there is no clear link between BPH and prostate cancer, other than difficulty peeing, too many men avoid going to see their doctor when they have symptoms. In both cases, the earlier you know what's happening the better. (See Prostate Cancer on page 316.)

Good medicine solutions

1. Look into screening tests and diagnosis

If you are more than 50 years old and male, there's a good chance you might have an enlarged non-malignant prostate or BHP. This carries with it certain symptoms, which are virtually identical to those of prostate cancer:

- Difficulty or pain when passing urine.
- The need to pass urine more often.
- Broken sleep due to the need to pass urine.
- Waiting for long periods before the urine flows.
- The feeling that the bladder has not completely emptied.

With prostate cancer you may also suffer with blood in the urine, and/or lower back pain and/or dribbling. Be aware, however, that many of the above symptoms can be caused by other factors, such as bacterial infection.

Your doctor can simply feel if you have an enlarged prostate (by a digital rectal examination). If he or she finds such an enlargement they will probably send you for a PSA test (prostate-specific antigen). PSA is an enzyme produced in the prostate. If your score is higher than 4ng/ml, you might be encouraged to have a biopsy, because this test is thought to be a reliable indicator of prostate cancer risk.

A high PSA level doesn't automatically mean you have prostate cancer. There are many other factors that can raise your level. Also, the usual cut-off point, 4ng/ml, is quite conjectural. A study at Stanford University in California compared PSA scores with tumour size in men with prostate cancer and found that a PSA of 9 was no more predictive of a large, aggressive tumour than a score of 2.

The test does not seem to distinguish fully between enlarged malignant prostates and non-malignant ones, and some studies show that half of those testing positive, probably are not. Over-diagnosis is a real concern. Roughly 12 per cent of the men told they have prostate cancer after PSA testing do not have it at all.

One way to minimise over-diagnosis is never to rely on a single test, but have three to six across a two-month period.

2. Don't drink milk; do reduce animal fats

The strongest dietary risk factor for prostate enlargement and cancer is dairy consumption. Switzerland, for example, has the highest dairy intake and the highest numbers of deaths from prostate cancer. This is almost certainly due to a hormone in milk called insulin-like growth factor (IGF). Prostate tissue has receptors for IGF-1 and IGF-2. Research shows clearly that men with high levels of circulating IGF-1 are at greater risk of suffering from prostate cancer than those with lower levels. Research also shows that circulating levels of IGF-1 in the blood correlate with high dairy consumption. A pint of milk a day, or the equivalent in other dairy products, quadruples risk.

Fats from dairy products, meat, fish and eggs are the highest sources of hormone-disrupting chemicals, and a high consumption of these foods is more likely to increase risk. So, moving more towards a vegetarian diet, using beans, lentils, nuts and seeds for protein, is consistent with keeping your prostate healthy. As there are other health benefits from eating fish and eggs, try to source organic or wild fish, or omega-3-rich eggs.

3. Increase omega-3 fats

Fish oils may be protective against prostate problems. Fish eaters at least halve their risk compared to non-fish eaters, especially if they eat oily fish (salmon, mackerel, herrings and sardines),[1] suggesting that the overall benefit outweighs a potential detriment of hormone-disrupting chemicals found in fish. Supplementing purified omega-3 fish oils (EPA and DHA) provides a guaranteed polychlorinated biphenyl (PCB)-free source of these powerful anti-inflammatory agents. If you're suffering from BPH or prostatitis, supplement the equivalent of 1,000mg of EPA a day.

4. Eat more fruit and veg, beans, lentils, nuts and seeds

The higher your consumption of fruit and veg, pulses, such as beans and lentils, nuts and seeds, the lower your risk of BPH. Particularly beneficial are tomatoes, which are rich in lycopene, and kale, cabbage, broccoli and cauliflower. These are profoundly cancer protective.

Soya is particularly protective, because it prevents excessive oestrogenisation. You need 15mg of phytoestrogens a day from soya foods for maximum protection. This is easily achieved by having a small portion of tofu – a 100g (3½oz) serving provides 78mg, a 100ml (3½fl oz) glass of soya milk or soya yoghurt, giving you 11mg, and a portion of chickpeas, perhaps as hummus, providing 2mg. Eating rye bread, beansprouts, beans, lentils, nuts and seeds also helps to boost your levels. Alternatively, you can supplement these.

5. Take an antioxidant supplement

Although individual antioxidants haven't always come up trumps, a trial giving over 5,000 men a combined antioxidant supplement containing vitamins C and E, beta-carotene, selenium and zinc daily for eight years proved protective.[2] However, the protective effect was far higher in those men with a normal PSA level (below 3mcg/l).The antioxidants did not, however, appear to lower either PSA or IGF levels.

6. Supplement saw palmetto and/or pygeum

Saw palmetto has been proven to help inhibit cancer growth and to reduce inflammation. This makes it the perfect supplement for both BPH and prostatitis as well as prostate cancer. Studies have shown a reduction in enlargement of the prostate with daily supplementation. In addition, saw palmetto inhibits an enzyme, called 5-alpha reductase, which turns testosterone into dihydrotestosterone (DHT), a form of testosterone that promotes prostate cancer.[3] Recent research has also shown that saw palmetto inhibits the growth-promoting effects of IGF-1 in milk, so that's an additional benefit.[4]

I recommend 120mg a day of saw palmetto for prevention and 360mg a day if you have BHP or prostate cancer. It's the fatty acids in saw palmetto that seem to be most biologically active, so choose a supplement that is standardised to 45 per cent fatty acids. This means it's high quality.

The other prostate-friendly herb that shows many similar beneficial properties is the African bark pygeum. It also lessens the harmful effect of too much IGF-1 and, in animal studies, is anti-cancer.[5] This is because pygeum is an excellent source of B-sitosterol, a plant sterol. When supplementing pygeum it's worth buying a high-quality standardised extract with up to 5 per cent B-sitosterol. I recommend 40mg a day for prevention and 120mg a day if you have BPH or prostate cancer.

Best foods

- Organic oily fish (salmon, mackerel, herring including kippers, sardines)
- Vegetables, especially tomatoes
- Fruits, especially berries
- Beans and lentils (pulses)
- Raw nuts and seeds

Worst foods

- Dairy products
- Animal fats
- Alcohol (in excess is associated with increasing cancer risk)
- Sugar (which is devoid of nutrients)

Best supplements

- 2 × high-potency multivitamin–minerals providing at least 10mg of zinc and 15mcg of vitamin D

- 2 × high-potency omega-3-rich fish oil capsules (choose products with the most EPA)
- 1 × antioxidant complex (containing beta-carotene, vitamin E and selenium, plus other antioxidant nutrients such as glutathione, alpha lipoic acid, co-enzyme Q_{10} (CoQ_{10}). and resveratrol)
- 1 × 360mg saw palmetto, plus 120mg pygeum

SCHIZOPHRENIA

General information

About one in a hundred people has schizophrenia. There are a variety of symptoms, including hallucinations, delusions or disordered speech/behaviour, as well as problems with fluency of language and thoughts or with expression of emotions. Conventional treatment is with tranquillising drugs. None of the recommendations below is contradicted with such medication.

Good medicine solutions

1. Improve your blood sugar balance

The incidence of blood sugar problems and diabetes is much higher in people who have schizophrenia, and the commonly prescribed antipsychotic medication may also further disturb blood sugar control. It is therefore very important to follow a low-GL diet, which will stabilise your blood sugar. Essentially, a low-GL diet focuses on: (a) avoiding sugar and refined carbohydrates; (b) eating at regular intervals; and (c) including protein with every meal and snack; for example, eating fish with brown rice, or an apple with some almonds. Also, avoid strong stimulants such as coffee, tea and energy drinks, and drink mild stimulants such as green tea only occasionally. Keep alcohol to a minimum; for example, no more than one unit per day, three to four times per week maximum.

2. Increase your intake of essential omega-3 and -6 fats

Our brains are built from specialised essential fats in a continuing process. Our bodies are always building membranes, then breaking them down, and building new ones. This breaking down – or stripping of essential fats from the brain membranes – is controlled by an enzyme called phospholipase-A2 (PLA2). This enzyme, however, is often overactive in people who have schizophrenia, and this leads to a greater need for these essential fats, which are quickly lost from the brain.

A number of studies have shown that taking omega-3 fish oil supplements, high in brain-supportive eicosapentaenoic acid (EPA), with other key vitamins, improves symptoms and prevents the development of schizophrenia in those at risk.

The best way to increase your intake is to eat fish at least twice a week, seeds on most days and supplement omega-3 oils. The best fish for EPA are (for a 100g/3½oz portion): mackerel (1,400mg); herring/kipper (1,000mg); sardines (1,000mg); fresh tuna (900mg); anchovies (900mg); salmon (800mg); and trout (500mg). Most tuna is high in mercury and should therefore be eaten no more than three times a month.

The best seeds are chia, flax and pumpkin. Flax seeds are very small and have a hard outer husk, so are best ground before sprinkling onto cereal. Chia seeds don't need grinding. Technically, these seeds provide omega-3, but only about 5 per cent of the type of omega-3 (alpha linolenic acid – ALA) contained in them is converted in your body into EPA.

When supplementing omega-3 fish oils aim for about 1,000mg of EPA a day for a mood-stabilising effect. That means supplementing a concentrated omega-3 fish oil capsule providing 500mg once or twice a day and eating a serving of any of the above fish three times a week. Alternatively, supplement a combination of omega-3 (containing EPA and DHA) and omega-6 (containing GLA). These essential fats can be found in combination supplements.

3. Increase antioxidants, especially vitamin C

Essential fats form a vital part of the brain, but are prone to damage by oxidants. Oxidants are formed, rather like exhaust fumes, whenever our cells turn food into energy. They are also created when something is burned, be it a cigarette or fried food or the petrol in cars. Oxidants have to be disarmed by anti-oxidants because the damage they cause in the body, oxidation, is harmful and similar to rusting or burning.

There is evidence of more oxidation in the frontal cortex of people with schizophrenia than in those who are not affected. Therefore, as well as increasing the intake of essential fats, it makes sense to follow a diet that minimises oxidants from fried or burned food, and by not smoking, as well as maximising your intake of antioxidant nutrients such as vitamins A, C and E.

To ensure you are getting the correct types and amounts of antioxidants, eat lots of fresh (or frozen, but not tinned or dried) fruit and vegetables in a variety of colours, and also supplement daily with 2,000mg of vitamin C, taken in two divided doses, plus 400iu (300mg) of vitamin E, as part of an all-round anti-oxidant that contains N-acetyl-cysteine (NAC) and/or reduced glutathione, as well as co-enzyme Q_{10} (CoQ_{10}).

Vitamin C has been shown to reduce the symptoms of schizo-phrenia in research trials, and a number of studies have shown that people diagnosed with mental illness may have much greater requirements for this vitamin – often ten times higher – and are frequently deficient.

4. Consider supplementing niacin

The classic symptoms of this condition are dermatitis, diarrhoea and disturbed mental health. A more extensive list of symptoms might include headaches, sleep disturbance, hallucinations, thought disorder, anxiety and depression. One of the classic vitamin-deficiency diseases in schizophrenia is pellagra – a niacin (vitamin B_3) deficiency.

Some people need more niacin than others to stay well. If you have the above symptoms, you may need a lot more niacin than the basic recommended daily allowance (RDA), sometimes as much as 2,000 – 100 times the RDA. Some people need more than others, perhaps for genetic reasons, and feel much better on large amounts of niacin, such as 1,000mg and above a day. Very large amounts, ten times these levels, can be liver toxic, however, especially from sustained-release supplements. Non-blushing niacin (inositol hexanicotinate) has lower toxicity than sustained-release formulations. In any event, I recommend that anything over 1,000mg is best taken under the supervision of a qualified practitioner.

Niacin is available in different forms. Niacin (formerly known as nicotinic acid) causes a harmless blushing sensation, accompanied with an increase in skin temperature and slight itching. This effect can be quite severe, and lasts for up to 30 minutes; however, if 500mg of niacin is taken twice a day at regular intervals, the blushing soon reduces.

Some supplement companies produce a 'no-flush' niacin by binding niacin with inositol. This also works, so it's probably the best form, but it is more expensive. Niacin also comes in the form of niacinamide, which doesn't cause blushing either, but it may not be as effective.

5. Check your homocysteine level and have enough B vitamins

For the brain to maintain the correct chemical balance, a critical process called methylation has to work efficiently. An indicator of faulty methylation is having a high level of a toxic amino acid in the blood called homocysteine, caused by a lack of B vitamins (B_2, B_6, B_{12} and folic acid). Many people with schizophrenia, especially young men, tend to have a high level of homocysteine, despite no obvious dietary lack of these vitamins. These unusually high levels, often above 15, don't appear to relate to diet or lifestyle factors, such as smoking, but are linked to genetic predisposition.

Homocysteine is lowered, and methylation improved, by taking a combination of the B vitamins listed above. You can test your homocysteine level using a home test kit or through your doctor or health-care practitioner. (See Chapter 4, Part 2 for more on homocysteine.)

Also, eat whole foods rich in B vitamins, including whole grains, beans, nuts, seeds, fruit and vegetables. Good sources for folic acid are green vegetables, beans and lentils (pulses), nuts and seeds. Vitamin B_{12} is found only in animal foods: meat, fish, eggs and dairy produce. A good starting point is to supplement a multivitamin providing optimal levels of B vitamins: which means 25–50mg of B_1, B_2, B_3 (niacin), B_5 (pantothenic acid), B_6 (pyridoxine or pyridoxal-$_5$-phosphate) and at least 100mcg of folic acid and 10mcg of B_{12} and biotin.

6. Check for pyroluria and an increased need for vitamin B_6 and zinc

Possibly one of the most significant 'undiscovered' discoveries in the nutritional treatment of mental illness is that many mentally ill people are deficient in vitamin B_6 and zinc. But this is no ordinary deficiency: you can't correct it by simply eating more foods that are rich in zinc and B_6. It is connected to an abnormal production of a group of chemicals called 'pyrroles' – now known to be hydroxy-hemopyrrolin-2-one (HPL) – which can be tested for by a nutritional therapist or doctor (see Resources).

Pyroluria is often a stress-related condition, with symptoms usually beginning in the teenage years after a stressful event such as exams or the break-up of a relationship. People with pyroluria often have weak immune systems and may have suffered from frequent ear infections as a child, as well as colds, fevers and chills. Other symptoms include fatigue, nervous exhaustion, insomnia, poor memory, hyperactivity, seizures, poor learning ability, confusion, an inability to think clearly, depression and mood swings. In girls, there can also be irregular periods. Other symptoms include bad breath and a strange body odour, a poor tolerance of alcohol or drugs, early morning nausea, cold hands and feet, and abdominal pain. A lack of dream recall is also very common.

It is important that people with pyroluria eat a healthy diet and supplement relatively large amounts of zinc, perhaps 25–50mg a day, as well as vitamin B_6, perhaps 100mg daily.

7. Investigate food intolerances

Some people with mental health problems are sensitive to gluten, especially wheat gluten, which can produce many of the symptoms of mental illness. You may suspect some foods are contributing to your symptoms. If this is the case, you could try an exclusion diet where the food or foods are eliminated for a brief trial period. The usual suspects are: gluten (in wheat, rye and barley), wheat, dairy (all types – cow, sheep, goat, milk, cheese, cream, and so on), soya, yeast and eggs. It's worth noting, however, that it is possible to be intolerant to any food. (See Allergies on page 31 for more details on testing and treatment.)

Best foods

- Vegetables
- Fruit
- Raw nuts and seeds
- Oats (which have a low allergenic potential and stabilise blood sugar)
- Oily fish (salmon, mackerel, herring, kippers, sardines)
- Eggs

Worst foods

- Alcohol
- Sugar
- Caffeinated drinks
- Refined foods
- Wheat (for some)

Best supplements

- 2 × high-potency multivitamin–minerals providing at least 20mg of B_6, 10mcg of B_{12}, 200mcg of folic acid, 15mcg of vitamin D, 10mg of zinc and 150mg of magnesium

- 2 × vitamin C 1,000mg

- 2 × essential omegas with fish-oil-derived omega-3, plus omega-6 from borage or evening primrose oil (supplying EPA, DPA, DHA and GLA)

Or

- 2 × high-potency omega-3-rich fish oil capsules (providing close to 1,000mg of EPA)

Optional

- 2 × antioxidant complex (containing beta-carotene, vitamin E and selenium, plus other antioxidant nutrients such as glutathione, alpha lipoic acid, co-enzyme Q_{10} (CoQ_{10}) and resveratrol)

- X* × homocysteine-modulating nutrients, B vitamin formula (* dose and need dependent on your homocysteine score, as explained in Chapter 4, Part 2)

- 2 × niacin 500mg (non-blushing form preferable) (note: *not* niacinamide)

- 2 × vitamin B_6 50mg and 1 × zinc 25mg, if tested pyroluric

CAUTIONS

If you become nauseated taking high doses of niacin (B$_3$), it is an indication to stop supplementation and resume three days later, with a lower amount. If you have a history of liver problems, or a high liver load due to medication, drugs or alcohol, you should have your liver enzymes monitored regularly by your doctor if you are taking a high dose of niacin (above 2,000mg a day).

Vitamin B$_6$ can be toxic at high doses, the key symptom of which is tingling hands or fingers. If this occurs, stop the B$_6$ immediately and the tingling will stop within one to three days. Once it has stopped, you could restart the B$_6$ at half the previous dose.

DIG DEEPER

To find out more on this subject read *Optimum Nutrition for the Mind* (Patrick Holford), which includes key referenced studies. The team of nutritional therapists and psychiatrists at the Brain Bio Centre, near London, offers support for people with mental health problems, both in the UK and all over the world via Skype. (See Resources.)

SHINGLES

see HERPES AND SHINGLES

SINUS PROBLEMS

Good medicine solutions

1. Increase vitamin C and other natural anti-inflammatories

Sinus problems can be the result of an infection or an allergic-type reaction that results in excessive mucus production. Vitamin C is profoundly anti-viral and antibacterial when taken at bowel-tolerance level (the level just below that which causes loose bowels). This is usually about 1,000mg an hour during an infection. Vitamin C is also anti-inflammatory and a natural antihistamine, immediately calming down allergic reactions, a common contributor to chronic sinus problems.

Antibiotics are inappropriately prescribed for three in four sinus infections despite the fact that viruses (and not bacteria) are by far the most frequent cause of this condition.[1] If you are given a course of antibiotics, also supplement probiotics for two weeks after the end of the course.

I also advise increasing your intake of other anti-inflammatory nutrients, including omega-3 fish oils, quercetin (found in red onions) and bromelain (an enzyme found in pineapples). Vitamin A also strengthens the sinus membranes and protects against infection. Drinking strong ginger tea and avoiding dairy products can also help.

2. Investigate hidden food allergies

It is common for people who have chronic sinusitis to have an allergic background, and the fact that anti-histamines are the second most prescribed drug for sinus sufferers would bear this out, since histamine is released in response to exposure to an allergen. Among children with sinus problems such as chronic rhinitis or frequent ear infections, as many as one in three has been shown to react allergically to either milk or wheat, the most common food allergens.[2]

I strongly recommend allergy testing for anyone with persistent nasal congestion or long-term sinusitis. You can buy a simple home test for food intolerances (see Resources, and Allergies on page 31 for more details).

Apart from food allergies it is possible that a majority of chronic sinus sufferers may be sensitive to pollution and other airborne particles. These can be moulds and house dust mites. If this is the case, expect to find relief in a hot, dry, unpolluted environment.

3. Try daily sinus washing

Washing the sinuses out with salt water on a daily basis also makes a big difference. One way is to use a saline nasal spray, available from pharmacists. Sterimar is a good product.

There is a limit as to how much these sprays penetrate into the deeper sinus cavities, however. A more advanced method of sinus irrigation involves buying a device called SinuPulse (available on the internet), and it helps considerably if you irrigate your sinuses every day.

There is also a yogic technique using a neti pot (also available on the internet), which is like a teapot with a long spout. You fill the neti pot with a light salt solution in warm water and, leaning over a washbasin, you pour the liquid into one nostril, holding your head at an angle so that the water washes through the sinuses and comes out of the other nostril. Buy a neti pot with a long fine spout. You will find a number of videos on YouTube demonstrating how to use it, and the pot will come with instructions.

Yoga is also good for the sinuses. It's best to attend a class and tell your teacher that you have sinus problems so that he or she can find the best ways for you to practise the postures. Iyengar yoga is best for this because some teachers are specially trained to advise on health issues.

4. Use steam inhalations

Local applications of heat have been shown to be effective in alleviating both short- and long-term symptoms of allergic rhinitis.[3] Make a steam inhalation by putting six drops of Olbas oil or eucalyptus and/or white sage oil into a bowl of steaming water. Cover your head and the bowl with a towel. Inhale deeply through both nostrils.

General advice

The net consequence of years of nasal irritation is that the tissue within the nose and sinuses becomes permanently inflamed and hardened. This narrows the breathing passages and makes inflammation more likely to lead to a blockage, which increases the chances of infection. (A sinus infection can be bacterial, viral or fungal.) All this is more likely in people with either a deviated septum or poor drainage from the sinus cavities caused by small holes. By this stage you'll probably be offered one of two operations, the lesser of which involves burning away the excess tissue that accumulates around the 'turbinates' (the three ridges along vents in the septum, the central cartilage along the nose, designed to maximise exposure of air to surfaces on its way into your lungs). The more extreme operation involves reconstructing the nasal passages, and maybe increasing the size of the holes for sinus draining. These operations can make a big difference but they don't address the underlying cause of the nasal/sinus inflammation.

Best foods

- Ginger and ginger tea
- Turmeric
- Oily fish (salmon, mackerel, herring, kippers, sardines)
- Water
- Carrot or watermelon juice

Worst foods

- Dairy products
- Alcohol (especially beer, which is high in yeast)
- Wheat and yeast (for some)
- Refined and sugary foods

Best supplements

- 2 × high-potency multivitamin–minerals with at least 5,000iu (1,500mcg) of vitamin A

- 1 × vitamin C 1,000mg every 1 or 2 hours during an infection, otherwise 2,000mg a day

- 2 × essential omegas with fish-oil-derived omega-3, plus omega-6 from borage or evening primrose oil (ten times more omega-3 than -6)

- 2 × anti-inflammatory formula containing a combination of quercetin, vitamin C, glutamine, MSM (sulphur), bromelain

Or

- 2 × quercetin 250mg

Optional

- 1–2 × probiotic supplements with *Lactobacillus acidophilus* and bifidobacteria, if you've been taking antibiotics (you need 5 million viable organisms)

SKIN CANCER

General information

There are two main kinds of skin cancer: basal, or squamous cell carcinoma, and melanoma. Skin carcinoma is both common and relatively easy to treat; melanoma, by comparison, is rare and highly malignant, and represents more of a risk. Excessive exposure to strong sunlight is the main risk factor for both kinds of skin cancer. Follow the general advice given for Cancer (see page 74) as well as the following specific factors to help with prevention as well as treatment.

Good medicine solutions

1. Protect your skin

Excessive exposure to ultraviolet radiation from sunlight or sun lamps causes both malignant melanoma and non-melanoma skin cancers – especially in fair-skinned people with red or blond hair, and those who have a lot of moles. Although UVB rays are the most damaging to our DNA, UVA rays also damage DNA through the generation of free radicals or oxidants, which effectively burn the skin. Ideally, you should limit your exposure to both, since UVA rays can weaken the body's immune responses, which are vital for dealing with damaged cells.

Be aware that not all sunscreens are equally effective, too. With many, some UV radiation still passes through to the skin. The key is to filter the harmful rays *and* protect the skin cells themselves with antioxidants. (Antioxidants are substances that remove or disarm potentially damaging oxidising agents, such as UV radiation, in the body.)

I am particularly impressed by the Environ products, which are rich in vitamins A and C, and their sunscreen RAD. Vitamins A and C are the nutrients that protect your skin from damage. I apply Environ's AVST vitamin A-rich skin cream most days to give my skin optimal protection from sun damage, and I use their RAD sunscreen when exposed to strong sunlight. The sunscreen contains natural antioxidants that increase sun protection and help to neutralise free radicals before they have a chance to do damage. Don't forget your feet if you wear sandals.

2. Care for your skin from the inside out

During strong sunlight exposure, the risk of oxidant damage to the skin (through burning) is at its highest. To help protect your skin from the damage by oxidants it's important to look at other lifestyle factors that are harmful. Smoking, for example, introduces oxidants into the lungs and bloodstream, and alcohol suppresses the immune system, weakening the body's natural defences. Fried food also introduces oxidants into the body, because the high temperatures involved in frying food cause it to oxidise. To fight the oxidants you should eat plenty of fruit and vegetables, which contain antioxidants.

Some of the best skin protectors are tomatoes, which contain the antioxidant lycopene. Lycopene is a member of the carotenoid family of phytochemicals and is the natural pigment responsible for the deep red colour of several fruits. In addition to its antioxidant activity, lycopene has been shown to suppress the growth of tumours and protect against skin cancer. Other foods high in lycopene include pink grapefruit, watermelon and guava. Other foods containing small amounts of lycopene include persimmon and apricots.

Levels of vitamin A and beta-carotene (known as a precursor of vitamin A) in the blood tend to be lower in people who have certain types of skin cancer. The antioxidant vitamins (which are often contained within high-quality daily multivitamin-minerals) help to protect against skin damage, but of particular importance are vitamins A and E, and beta-carotene nutrients.

3. Increase plant polyphenols

Polyphenols are antioxidant phytochemicals that prevent free-radical damage and protect the skin. Polyphenols are prevalent in foods such as nuts, seeds, onions, green tea, pomegranates, apples, berries, cherries and other fruits, also grape seeds, as well as vegetables and pulses such as beans and lentils. They are also found in the spice turmeric and the supplements resveratrol and silymarin (milk thistle extract). Polyphenols have many anti-cancer actions, such as reducing inflammation, reducing oxidative stress and preventing damage to DNA. They also boost the immune system and can directly inhibit tumour progression. Most research has focused on green tea extract and other polyphenols, such as grape seed proanthocyanidins, which have been shown to inhibit skin-cancer cell growth. Green tea has long been suspected of possessing anti-cancer properties, and the extract, called epigallocatechin gallate (EGCG), has been shown to be effective at shrinking skin tumours. Although you can obtain reasonable levels of EGCG from drinking green tea, you will also be taking in a lot of caffeine to reach the desired amount, so it may be worth taking green tea extract instead; it is often included in antioxidant complexes.

Resveratrol, a potent antioxidant found in the red skin of grapes and peanuts, has also been shown to reduce skin cancer tumours and help reduce the risk of cancer spreading. Although most research has been carried out on animals, I would certainly increase my intake of resveratrol, if it were necessary. The key feature of resveratrol is that it is activated only inside the cancer cells, which it arrests or kills.

Although some resveratrol can be obtained by eating large amounts of organic fruit and vegetables, extra virgin olive oil and unfiltered juices, it is difficult to get sufficient from diet alone. The concentration of resveratrol in foods varies enormously, so to benefit from higher amounts you need to take supplements. This could be in an antioxidant formula containing resveratrol. If you have cancer, you may want a higher therapeutic dose (see Cancer on page 74). Other polyphenols that can retard the growth of skin cancer include the isoflavones found in soya beans.

Best foods

- Tomatoes
- Garlic
- Turmeric
- Green tea

Worst foods

- Burned, fried and processed meat (associated with increased cancer risk)
- Dairy products (which promote the growth of cancer cells)
- Alcohol

Best supplements

- 2 × high-potency multivitamin–minerals
- 2 × high-potency omega-3-rich fish oil capsules (choose products with the most EPA)
- 5,000mg or more vitamin C or as much orally as you can tolerate before it induces diarrhoea (known as the bowel-tolerance level)
- 1 × antioxidant complex (containing beta-carotene, vitamin E and selenium, plus other antioxidant nutrients such as glutathione, alpha lipoic acid, co-enzyme Q_{10} (CoQ_{10}) and resveratrol)
- 2 × salvestrol 2,000 units for recovery; 350 units for prevention
- 1 × 1,000iu (25mcg) vitamin D

> **CAUTIONS**
>
> Some chemotherapy agents act as oxidants, and during treatment, depending on the drug you are being given, it may be advisable to avoid supplementing antioxidants. (Vitamin C in high doses acts as a pro-oxidant, so it is unlikely to interfere.) Please seek the advice of your oncologist.
>
> You must not undertake an extensive nutritional strategy on your own. It is important to ensure that you get the correct guidance from a nutritional therapist.

DIG DEEPER

To find out more on this subject read *Say No to Cancer* (Patrick Holford), which includes key referenced studies.

SLEEP APNOEA AND SNORING

General information

Sleep apnoea is a condition that interrupts your breathing when you are asleep. It is usually caused by an obstruction blocking the back of the throat so that the air cannot reach your lungs. This can be caused by being overweight or producing too much mucus. The cessation of breathing makes you wake up in order to start breathing again. This can happen many times during the night, depriving you of oxygen and a good night's sleep.

Good medicine solutions

1. Stop smoking and reduce alcohol

Both smoking and drinking too much alcohol contribute to sleep apnoea and snoring: alcohol relaxes the muscles of the upper airway, and you are three times more likely to develop sleep apnoea if you smoke. The oxidants in each toxic puff of a cigarette not only damage your lungs and age your skin but they also affect the internal 'skin' of your throat. This makes the throat lose its elasticity – giving you an internal 'turkey neck' that wobbles as you breathe. This is what makes the snoring sound.

The other cause of snoring is the mucus that coats the throat and nose. Smokers are allergic to cigarette smoke, so the body does its best to protect itself from the damage by producing a layer of mucus. This then vibrates as the smoker sleeps, causing more of the snoring sound. It's obviously important to give up smoking.

Also, take a strong antioxidant supplement containing vitamins A, C and E and beta-carotene, plus zinc, selenium, glutathione and cysteine. These help to reduce inflammation, as do omega-3 fish oils. (See Chapter 2, Part 2 on how to increase your antioxidants.)

2. Lose weight

Sleep apnoea and snoring are associated with being overweight. Excessive body fat increases the bulk of soft tissue in the neck, which can place a strain on the throat muscles. Excess stomach fat can also lead to breathing difficulties, which can make the condition worse. Diabetics are also three times more likely to develop sleep apnoea, so following a diet that helps to reduce your risk is wise. A low-GL diet is an effective way to lose weight, and it also reduces the risk of, and can reverse, diabetes. (See Chapter 1, Part 2 for details on how to follow a low-GL diet.)

3. Replace sleeping medication with good sleep practice

If you are having problems sleeping, look to natural methods to help improve your sleep rather than taking sleeping tablets, as they can contribute to sleep apnoea. Practise good sleep hygiene to help you breathe less heavily: (a) ensure your room is dark – keep artificial light to a minimum; (b) wear comfortable clothing; (c) avoid caffeine and alcohol after noon – caffeine depresses melatonin, required for sleep, for up to ten hours; alcohol promotes inflammation; (d) don't eat for two hours before going to bed; (e) keep your room cool and airy; and (f) try to sleep on your left-hand side. (For further advice on how to sleep well without medication see Insomnia on page 236.)

4. Test and identify your allergies

Allergies that cause nasal congestion, sneezing and a runny nose (what doctors call allergic rhinitis) lead to more frequent and louder snoring. Several studies have shown that people with moderate to severe allergic rhinitis are more likely to have sleep disorders, such as sleep apnoea. Wheat and dairy are two of the most common allergenic foods, so you could try cutting these out to see if it makes a difference. It is also worth taking an IgG food intolerance test, which you can do using a home test kit (see Resources), but if you decide to do this don't cut out any foods prior to the test. Alternatively, contact a nutritional therapist to arrange an allergy test. (See Allergies on page 31 for more information.)

5. Practise the Buteyko method

Although most treatments – nasal decongestants, nasal strips, surgery, dental appliances, and so on – are aimed at expanding the airways, the goal of the Buteyko method is to unblock the nose and correct the breathing volume to normal levels. (The

Buteyko method was developed almost 50 years ago by Dr Konstantin Buteyko.) Mouth snoring stops when you learn to breathe through your nose during sleep. By learning how to unblock your nose, thereby switching to nasal breathing and normalising breathing volume, your breathing will be quiet, calm and still throughout the night, and nasal snoring will cease. For more information on this method, see Resources.

Best foods

- Organic fruit and vegetables (high in natural anti-inflammatories)
- Low-GL foods such as cottage cheese, lean meats, beans and pulses

Worst foods

- Dairy and wheat (if allergic)
- Alcohol
- Coffee and tea
- Refined and processed foods (high-GL foods make you gain weight)

Best supplements

- 2 × antioxidant supplements containing vitamins A, C and E and beta-carotene, plus zinc, selenium, glutathione and cysteine
- 2 × vitamin C 1,000mg
- 2 × high-potency omega-3-rich fish oil capsules (choose products with the most EPA)

DIG DEEPER
Read *Sleep with Buteyko* (Patrick McKeown).

SMOKING

see **NICOTINE DEPENDENCE**

SORE THROAT

General information

Over 90 per cent of sore throats are caused by viruses, although without testing you can't tell the difference between viral or *Strep.* throat (*Streptococcus pyogenes* or bacterial tonsillitis), a bacterial infection. Studies have shown that antibiotics don't really work for sore throats, but if you are considering taking them, make sure your doctor tests you first, because viral diseases don't respond to antibiotics and it's advisable for several reasons not to take antibiotics unnecessarily. The following guidelines are general and can treat either a sore throat caused by a virus or a *Strep.* throat. If you have a viral infection, however, also refer to Colds and Flu on page 101.

Good medicine solutions

1. Take high-dose vitamin C

Whether your sore throat is caused by a virus or bacterium, vitamin C helps boost your immune system and fight off infection. Vitamin C works, but you have to take a lot – ideally 1,000mg (that's 20 oranges' worth) an hour. The amount needed depends very much on the individual. Some people experience loose bowels on high doses, but that is all; there's no harm in taking large amounts of vitamin C for a few days. Preferably, take the prescribed amount of vitamin C to just below 'bowel tolerance', which means the maximum level you can take before it causes loose bowels. What really works is to dramatically increase your blood level of vitamin C as soon as you get the first hint of symptoms and keep it up until the sore throat has gone. (To find out more about vitamin C, see Colds and Flu page 101.)

The effectiveness of vitamin C is increased by taking it with other antioxidants (substances that remove or disarm potentially damaging oxidising agents in the body). Most people think of blueberries as the best source of antioxidants, but one of the richest sources is cherries, particularly Montmorency cherries. During an infection, it's worth having two or three shots a day of either Cherry Active or Blueberry Active – for example, in a hot drink with some thin slices of fresh ginger – to soothe a sore throat.

2. Try helpful herbs

Goldenseal is one of the most popular herbs to treat *Strep.* throat. The berberine component of goldenseal extract has an antibiotic activity against streptococci and has been shown to prevent bacteria and viruses attaching to the lining of the throat. Goldenseal also directly stimulates the immune system. You can buy it as a tea, a tincture or drops of fluid extract (usually 20 drops are taken three times a day). I would recommend looking for a product that is also combined with echinacea to enhance the effects.

Echinacea is a powerful agent against both viruses and bacteria. To promote the spread of colonies, microbes secrete large amounts of hyaluronidase, an enzyme that makes them more invasive. Echinacea blocks this enzyme. It also increases the amount of white blood cells and enhances their movement into infected areas. It is best taken either as capsules of the powdered herb (2,000mg a day) or as drops of an extract (usually 20 drops three times a day).

Ginger works as an anti-viral and antibacterial agent, as well as having a strong antioxidant effect, but perhaps its main benefit for sore throats is its ability to reduce inflammation. This action can really help to soothe and prevent irritation. Most studies on ginger have used the powdered ginger root at about 1,000mg a day. Fresh root ginger may have even better results, however, because it contains higher levels of the active ingredients. Use about a 5mm (¼in) piece, sliced, in teas throughout the day. A particularly throat-soothing tea is made with grated ginger, lemon juice and manuka honey with hot water. Manuka honey has recently come under the spotlight for its potential antibacterial effects. For sore throats, three teaspoons a day has been found to retard the bacteria that cause infection. I would recommend drinking this tea throughout the day to calm the irritation.

Elderberry is also useful for upper-respiratory infections by preventing viruses from penetrating the cell membranes. (For more on elderberry, see Colds and Flu on page 103.)

3. Increase your intake of zinc

Zinc is an essential mineral found in the 'seeds' of things – from eggs to nuts, seeds themselves and beans (pulses). Meat and fish are also high in zinc. The ideal intake is about 15mg a day, but most people achieve only half this amount from their diet. In times of illness, much higher doses (50–100mg a day) have been shown to make the body's immune-responsive T cells much more effective, hence boosting immunity. In addition to promoting strong immunity, zinc appears to stop the replication of the virus responsible for cold symptoms (such as sore throats), giving your immune system a chance to fight it off sooner. Zinc is most effective for sore throats during the first day of throat pain, so it's essential to act fast. Using zinc lozenges is believed to target the infection where it lives: in the nose and sinuses. Take zinc lozenges (containing 15–20mg zinc) every three hours for up to three days while suffering from a sore throat. Discontinue as soon as the throat feels better. Note that long-term use of zinc lozenges can cause an imbalance of other nutrients in the body.

Another reason why zinc may be helpful when you have an infection is because it helps vitamin A (which is stored in the liver) to be used. To fight infections, your body needs to have sufficient vitamin A. Although you should eat lightly when you have any infection, foods rich in vitamin A – such as dark green vegetables and yellow/orange fruit and vegetables (carrots, sweet potatoes, squashes, apricots, peaches) – give your immune system a boost.

4. Check for, and avoid, food allergies or intolerances

If you don't have a fever or other cold and flu symptoms, the cause of your sore throat may be a food allergy or intolerance. These are often overlooked in the diagnosis, but studies show that allergies are a common cause of sore throats. Typical symptoms in the upper respiratory tract of a delayed food allergy (that is, an IgG sensitivity) include chronic sore throats, a runny nose, sinusitis, tonsillitis and laryngitis.

IgG sensitivities to foods are not obvious because they don't cause immediate or severe reactions unlike IgE allergies which have immediate and severe reactions. Common foods that cause IgG reactions are milk products, gluten, cereals (wheat, rye, barley, oats), eggs and yeast. I recommend testing. Once you know what you are reacting to, you should strictly avoid your allergens for up to six months. (See Allergies on page 31 to find out how to test and avoid other potential food allergens or intolerances.)

5. Take probiotics

Beneficial bacteria (called probiotics) in the body protect against pathogenic bacterial infections by priming the immune system and producing natural antibiotics. They also reduce your body's inflammatory response, which experts believe helps relieve sore throats. We have colonies of beneficial bacteria throughout our bodies, including in our throats, but the delicate balance of bacteria can easily be disrupted by antibiotics, mouthwashes, a high-sugar, low-fibre diet and alcohol. Supplementing beneficial bacteria also lessens viral cold symptoms, including sore throats.

I would also recommend that you avoid all alcohol, sugar, refined carbohydrates and mouthwashes, as these kill off the good bacteria and/or feed pathogenic ones. The trick is to include good food sources for the beneficial bacteria as well as supplementing a probiotic. Our two main beneficial bacterial species – lactobacilli and bifidobacteria – need us to eat a diet rich in the fibre found only in fresh, unprocessed fruit, vegetables and grains. These are the hard-to-digest carbohydrates known as probiotics – factors that nourish gut bacteria. Foods rich in prebiotics, which feed the probiotics, include chicory, Jerusalem artichokes, leeks, asparagus, garlic, onions, oats and soya beans. The best probiotic supplements also include some prebiotics in the form of fructo-oligosaccharides (FOS) in the capsules. When you take them, you are giving the good-bacteria population a boost as well as an added food supply.

Best foods

- Ginger
- Garlic
- Berries
- Montmorency cherry juice (Cherry Active)
- Blueberry juice or concentrate (Blueberry Active)
- Carrots

Worst foods

- Sugar
- Refined carbohydrates
- Alcohol

Best supplements

- 2 × a high-potency multivitamin–minerals providing at least 15mcg of vitamin D and at least 1,500mcg of vitamin A

- 1,000mg vitamin C (ideally with berry extracts) every hour

- 1 × zinc lozenge (15–20mg) dissolved in the mouth every three waking hours for up to 3 days

- 10 drops of echinacea and goldenseal combination every three hours

- 2 × probiotics (containing FOS and providing at least 15 billion active organisms)

CAUTIONS

If antibiotics have been taken, it is important to use a probiotic supplement at a dose of at least 15–20 billion active organisms per day. Take the probiotic as far apart in time from the antibiotic as possible, and continue with the probiotics for two weeks after the course.

DIG DEEPER

To find out more on this subject, read *Boost Your Immune System* (Patrick Holford & Jennifer Meek), which includes key referenced studies.

STOMACH BUGS

see **GASTROENTERITIS (STOMACH BUGS)**

STOMACH ULCERS AND *HELICOBACTER PYLORI* INFECTION

Good medicine solutions

1. Check for *Helicobacter pylori* and treat it

Most, but not all, stomach ulcers are caused, in part, by infection by the bacterium *Helicobacter pylori* and are usually treated with a combination of two antibiotics, plus a proton-pump inhibitor (PPI) drug, which stops you making stomach acid. PPI drugs should be for short-term use only, as the suppression of stomach acid is extremely bad for nutrient absorption and leads to all sorts of complications as a result, including increased risk of osteoporosis, brain shrinkage and infections.

Natural remedies that help treat this infection are:

Probiotics (beneficial bacteria) *Acidophilus and Bifidus* bacteria slow the growth of *H. pylori* in six weeks,[1] and can even kill it. Probiotics can also significantly reduce side effects and improve the effectiveness of conventional treatment. I recommend taking a high-strength probiotic providing 10 billion CFUs daily a week before, and for three months after, antibiotic therapy. (Probiotics are graded by the number of colony forming units (CFUs) contained in them – it's a fancy way of saying 'live and healthy microbes'.)

Oregano is one of the best natural agents against *H. pylori*, and is thought to work by inhibiting the way *H. pylori* produces chemicals that neutralise acid in their vicinity, allowing them to survive, so it is effectively a natural antibiotic. You can buy capsules or tinctures. Take 15–45mg a day.

Deglycyrrhised liquorice root (DGL) also suppresses *H. pylori* growth and helps to repair and strengthen the stomach lining.

Take 500–1,500mg a day. Make sure you take the DGL form, since liquorice can raise blood pressure if taken in the long term.

Mastic gum Another remedy that's making the headlines is mastic gum, although the evidence is not conclusive. It has been used in traditional Greek medicine for thousands of years for various gastrointestinal disorders, including peptic ulcers. Researchers in Greece in 2012 found that although it did not completely eradicate *H. pylori*, it reduced numbers.[2] It's worth trying, although it's not proven to have no side effects. Take 1,000mg twice a day for three months.

I would recommend taking probiotics before having the usual triple therapy (two antibiotics, plus a PPI drug, as mentioned above), then having the triple therapy, followed by natural remedies for three months under the guidance of a nutritional therapist.

2. Reduce acid-stimulating foods and gastric irritants

The stomach produces acid to digest protein. Following a high-protein diet (high in meat, fish and eggs) is likely to aggravate inflamed stomach membranes further. Coffee and alcohol, as well as non-steroidal anti-inflammatory painkillers (NSAIDs), also aggravate the gut wall. The combination of painkillers and alcohol, if you have ulceration, is extremely dangerous, as it can cause internal bleeding.

Nevertheless, oily fish have the advantage of containing anti-inflammatory omega-3 fats, which help to calm down inflamed membranes, so eating oily fish in moderation is likely to do more good than harm.

Although spicy foods are thought to be acid forming, in fact they are alkaline and, provided you don't feel worse, evidence shows that they don't make ulcers worse.

3. Take vitamin A and glutamine to heal the gut

Vitamin A and the amino acid glutamine help to regenerate healthy epithelial cells, which line the digestive tract. Glutamine is best taken as a powder: take 1 heaped teaspoon (5g) in a glass of cold water last thing at night on an empty stomach. A generous supply of glutamine can help repair and maintain a healthy small intestinal lining. Taking this for a month can help to heal ulcers.

Vitamin A, in the animal form retinol, is also vital for healthy cells in the stomach. High doses are not recommended during pregnancy, but men, and women who are unlikely to become pregnant, may find that taking high doses for a month helps to speed up the healing of ulcers.

Vitamin C also helps healing, but too much, especially in the slightly acid ascorbic-acid form, can aggravate ulcers. Either limit your daily intake to 200mg or take an alkaline form of vitamin C such as a mineral ascorbate.

Although there are no human trials to date, animals with gastric ulcers have been helped by taking sea buckthorn, a rich source of omega-7 fats.[3] You might gain further benefits from supplementing sea buckthorn, as it also contains other ulcer-repairing antioxidant and anti-inflammatory substances, including carotenoids, vitamin E and omegas-3, -6 and -9.

4. Check for, and avoid, allergies and intolerances

Eating any food you are allergic or intolerant to will increase inflammation and aggravate an ulcer. An unidentified food allergy may even precipitate this condition, especially if you have undiagnosed coeliac disease (see page 95). See page 31 for how to check for and eliminate food allergies and intolerances.

Best foods

All these foods are low allergenic and high in nutrients:
- Vegetables
- Non-citrus fruits
- Oats
- Red onions
- Garlic
- Seeds
- Quinoa
- Oily fish (salmon, mackerel, herring, kippers, sardines – unfried)

Worst foods

- Red meat
- All animal protein in excess
- Dairy products
- Alcohol
- Coffee

Best supplements

- 2 × high-potency multivitamin–minerals with at least 5mcg of B_{12} and 10mg of zinc, plus 200mg of vitamin C
- 1–2 × essential omegas with fish-oil-derived omega-3, plus omega-6 from borage or evening primrose oil
- 3 × vitamin A 5,000iu capsules (5,000mcg in total)
- 1 × digestive enzyme supplement with each main meal
- 1 × probiotic supplement giving 5–10 billion viable organisms
- 1 teaspoon (5g) glutamine powder in water last thing at night on an empty stomach

Or
- 3 × combined digestive enzyme, probiotic and glutamine formula

Optional

- 2 × omega-7 (sea buckthorn oil) 250mg

CAUTIONS

Proton pump inhibitor drugs (PPIs), whose names end in '-azole', inhibit the production of stomach acid and may provide relief. The long-term use of these drugs is dangerous, however, because stomach acid is needed for the absorption of vitamin B_{12} and minerals.

Vitamin C, although good for general health, can further aggravate a stomach ulcer, so it is better to limit your intake to 200mg a day until your ulcers are healed.

DIG DEEPER

To find out more on this subject, read *Improve Your Digestion* (Patrick Holford), which includes key referenced studies.

STROKE

General information

A stroke happens when there is a disturbance in the brain's blood supply, which starves cells of oxygen and leads to cell death and a loss of brain function. There are two main types of stroke: ischaemic and haemorrhagic. Ischaemic strokes are more common and occur when blood flow to or within the brain is blocked. This blockage could happen for a variety of reasons. A blood clot might form in one of the four main arteries carrying blood to the brain (the right and left carotid arteries, and the right and left vertebrobasilar arteries) or in smaller arteries and capillaries within the brain. Alternatively, a blood clot, fat globule or air bubble present in a blood vessel in another part of the body could be carried to the brain. Haemorrhagic strokes occur when a damaged or weakened artery bursts and there is bleeding into the brain. These damaged blood vessels could be located within the brain (causing an intracerebral haemorrhage) or on the brain surface (causing a subarachnoid haemorrhage).

Stroke is the third most common cause of death in the UK. While men are more likely to suffer a stroke, women are more likely to die from it. Known risk factors include age, high blood pressure, high cholesterol and smoking, so if you have a combination of these, your stroke risk is much increased. But the good news is that your overall risk can be reduced through simple changes in dietary and lifestyle habits.

Good medicine solutions

1. Eat choline-rich foods and lecithin

Much of the damage from strokes is believed to result from the activation of various enzymes that damage or deplete phospholipids and essential fats, both of which are key components of brain cell membranes. These enzyme-driven structural changes eventually result in brain-cell death.

Choline is an essential nutrient that is used to make phospholipids. It also has other functions in the central nervous system. As well as a structural role, choline is used to form the brain chemical acetylcholine, which is involved in muscle control and memory, both of which are affected by stroke.

The best food sources are liver, eggs, fish, chicken, beans, nuts, cauliflower and greens. Eating an egg, two servings of greens and a serving of beans (pulses, especially soya – such as in tofu), quinoa, almonds or peanuts each day would give you significant amounts.

Good amounts of choline in the diet can be neuro-protective, and there's also compelling evidence to support supplementing choline after a stroke – particularly in acute ischaemic stroke, where blood flow to the brain is blocked. Studies giving stroke patients cdp-choline (the brand name of which is Citicholine) have shown a halving of brain damage. It is likely that other forms of choline will have similar benefits.

Alternatively, you can take a lecithin supplement, which will provide you with the most common type of choline found in food called phosphatidylcholine (PC). As well as its role in supporting brain health, lecithin also helps your body process cholesterol, so it is good for your cardiovascular health too. Three teaspoonfuls of lecithin provides 1,000mg of PC. You can also buy high-PC lecithin, which provides this amount in 1 teaspoonful. This is enough for prevention, but two to three times this amount is ideal for maximising recovery.

2. Take the vitamins that will support methylation

Methylation is a critical biochemical process in the brain and body, which requires B vitamins and other nutrients to function properly. As well as indicating poor methylation, raised homocysteine levels in the blood damage arteries. Low methylation is associated with an increased risk of heart disease and stroke, as well as death in previously healthy people. The combination of B vitamins along with tri-methyl-glycine (TMG) and N-acetyl-cysteine (NAC) will encourage a healthy methylation process.

You can assess the level of your methylation by measuring your homocysteine level, as this will rise if methylation is poor. Ask your doctor or buy a home test kit (see Resources). Stroke risk increases with a homocysteine level of 10mcmol/l.

Lowering homocysteine makes a big difference as far as lower stroke risk is concerned. One key homocysteine-lowering nutrient is folic acid. According to a recent analysis of all trials published in the *Lancet*, taking folic acid alone for three years can lower stroke risk by almost a third.

I would suggest you avoid taking a single folic acid supplement, however, because it can mask a B_{12} deficiency – which is very common in the elderly due to a decline in the body's ability to absorb nutrients. I'd therefore advise you to take a combination supplement designed to normalise homocysteine and provide folic acid, vitamins B_{12} and B_6, together with TMG and zinc, and to continue doing so in the long term, as homocysteine levels tend to revert to their original values after ten weeks without supplementation. The best homocysteine-modulating formulas contain all of these. In older people, also supplementing NAC offers further homocysteine protection.

3. Increase your antioxidant intake

You'll get the broadest variety of antioxidants by eating fresh vegetables and fruits as many colours as possible – for example, garlic (white), tomatoes (red), squashes (orange), kale (green), red grapes (purple), blueberries (blue). Even better is to know a food's ORAC value, which is a simple way of rating antioxidant capacity. (See Chapter 2, Part 2 for an in-depth explanation.)

Your body is under much more oxidative stress both during and following a stroke, and you'll need more antioxidants to effect repair. After an ischaemic stroke there are significantly lower levels of antioxidants and antioxidant activity in the blood.[1] Excessive oxidation leads to cell damage, but having a high level of antioxidants (which remove or disarm potentially damaging oxidising agents in the body) prior to a stroke will presumably offer a greater degree of neuro-protection; there are animal studies showing just this.[2]

Similarly, benefits are gained by increasing antioxidants after an event. Excess oxidation and cell death occur for as many as six days following a stroke. Antioxidant supplements decrease the severity and help to support post-stroke recovery. Studies using vitamins C and E and alpha lipoic acid have shown positive benefits in reducing inflammation, healing blood vessels, improving memory and/or reducing risk of a second stroke.

When taking a supplement, it's better to look for a complex

rather than just focusing exclusively on one or two antioxidants. This is because antioxidants work more effectively in combination, recycling each other, and therefore prolonging their antioxidant activity. Other potent antioxidants include vitamin A, selenium, glutathione and co-enzyme Q_{10} (CoQ_{10}).

Take a good antioxidant complex that contains all of the above each day, along with an extra 1,000mg of vitamin C.

4. Eat oily fish and seeds for omega-3

Increasing your intake of oily fish, or including a daily fish oil supplement, will provide you with the healthy omega-3 fats, EPA and DHA that have several stroke-minimising actions in the cardiovascular system. Not only do omega-3 fats decrease inflammation and regulate the amount of undesirable blood fats, called triglycerides, but they also decrease blood clotting and stickiness by 'thinning' the blood and improving blood pressure. It's certainly desirable to have more fluid and less sticky blood circulating in your body at a reduced pressure.

The smaller cold-water fish, such as herrings, sardines, mackerel and pilchards, are excellent sources of omega-3 oils. Aim to have at least two servings each week. You don't have to focus on just the oily fish. You can reduce your risk of stroke by eating any type of fish or supplementing omega-3 oils. Strict vegetarians and vegans will need to eat chia seeds every day as their main source of omega-3, although these are not as powerful as fish oils.

If your stroke risk factors are high, or if you are recovering from a stroke, you need to be eating these foods and also supplementing 1,000mg of fish oils every day. Omega-3 fish oils also help to alleviate depression, which is very common after stroke.

5. Reduce your risk factors

Stroke risk increases with age, and other factors include high blood pressure, high cholesterol and smoking.

High blood pressure is one of the top risk factors and is linked to three-quarters of strokes. Fortunately, there are lots of ways to reduce it without taking drugs, which have their own associated side effects. A low-GL diet and nutrients including magnesium, potassium and vitamin C are all effective in reducing blood pressure (see High Blood Pressure on page 195).

You'll also need to check your cholesterol. LDL cholesterol, commonly called 'bad' cholesterol, can promote atherosclerosis (where fat and cholesterol accumulate and block your blood vessels) increasing blood pressure and increasing your risk of stroke. Having high HDL cholesterol, the 'good' cholesterol, however, reduces your stroke risk. It's obviously best to work on lowering your LDL cholesterol and increasing your HDL cholesterol. The B vitamin niacin, for example, in doses of 1,000mg, effectively raises HDL and lowers LDL cholesterol. (See High Cholesterol on page 202 for more advice on improving your cholesterol through diet, supplements and exercise.)

Stopping smoking is essential for reducing risk (see Nicotine Dependence on page 280).

Best foods

- Liver
- Eggs
- White and oily fish (salmon, mackerel, herring, kippers, sardines)
- Fresh vegetables, especially cauliflower and greens
- Fruit, especially berries
- Almonds
- Walnuts
- Peanuts
- Chia or flax seeds

Worst foods

- Deep-fried and high-fat processed foods (which increase oxidation)
- Salt (which raises blood pressure)
- Sugar (which promotes triglycerides)

Best supplements

- ◾ 2,000mg of cdp-choline or 2–3 teaspoons of high-PC lecithin (for stroke recovery)

- ◾ 1 teaspoon of high-PC lecithin or 3 teaspoons of regular lecithin (for stroke prevention)

- ◾ 1 × antioxidant formula providing a combination of ALA, glutathione, vitamin E, resveratrol and CoQ_{10}

- ◾ 2 × vitamin C 1,000mg

- ◾ X* × homocysteine-modulating B vitamin formula (*dose and need dependent on your homocysteine score, as explained in Chapter 4, Part 2)

Or

- ◾ 2 × high-potency multivitamin–minerals providing at least 200mcg of folic acid, 20mg of B_6, 10mcg of B_{12} and 10mg of zinc, if your homocysteine level is below 7

CAUTIONS

Cholesterol also has a role in stroke recovery. It helps by transporting the essential fats that are needed to create nerve pathways and repair or replace damaged cells. What is more, having too low a cholesterol level can actually result in muscle and nerve degeneration and an increased stroke risk. So bear this in mind, especially if you've been prescribed a cholesterol-lowering drug as part of your stroke rehabilitation programme.

DIG DEEPER

To find out more on this subject read *Say No to Heart Disease* (Patrick Holford), which includes key referenced studies.

TOOTH DECAY AND PERIODONTAL (GUM) DISEASE

General information

Periodontal disease is a term describing disease of either the gums or the bones supporting the teeth. Alongside tooth decay, this is a degenerative condition that will affect dental health.

Good medicine solutions

1. Sweeten your food with xylitol

Xylitol, which is the principal sugar found in plums, cherries and most berries, has been shown in a recent study to effectively prevent tooth decay by acting as an antibacterial agent against organisms that cause cavities. Bacteria that feed off xylitol become unable to stick to teeth and cause rotting. Xylitol contains 40 per cent fewer calories than conventional sugar, is sweeter than most other sugar substitutes but, unlike artificial sweeteners such as aspartame or saccharin, it doesn't contain any unnatural chemicals or have an unwanted aftertaste. You can eat xylitol just as you would regular sugar and, unlike other sweeteners, which break down with heat, xylitol can be used in cooking. Use it in almost any recipe that calls for sugar (the substitution is 1:1). It's a great guilt-free sweetener for cereals, baking and puddings. But since yeast cannot metabolise it, it is not recommended for bread recipes using yeast.

Xylitol is also used in some mouthwashes, toothpastes and chewing gums.

2. Floss and brush your teeth regularly, and drink plenty of water

Periodontal disease has been associated with heart disease, type-2 diabetes, respiratory and kidney disease, and problems in pregnancy, such as miscarriage and premature birth. Around 10 per cent of the population is believed to have severe periodontal disease. Regular brushing and flossing of teeth is the best way to prevent it. It is best to floss your teeth twice a day, after meals, or at least twice a week if you cannot face doing it every day.

Drinking water keeps the gums hydrated and helps wash away trapped food particles that decompose in the mouth and cause bad breath. Water also helps your saliva to nourish your teeth, hydrate your gums, and remove some of the trapped food particles that can create plaque.

3. Drink green tea

Green tea contains natural antioxidant compounds which prevent plaque from accumulating, therefore reducing the risk of cavities and bad breath. A recent study suggests that drinking just one cup of green tea a day may decrease the risk of tooth loss. Plant chemicals in green tea, known as catechins, may combat bacteria that lead to cavities and gum disease. These same chemicals may also help prevent tooth loss.

4. Eat your onions and chew your celery

Researchers in Russia found that raw onion helps to kill unwanted bacteria in the mouth and that consuming one raw onion daily by thorough mastication helps to protect teeth from a number of dental diseases. If a raw onion a day sounds a bit much, at least include raw onion in salads and chew it well. Additionally, toothache can often be soothed by placing a small piece of onion on the bad tooth or gum.

Chewing celery also produces lots of saliva, which neutralises different bacteria that cause cavities, and it massages the gums and cleans between the teeth, keeping them healthy.

5. Take vital vitamins

Vitamins C and A are vital for the health of your teeth and gums. Vitamin C is the cement that holds all of your cells together, so it's vital for the health of your gum tissue. If you don't get enough vitamin C, research shows that the collagen network in your gums can break down, making your gums tender and more susceptible to the bacteria that cause periodontal disease. Foods high in vitamin C include peppers, leafy green vegetables, berries, oranges and tomatoes.

Vitamin A is vital for the formation of tooth enamel. The best sources of vitamin A are liver, carrots, sweet potatoes and squash.

6. Have sufficient dairy and protein

Unsweetened yoghurt and milk have low acidity, which helps to reduce dental erosion. Cheese and milk contain calcium, the main component of teeth, and cheese also has a high phosphate content, which helps balance your mouth's pH. It also preserves and rebuilds tooth enamel, helps to produce saliva and kills the bacteria that cause cavities and gum disease.

Protein foods, such as meat, poultry and eggs, are rich in phosphorus. Calcium combines with phosphorus and vitamin D to produce our teeth and bones, so it's important to eat good-quality protein for healthy teeth. Contrary to popular opinion, dairy products are not the best overall source of minerals, including calcium. Beans (pulses), nuts and seeds are great sources of calcium and other tooth- and bone-friendly minerals.

Best foods

- Berries
- Xylitol
- Leafy green vegetables
- Green tea
- Oranges
- Onions
- Carrots
- Celery
- Sweet potatoes
- Eggs
- Plain yoghurt and milk
- Turkey

Worst foods

- Sugar
- Processed foods (high in sugars)
- Sweetened drinks, including natural fruit juice (except unsweetened cherry, plum or berry juice)

Best supplements

- 2 × high-potency multivitamin–minerals with at least 300mg of calcium and 150mg of magnesium, plus 7,500iu of vitamin A and 600iu (15mcg) of vitamin D
- 2 × vitamin C 1,000mg

ULCERATIVE COLITIS

see **CROHN'S DISEASE AND ULCERATIVE COLITIS**

UNDERACTIVE THYROID

General information

The thyroid gland, which sits at the base of the throat, produces a hormone called thyroxine (T4), which is then converted into an active form of thyroxine (T3) by enzymes requiring iodine, zinc and selenium. These control your rate of metabolism. If you produce too little you may develop the symptoms of an underactive thyroid, described below. An overgrowth of thyroid tissue can result in a hyperactive thyroid or hyperthyroid, with too fast a metabolism, anxiety and even bulging eyes. This usually requires either surgery or treatment involving radioactive iodine, which reduces the size of the thyroid. Since it is an overgrowth, the same guidelines for Cancer (see page 74) apply for reducing the risk. Sometimes, a person's thyroid function can go high then low due to the imbalances discussed below.

Good medicine solutions

1. Test for an underactive thyroid

Symptoms of an underactive thyroid range from fatigue, low energy, cold hands and feet to a low metabolism, goitre – in which the throat region swells – and weight gain. The first thing to do if you are worried about your thyroid levels and have had them tested by a doctor is not to accept vague phrases describing them as 'high' or 'low'. Instead, ask for actual numbers and ask what the testing lab considers to be a normal range. If possible, ask for a copy of the actual report. This will show you two things: your level of thyroxine, the thyroid hormone, and your level of thyroid stimulating hormone (TSH), which is the brain's signal to the thyroid gland to produce more thyroxine. If the report shows that your TSH level is below 5, or even below 10, you may be told that this is normal. However, the American Association of Clinical Endocrinologists (AACE) now recommends treating when TSH goes above 3, and some thyroid experts consider anything above 2.5 to be abnormal, indicating that your thyroid is potentially underproducing thyroxine.

A more detailed test, including testing your levels of T3 (the active thyroid hormone) and T4, as well as the presence of anti-thyroid antibodies (see below), can be run by Genova Diagnostics (see Resources, or consult your health-care practitioner or a nutritional therapist).

2. Boost your thyroxine

Your doctor may give you thyroxine to compensate for your symptoms, but you can boost your thyroid gland nutritionally to help it make its own thyroxine. The key duo is the minerals iodine and tyrosine. Seaweeds, such as dulse or kelp, are very rich in iodine, as are sea vegetables, such as nori and arame, mushrooms, Swiss chard, butter beans and sesame seeds. Tyrosine is also found in butter beans, and in fish, almonds, bananas, avocados and pumpkin seeds. To supplement, take 200mcg of iodine a day and 500mg of L-tyrosine twice a day.

Essential fats are also vital for proper thyroid function, so include oily fish such as salmon and mackerel, seeds and cold-pressed oils in your regular diet.

A range of nutrients is needed for full thyroid and adrenal support. In addition to tyrosine and iodine, these include essential fatty acids, zinc, selenium, vitamins C and B complex and manganese. Make sure you take a comprehensive supplement programme or a specialised thyroid supplement formula (ask in your health food store). If you are on medication, have your needs monitored by your doctor once you start to support your thyroid nutritionally, as your medications may change.

3. Check out your adrenals and reduce stress

Your adrenal glands are responsible for producing the short-acting adrenalin and the long-acting cortisol, two hormones that prepare your body for stress (action) as part of what is known as the 'fight or flight' response. Adrenal hormones speed up the body's metabolism to respond to stress by activating the thyroid gland. Cortisol, if raised too much or for too long, interferes with thyroid function. Excessive stress hinders thyroid function, because the stress hormone cortisol blocks the receptors for thyroxine. If you are adrenally burned out, it is common for this to go with thyroid dysfunction and is possibly due to the prolonged effect of too much cortisol. You may therefore need to consider nutritional support for your adrenal glands, including following a low-GL diet, avoiding stimulants and supplementing with vitamin C and B complex. (See Chapter 1, Part 2 for details on how to follow a low-GL diet.) Also look at ways to reduce your stress load; for example, by practising meditation or yoga, or by walking or just giving yourself time to chill out. (See Chapter 6, Part 2 on reducing your stress levels.)

3. Check for, and avoid, food allergies or intolerances

Some people produce 'anti-thyroid antibodies' which destroy thyroid tissue. This can be caused by a cross-reaction in which your body reacts to a food and mistakenly attacks the thyroid. Gliadin (a type of gluten), contained in grains such as wheat, rye and barley, is strongly associated with many autoimmune disorders, so you could try eliminating these foods from your diet and see how you feel. Even better is to test yourself for food intolerances. Coeliac disease (gliadin sensitivity) is much more common in people with anti-thyroid antibodies. It would also be wise to consult a nutritional therapist to investigate what is causing your immune system to overreact in this way. (See Allergies on page 31.)

4. Limit problem foods

The brassica family (cabbage, Brussels sprouts, broccoli and kale) contains small amounts of thiouracil, which inhibits the formation of thyroid hormone within the thyroid gland itself. Soya contains phytoestrogens, which also interfere with the ability of the body to use the thyroid hormone. Therefore, it may be wise to limit these foods, although total avoidance is probably unnecessary.

Sugar, refined foods, alcohol and cigarettes also interfere with thyroid function, and dairy products contain a lot of oestrogen, which competes with thyroxine, so avoid or eat these foods only in moderation. If you cut down on dairy products, ensure you increase your intake of nuts and seeds to get adequate calcium. The best diet to follow is my low-GL diet, which will cause minimum stress to your body. (See Chapter 1, Part 2 for details on how to follow a low-GL diet.)

5. Take exercise

When you have an underactive thyroid, exercise may be the last thing you want to do, but in fact exercise helps to boost thyroid function, so try to find an exercise that you enjoy and gradually build up how much you can do each day. Aim for 30 minutes exercise a day.

Best foods

- Seaweeds, such as dulse and kelp
- Sea vegetables, such as nori and arame
- Mushrooms
- Swiss chard
- Butter beans
- Sesame seeds
- Oily fish (salmon, mackerel, herring including kippers, sardines)
- Almonds

- Bananas
- Avocados
- Pumpkin seeds

Worst foods

- Brassicas – cabbage, Brussels sprouts, broccoli and kale, in excess
- Soy, in excess
- Refined and sugary foods, such as white bread, cakes and biscuits
- Caffeine (raises adrenalin and cortisol)
- Alcohol
- Dairy

Best supplements

- 2 × high-potency multivitamin–minerals providing magnesium 200mg, manganese 10mg, selenium 200mcg and zinc 15mg, plus B vitamins

- 2 × vitamin C 1,000mg

- Kelp with iodine 200mcg and L-tyrosine 1,000mg

- 2 × essential omegas with fish-oil-derived omega-3, plus omega-6 from borage or evening primrose oil

Or

- A special thyroid blend (see page 372)

DIG DEEPER
To find out more on this subject, read *The Great Thyroid Scandal and How to Survive It* (Dr Barry Durant-Peatfield).

URTICARIA

see **HIVES (URTICARIA)/RASHES**

WEIGHT GAIN AND OBESITY

General information

One of the prevailing myths still quoted like a mantra by so-called health experts is that weight gain is just to do with calories in from food and calories out through exercise, and that a calorie is a calorie, regardless of the food it comes from. Although calorie intake and exercise are important, complex metabolic processes are happening continually in your body, and they treat fat and sugar differently from protein. Of these food types, sugar is the most easily converted into fat, followed by alcohol.

Also, many psychological issues lead to emotional eating, and factors such as stress promote the use of sugar and caffeine for energy lifts. Also, if you are depressed, you are more likely to crave sweet foods.

Some people are more genetically prone to gaining weight and, to some extent, your total amount of fat cells determines how much you can store, so childhood obesity will set a pattern for life, although it is possible to lose weight nevertheless.

Good medicine solutions

1. Eat less, exercise more

At a basic level the more calories you eat and the less you exercise, the more weight you are going to gain. Exercise, particularly resistance exercise (using weights, for example) also builds muscle and muscle burns fat; therefore, the more lean muscle you have, the more you are able to burn fat.

It is especially important to do exercise that builds abdominal (core) and upper-body strength because this will help to build muscle on the top of your body, giving a toned appearance. Aerobic or endurance exercise that gets you huffing and puffing is also essential, because both kinds of exercise (resistance and aerobic) speed up the body's metabolism for several hours, which helps to burn fat.

It's easy to take in too many calories from sweetened drinks and larger portion sizes. Many people also make the mistake of choosing 'low-fat' foods, not realising that they are full of sugars, which really pile on the pounds because of the way your body has to process sugar in the blood, as explained below.

2. Follow a low-GL diet

Your appetite and weight are largely controlled by how your body deals with blood sugar balance. If your blood sugar level goes too high, which is the direct consequence of eating or drinking too much fast-releasing carbohydrate (such as sugar or foods made with white flour) in a meal or snack, the excess is converted into fat. Your blood sugar level then dips, which triggers hunger. Before long, you are gaining weight but also feeling hungry a lot of the time. You then become less sensitive to the effect of insulin, the key hormone that controls blood sugar, a condition that is called 'insulin resistance'. This eventually leads to diabetes (see page 137).

The solution is to eat a low-GL diet. GL means glycemic load, and it is a unit of measurement, rather like grams, litres, centimetres and calories, except that it is used to measure the amount of sugar and starch in a food and their impact on the body. Foods with a low GL have little effect on blood sugar, while foods with a high GL raise blood sugar. There is a wealth of evidence to support the positive benefits of a low-GL diet as a superior way to lose weight than a conventional low-fat, low-calorie diet.

There are two ways of eating low GL. One, first proposed by Dr Robert Atkins, involves eating very little carbs, with much more protein and fat. This does result in weight loss, but it is not healthy in the long term, so I would only recommend it for the short term.

The other, which is explained in detail in Chapter 1, Part 2, involves eating fewer carbohydrates, and only slow-releasing carbohydrates, which have less of an effect on blood sugar, in combination with protein, which slows down the release of sugars from the carbs – and eating little and often.

The beauty of eating a low-GL diet is that people say they just don't feel hungry. This is because you eat regularly and can have decent-sized portions. A low-GL diet is also easy to follow. You just need to follow three golden rules:

1 Eat no more than 40GLs a day (different foods have different GL scores).

2 Eat protein with carbohydrate.

3 Graze don't gorge.

Your daily GL intake breaks down as 10GLs each for breakfast, lunch and dinner, plus 5GLs each for a mid-morning and a mid-afternoon snack – so you eat (or graze) regularly instead of gorging at one or two big meals.

The easiest and most visual way to make protein–carb combining a part of your daily life is to keep your food in the following proportions:

- A quarter of each main meal should be protein.

- A quarter of each meal should be carbohydrate: starchy vegetables or other starchy foods.

- Half of each meal should be non-starchy vegetables.

Chapter 1, Part 2 shows you which foods to eat and in what proportions for a weight-loss result.

One particularly effective way to lose weight and cut calories is to eat an 'alternate day' diet, with much lower calories two or three days a week. This is very effective if combined with a low-GL diet. (See page 400 to find out more about alternate-day dieting.)

3. Eat sufficient fibre

Soluble fibre, which absorbs more water, helps you to lose weight, because you feel fuller and crave less food, plus it slows down the release of sugars in food. This healthy fibre will be present in the foods recommended in the low-GL diet, but you can also benefit from supplementing other particular forms of fibre. Glucomannan, a fibre found in a tuber vegetable called konjac, is many times more effective than the fibre in whole grains. It absorbs a large amount of water and makes you feel full, also lowering the GL of any meal. Taking 3g of glucomannan, roughly 1 teaspoonful, has been shown to reduce appetite in several studies.

In the US one of the top-selling diet-support supplements is PGX. It is made by combining three fibres, one of which is glucomannan. Many studies have shown it to reduce appetite, making you feel fuller for longer. It also lowers the GL of a meal.

Glucomannan absorbs several times its own weight in water, so it is essential to take it with a glass of water a few minutes before a meal. It comes in capsules or powder, which can be stirred into the water. Drink it quickly before it turns into a porridge-like gel.

4. Try weight-losing supplements

Slimming pills rarely work, and those that do often act like stimulants, speeding up your metabolism. This may give you short-term weight loss but also long-term problems. But there are three nutritional supplements that are extremely effective and are therefore recommended to support weight loss. They are hydroxycitric acid (HCA), 5-hydroxytryptophan (5-HTP) and the mineral chromium.

HCA is extracted from the dried rind of the tamarind fruit (*Garcinia cambogia*), which you may know from Asian cuisine. HCA is not a vitamin, but it will help you to lose weight. It works by inhibiting the enzyme – ATP-citrate lyase – that converts sugar (or glucose) into fat, thereby slowing down the production of fat and reducing appetite. It has been extensively tested and found to have no toxicity or safety concerns.

I recommend taking HCA, especially during the first three months of any weight-loss diet. You need 750mg a day. Most supplements provide 250mg per capsule, so take one capsule three times a day, ideally between 30 minutes and just before eating a main meal. It is widely available as a supplement.

5-HTP The two most powerful controllers of your appetite are your blood sugar level and your brain's level of serotonin, the 'feel-good' neurotransmitter. Serotonin is often deficient, especially in those on weight-loss diets. A low level can lead to depression and an increased appetite (which is why many depressed people overeat).

If your body is low in serotonin, one of the quickest ways to restore normal levels, and normal mood and appetite, is to supplement your diet with 5-HTP. It is proven to be effective for both weight loss and sugar cravings.

Chromium is a mineral that is essential for insulin to work properly. Many people struggling with weight are insulin resistant, which makes you more prone to storing sugar as fat. The average daily intake of chromium is below 50mcg, although an optimal intake – certainly for those with weight and blood sugar problems – is around 200mcg or more.

Chromium is found in whole foods and is therefore higher in wholemeal flour, bread or pasta than refined products. (Refined carbs can have up to 98 per cent of the chromium removed in the refining process – another reason to stay away from over-processed products.) Beans (pulses), nuts and seeds are other good sources, and asparagus and mushrooms are especially rich in chromium.

Most good multivitamins will contain 30mcg of chromium, but you can help maintain blood sugar control, and hence reduce sugar cravings, more quickly by taking 200mcg twice a day for the first three months of a weight-loss regime (ideally with your mid-morning and mid-afternoon snacks).

'I used to have . . . '

'I've lost 16 pounds [7.2kg/1 stone 2lb] in six weeks. My blood sugar is well under control (I'm diabetic) and I've been able to halve my medication. It's been so easy and I no longer have any unhealthy cravings,' says Linda.

'Your diet has enabled me to lose 17½lb [8kg/1 stone 3½lb] in only eight weeks with little change to my diet and eating habits, and no change to my exercise routine. An added benefit was that I did not feel hungry and I did not crave any foods. Now I have more energy, lower cholesterol and stable blood sugar,' says Tony.

'With the help of the [low-GL] diet and exercise I've managed to lose 7 stones [44.5kg/98lb] in seven months. The amazing thing is you never feel hungry on the low-GL diet,' says Eamon.

Best foods

- Whole foods
- Oats and barley (which are low GL and high in soluble fibre)
- Vegetables
- Beans and lentils (pulses)
- Berries, cherries and plums (the lowest-GL fruits)
- Lean meat and fish
- Wholegrain pasta
- Brown rice
- Quinoa

- Oatcakes
- Pumpernickel bread (in moderation)

Worst foods

- Sugar and sweetened drinks
- Refined carbs (white bread, pasta, rice)
- Chips and potatoes (in excess)
- Fried and fatty foods (damaged fats are harder for the body to process)
- Bananas and grapes (high in sugar, high GL)

Best supplements

- 2 × high-potency multivitamin–minerals providing 10mg of zinc and 150mg of magnesium, plus B vitamins, including at least 10mcg of B_{12}

- 2 × vitamin C 1,000mg

- 2 × essential omegas with fish-oil-derived omega-3, plus omega-6 from borage or evening primrose oil

- 2 × chromium 200mcg

- 3 × HCA 250mg

- 2 × 5-HTP 50mg

Or

- 3 × combination supplements containing all three (chromium, HCA and 5-HTP)

- 1 heaped teaspoon of PGX or glucomannan powder in water before each main meal, or 3 capsules

CAUTIONS

If you are on SSRI antidepressants and you also take large amounts of 5-HTP, this could theoretically make too much serotonin. I therefore don't recommend combining the two.

Some people get mild nausea when starting 5-HTP. If so, lower the dose. 5-HTP doesn't suit everybody.

Always take glucomannan with a large glass of water.

If you fail to lose weight, check your thyroid (see page 371) and for food allergies (see page 31).

DIG DEEPER

To find out more on this subject, read *Burn Fat Fast* (Patrick Holford with Kate Staples) and *Low-GL Diet Bible* (Patrick Holford). See also Resources for details of my website.

PART 2

Putting Good Medicine into Action

In this part you will find the cornerstones of health that will help you to prevent or reverse a number of health issues. These are: following a low-GL diet for optimum health, weight loss or weight maintenance; understanding the role of antioxidants in fighting the damaging effects of oxidation in the body and slowing the body's ageing process; ensuring good health by eating and supplementing the fats that are essential to maintain the body's processes; avoiding high homocysteine in the blood – a marker for a number of serious health issues; tailoring a supplement programme to suit your personal needs; and finding ways to de-stress.

Depending on your particular health concern, you'll be recommended to follow some of these cornerstones on Part 1 although, in truth, each one of us can benefit from following them all in any case.

The chapters that follow give you a blueprint for how to live free from disease, free from pain and without the need for drugs.

CHAPTER 1

The Low-GL Diet for Perfect Weight and Blood Sugar Control

My low-GL diet has been tried and tested for over a decade and is proven to be a workable weight-loss and weight-maintaining healthy diet. It is based on the principle that when you can control your blood sugar you can also stop weight gain and prompt weight loss. You can eat a wide variety of foods and you won't feel hungry. This is because the kinds of foods you will be eating will not upset your blood sugar balance, and you will be combining protein with carbohydrate and eating regularly to avoid blood sugar lows.

An even blood sugar is key to weight loss

GL stands for glycemic load and is a precise measure of what a food or a meal does to your blood sugar levels. Foods with a high GL (refined carbohydrates and sugar) have a greater effect on your blood sugar than foods with a low GL (whole foods, such as brown rice). Constant spikes in blood sugar, caused by high-GL foods, are what cause weight gain and a number of illnesses, particularly diabetes. When your blood sugar level goes high, insulin is released into the blood to remove the glucose (the sugar). Some of the glucose goes to the brain and the muscles, but if you've eaten more than you need, the remainder goes to the liver. The liver turns the excess glucose into fat and stores it in the nearest place possible, starting with your waist. Insulin, therefore, is the fat-storing hormone. Afterwards, the blood glucose levels go low, and this triggers hunger and also the release of stress hormones to get you 'hunting' for more food (see The sugar cycle below). Your appetite, sugar and carb cravings then kick in.

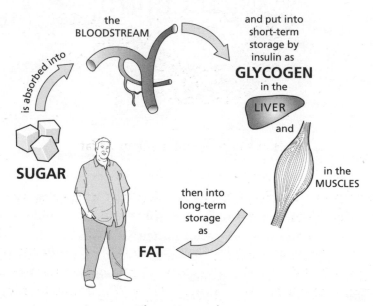

The sugar cycle

The more blood sugar highs (followed by lows) you have, the more blunted, or deaf, become the receptor sites for insulin that are inside your arteries and cells. In time, you become 'insulin resistant' with less and less sensitivity to insulin. Your body then has to produce even more insulin to achieve the desired effect of lowering blood glucose. You start to get 'rebound' blood sugar lows when the insulin finally kicks in.

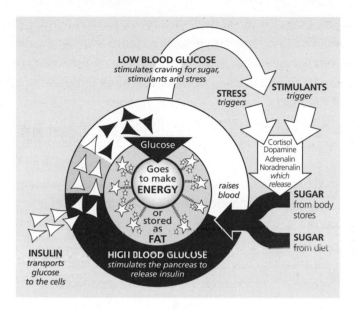

How the body stores energy as fat

Blood sugar fluctuations directly affect your health and mood

The symptoms of low blood sugar include poor concentration, irritability, nervousness, depression, sweating, headaches and digestive problems. But most of all you feel tired and hungry. If you refuel with fast-energy-releasing high-GL carbohydrates (sugary and carb-heavy foods), you then cause your blood sugar to rise rapidly. Your body doesn't need this much sugar, so, as before, it dumps the excess into storage as fat. Then your blood sugar level goes low again. This is how you enter the vicious cycle of yo-yoing blood sugar that leads to tiredness, weight gain and carbohydrate cravings.

An estimated three in every ten people have impaired ability to keep their blood sugar level stable. The result, over the years, is that you are likely to become increasingly fat and lethargic. If you can control your blood sugar levels, however, the result is stable weight and constant energy.

Through my associated weight-loss groups, we have shown

that many people lose 7kg (14lb) in a month without going hungry when following my low-GL diet. Thousands of people have benefited from following the low-GL principles over the years, reversing diabetes and heart disease, regaining health and losing weight.

High-fat and high-protein diets are not healthy

There are two extremes for achieving a low-GL meal. One, first advocated by the late Dr Robert Atkins, is to avoid carbohydrates, eating high protein and fat instead. This kind of diet is very high in meat and dairy products. The other, which is preferable for reasons I will explain, is to have some carbohydrates, but only those that release their sugar content slowly, and always to eat carbohydrate with protein; for example, the main sugar in berries is xylose, which has a very low GL, and, if you eat berries with seeds (which are high in protein), such as pumpkin or chia seeds, the net effect is very low GL.

One reason, but not the only reason, I prefer this approach is that meat, and especially dairy products, actually raise a type of insulin called insulin-like growth factor, or IGF-1. This, like too much insulin, is bad for your health, and is associated with an increased risk of cancer.

The three golden GL rules

The best way to achieve stable blood sugar balance is to control the GL of your diet. The reason I focus on the carbohydrate content of foods is because the other two main food types – fat and protein – don't have any appreciable effect on blood sugar. In fact, I recommend you eat some fat and protein with your carbohydrate, because this will further lessen the effect the carbohydrate has on your blood sugar, thereby lowering the GL of the meal. You'll find my food suggestions are balanced to give a protein-rich food, such as fish, with a carbohydrate-rich food, such as rice. I'll give you the GL values of a number of foods and explain how to choose the healthiest ones, with the lowest GL values.

For balancing your blood sugar, there are only three rules:

- **Rule 1** Eat 40GLs a day to lose weight, 60GLs to maintain it.
- **Rule 2** Eat carbohydrate with protein.
- **Rule 3** Graze, don't gorge.

The third rule means eating little and often, so always eat breakfast, lunch and dinner – and introduce a snack mid morning and mid afternoon. This way you'll provide your body with a constant and even supply of fuel, which means you'll experience fewer food cravings.

Understanding the glycemic load

The glycemic load combines the glycemic index with the concept of measuring carbohydrate intake to provide a scientifically superior way of controlling blood sugar. Put simply, the glycemic index (GI) of a food tells you whether the carbohydrate in the food is fast or slow releasing. It's a *quality* measure. It doesn't tell you, however, how much of the food is carbohydrate. Carbohydrate points, or grams of carbohydrate, tell you how much of the food is carbohydrate, but they don't tell you what the particular carbohydrate does to your blood sugar. It's a *quantity* measure. The glycemic load (GL) of a food is the *quantity times the quality*. It's the best way of telling you that you'll gain weight if you eat a certain amount of a particular food.

Here are some examples of high- and low-GL carbohydrates so that you can understand which kinds of foods to choose. Ideally, you want to eat 5GLs for a snack and 7–10GLs for the carbohydrate portion of a main meal. The low-GL foods are shown in bold, the moderate-GL in ordinary text, and the high-GL in italics.

→

FOOD	Serving looks like	GL
Fruit		
Blueberries	1 large punnet (600g)	5
Apple	1 small (100g)	5
Grapefruit	1 small	5
Apricot	4 apricots	5
Grapes	10 grapes	5
Pineapple	1 thin slice	5
Banana	1 small banana	10
Raisins	*20 raisins*	*10*
Dates	*2 dates*	*10*
Starchy vegetables		
Pumpkin/squash	1 large serving (185g)	7
Carrot	1 large (160g)	7
Beetroot	2 small	5
Boiled potato	3 small potatoes (60g)	5
Sweet potato	1 sweet potato (120g)	10
Baked potato	1 baked potato (120g)	10
French fries	*10 fries*	*10*
Grains, breads, cereals		
Quinoa (cooked)	65g (⅔ cup)	5
Pearl barley (cooked)	75g	5
Brown basmati rice (cooked)	1 small serving (70g)	5
White rice (cooked)	*½ serving (65g)*	*10*
Couscous (soaked)	*½ serving (65g)*	*10*

→

Rough oatcakes	2–3 oatcakes	5
Pumpernickel-style rye bread	1 thin slice	5
Wholemeal bread	1 thin slice	5
Bagel	*¼ bagel*	5
Puffed rice cakes	*1 rice cake*	5
White pasta (cooked)	1 small serving (75g)	10

Beans and lentils

Soya beans	3½ cans	5
Pinto beans	1 can	5
Lentils	1 large serving (200g, cooked)	7
Kidney beans	1 large serving (150g, cooked)	7
Chickpeas	1 large serving (150g, cooked)	7
Baked beans	1 large serving (150g)	7

For a complete list of foods and their GL scores, see my free GL counter at www.holforddiet.com.

Breaking the sugar habit

The taste for concentrated sweetness is often acquired in childhood. If sweet things are used as a reward or to cheer someone up, they become emotional comforters. The best way to break the sugar habit is to avoid concentrated sweetness in the form of sugar, sweets, sweet desserts, dried fruit and neat fruit juice. Instead, dilute fruit juice with water (and only have one small glass per day) and get used to eating fresh fruit instead of dessert. Sweeten breakfast cereals with fruit, and have fruit instead of sweet snacks. Also, by combining fruit, or diluted fruit juice (carbohydrate), with some nuts or seeds (protein), you'll further slow down the release of the sugars, thereby lowering the GL of the snack. If you gradually reduce the sweetness in your food, you will get used to the taste.

Sugar alternatives

Beware of switching to natural sugars, such as honey or maple syrup, as these still cause a rapid increase in blood sugar. Artificial sweeteners are not so great either. Some have been shown to have harmful effects on health, and all perpetuate a sweet tooth. One of the best sugar alternatives is xylitol, a vegetable sugar that has a very low GL. It tastes much the same as regular sugar but has little effect on raising blood sugar. Nine teaspoons of xylitol, for example, have the equivalent effect of just one teaspoon of regular sugar or honey. Another low-GL sweetener is agave syrup. This has the cooking advantage of being liquid, but it is mainly fructose, which the liver can easily process into fat, so it's not as good as xylitol. In any event I recommend you keep your use of both of these to a minimum.

Low-GL breakfasts

My three favourite simple low-GL breakfasts that balance protein with carbs are:

1 Oat flakes or porridge (5GL portion) with berries or apple (5GL portion) and chia seeds or almonds (for protein)

2 Two scrambled eggs (for protein) on a thin slice of rye or pumpernickel bread (a 10GL portion)

3 A serving of Get Up & Go, with 300ml (10fl oz/½ pint) oat milk, a handful of berries and 1 teaspoon of chia seeds (10GLs – balanced for protein and carbs)

Low-GL snacks

To keep your blood sugar level even throughout the day, it is best to have a mid-morning and a mid-afternoon snack. As before, snacks need to be balanced for protein and carbohydrate. Here are some examples:

- A piece of fruit, plus five almonds or three teaspoonfuls of pumpkin seeds
- A thin piece of bread or two oatcakes and half a small tub of cottage cheese (150g/5½oz)
- A thin piece of bread/two oatcakes and quarter of a small tub of hummus (50g/1¾oz)
- A thin piece of bread/two oatcakes and peanut butter
- Crudités (a carrot, pepper, cucumber or celery) and hummus
- Crudités and cottage cheese
- A small plain yoghurt (150g/5½oz), no sugar, plus berries or soya berry yoghurt (although bear in mind that the latter will contain a little sugar)
- Cottage cheese, plus berries

Lunches and dinners – a model low-GL meal

Here's a simple way to apply my low-GL principles to give you healthy, well-balanced and satisfying lunches and dinners. Protein should make up one-quarter of your meal; starchy carbohydrates (that is, rice, potatoes, pasta or bread) make up another quarter; and half your plate should contain fresh low-carbohydrate vegetables or salad. Here's what it looks like:

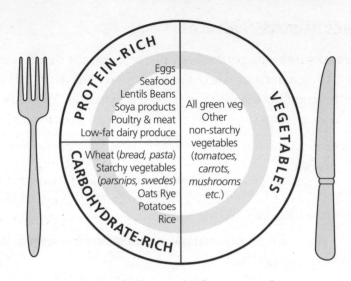

How to balance what's on your plate

Protein options

For optimal health, the message is to eat more vegetable protein and fish, and less red meat and dairy. Experiment with new foods such as tofu – which you can buy marinated and ready to toss into stir-fries or salads. The protein-rich grain quinoa is also easy to cook – just add double the quantity of water or vegetable stock and gently simmer for 15 minutes.

Lentils, chickpeas and beans (pulses) can be enjoyed in pâtés or dips (such as hummus) and can also be added to stews and pasta sauces for some high-fibre protein (Buy ready-to-eat in tins, or soak and cook your own from dried sources).

Fish is also easy to cook – steam, grill or bake with lemon and herbs. Tinned fish is also a cheap and easy way to add lean protein to a meal; for example, add some anchovies to a pasta sauce or mix wild salmon with cooked potatoes and onions to make a tasty fish cake (bind with an egg, add some seasoning and dust with flour or cornmeal before grilling).

Balancing carbohydrates

As you saw on the list of foods on pages 392–3, not all carbs are created equal. On the low-GL diet you will be eating slow-releasing carbohydrates – that is, those with the lowest GL scores. On pages 398–9 are some examples of starchy carbohydrates with a GL score of 7 (7GLs). The reason for 7GLs is that half a plate of vegetables or salad averages 3GLs, plus the starchy carbs, giving you 10GLs in total, which is the maximum you should eat in a meal if you want to lose weight. If you don't need to lose weight you can increase the starchy carb portion to a maximum of 10GLs, as shown, although many people find a 7GL portion suffices.

Starchy carb portions

Starchy carb	7GLs looks like	10GLs looks like
Pumpkin/squash	Large serving (185g/6½oz)	Double regular serving (265g/9¼oz)
Carrot	1 large (160g/5¾oz)	2 regular (265g/9¼oz)
Swede	Regular serving (150g/5½oz)	Large serving (215g/7½oz)
Quinoa	Regular serving (120g/4¼oz)	Large serving (185g/6½oz)
Baked beans	Large serving (150g/5½oz)	Double serving (215g/7½oz)
Lentils	Large serving (175g/6oz)	Double serving (300g/10½oz)
Kidney beans	Large serving (150g/5½oz)	Double serving (215g/7½oz)
Pearl barley	Small serving (95g/3¼oz)	Regular serving (135g/4¾oz)
Wholemeal pasta	Half serving (85g/3oz)	Large serving (110g/3¾oz)
White pasta	Third serving (65g/2¼oz)	Small serving (75g/2¾oz)
Brown rice	Small serving (70g/2½oz)	Regular serving (85g/3oz)
White rice	Third serving (45g/1½oz)	Half serving (65g/2¼oz)

chart continues →

Starchy carb	7GLs looks like	10GLs looks like
White rice	Third serving (45g/1½oz)	Half serving (65g/2¼oz)
Couscous	Third serving (45g/1½oz)	Half serving (65g/2¼oz)
Sweetcorn	Half a cob (60g/2⅛oz)	1 small cob (90g/3¼oz)
Boiled potato	2 small (75g/2¾oz)	3 small (100g/3½oz)
Baked potato	1 medium (60g/2⅛oz)	1 large (85g/3oz)
French fries	6–7 chips (45g/1½oz)	8–10 chips (70g/2½oz)
Sweet potato	Half (60g/2⅛oz)	1 small (90g/3¼oz)

Non-starchy vegetables

You can enjoy these vegetables in unlimited quantities as their starch (sugar) content is minimal. Aim to fill half your plate with foods from this list:

Alfalfa	Courgette	Peppers
Asparagus	Cucumber	Radish
Aubergine	Endive	Rocket
Beansprouts	Fennel	Runner beans
Beetroot (raw)	Garlic	Spinach
Broccoli	Kale	Spring onions
Brussels sprouts	Lettuce	Tenderstem
Cabbage	Mangetout	Tomatoes
Carrot (raw)	Mushrooms	Watercress
Cauliflower	Onions	
Celery	Peas	

You'll find that it soon becomes very easy to work out balanced meals with just the right amount of carbohydrates to stimulate weight loss or to maintain a steady weight by eating foods that will nourish you.

You can also incorporate alternate-day fasting, if you want to speed up your weight loss. On the fasting days you will eat a 7GL portion of starchy carbs and only one 5GL snack. On 'feast' days you can have up to a 10GL portion of carbs and two or three 5GL snacks.

SUMMARY

To balance your blood sugar, which will help you achieve stable energy and regulate your weight:

- Choose low-GL foods.

- Eat carbs with an equal amount of protein.

- Have half a plateful of vegetables (raw or cooked) for main meals.

- Avoid refined carbohydrates and sugary foods.

- Graze rather than gorge, with three main low-GL meals and two snacks. Or, if trying alternate-day fasting, have one snack on 'fast' days and two or three snacks on 'feast' days.

To find out more about the low-GL diet, read *The Low-GL Diet Bible* or *The Low-GL Diet Cookbook*, which will give you lots of recipes to choose from, all GL counted. *Food Glorious Food* gives you entertainment-level recipes and menu ideas for applying these principles. The *Ten Secrets of 100% Health Cookbook* combines low-GL recipes with those high in antioxidants, essential fats and B vitamins for all-round good health.

CHAPTER 2

Increase Your Intake of Antioxidants

What makes the body age? The process of ageing is largely determined by oxidation – the gradual damage to our cells produced by oxygen burning the fuel from our food. The fuel is glucose, and as it is burned with oxygen it creates 'exhaust fumes' through oxidation. Oxygen is our most vital nutrient, without which we die in minutes, and every cell depends on a steady supply of it. Yet, while the body uses oxygen to extract the energy from food, we make oxidants which cause damage to the body: our skin becomes less soft and flexible, and the membranes of all our cells become gradually less functional. The antidote to this process of ageing is to optimise your intake of nature's age defenders: antioxidants. These protect us from the DNA-damaging effects of oxidants.

Measuring food's antioxidant power

Some foods have higher levels of antioxidants than others, giving them more power to disarm damaging oxidants. These high-level antioxidant foods are naturally colourful, such as the yellow of turmeric, the blue of blueberries, the orange of carrots, the red of tomatoes and the dark green of vegetables such as broccoli. The different colours denote slightly different kinds of antioxidants, which in combination provide the most protection. Choosing a rainbow of colours when deciding on which foods to eat each day will give you a good range of these important antioxidants.

Although colour is a good indication of the antioxidant power of a food, however, there is a more precise way to measure it using a food's ORAC potential (meaning oxygen radical absorbency capacity). This is an objective measure of how good a food is at dealing with those oxidising exhaust fumes of life.

The oldest living communities consume at least 6,000 ORACs a day – the optimum amount for good health. Okinawa, Japan's most southerly island group, for example, is home to one of the longest-living communities in the world. In a population of 1.3 million, there are 900 centenarians – four times the proportion found in Britain or America. The Okinawans, in common with other peoples who enjoy a long life expectancy, include large amounts of antioxidant-rich fresh fruits and vegetables in their diets, and these prevent cell damage in the body.

According to Dr Richard Cutler, former director of the US Government Anti-ageing Research Department, 'the amount of antioxidants that you maintain in your body is directly proportional to how long you will live'.

6,000 ORACs a day keeps ageing at bay

The chart below shows the ORACs of 20 different foods that you can incorporate easily into your daily diet. Each serving contains approximately 2,000 units, so by choosing at least three of these daily you'll hit your anti-ageing target of 6,000.

- ⅓ tsp ground cinnamon
- ½ tsp dried oregano
- ½ tsp ground turmeric
- 1 heaped tsp made mustard
- 30g (1oz) blueberries
- ½ pear, grapefruit or plum

- 60g (2oz) blackcurrants, berries, raspberries or strawberries
- 75g (2¾oz) cherries or a shot of Cherry Active concentrate
- 1 orange or apple
- 4 pieces of dark chocolate (at least 70% cocoa solids)

- 7 walnut halves
- 8 pecan halves
- 30g (1oz) pistachio nuts
- 100g (3½oz) cooked lentils
- 150g (5½oz) cooked kidney beans
- ⅓ medium avocado
- 35g (1¼oz) red cabbage
- 200g (7oz) broccoli
- 1 medium artichoke or 8 asparagus spears
- ⅓ medium glass (150ml/5fl oz/¼ pint) red wine

Source: Oxygen Radical Absorbance Capacity of Selected Foods – 2007, US Department of Agriculture

Berries, cherries and plums rule

Fruits that have the highest levels of ORACs are those with the deepest colour, such as blueberries, raspberries and strawberries. These are particularly rich in powerful antioxidants called anthocyanidins. One cup, 115g (4oz), of blueberries will provide 9,697 units. You would need to eat 11 bananas to get the same benefit as a cupful of blueberries! Berries are rich in xylose, which keeps your blood sugar level even, whereas bananas contain a lot of glucose and, unless you are exercising a lot, will promote abdominal weight gain.

One of the simplest and easiest ways to achieve a guaranteed 6,000 ORACs a day is to have a daily shot of a Montmorency cherry concentrate, called Cherry Active, diluted with water. This measures 8,260 on the ORAC scale, which is the equivalent of around 23 portions of regular fruit and vegetables. Other juices, such as acai and pomegranate, also claim high ORAC scores, but this tops the lot. Other good options are Blueberry Active and Beet Active, which are both pure concentrates to which you add water. Blueberries are particularly good for immune support, whereas beetroot lowers blood pressure.

Seven of the best

The amount of fruit and vegetables you need per day in order to meet your ORAC quota really does depend on which ones you choose, as you can see in the menus for two days below. Both days have five portions selected, but Day 2's selection is 8,000 ORACs more than that for Day 1. If you aim for seven servings a day – that's three fruit servings over the day and two vegetable servings with each main meal – you'll easily achieve 6,000 ORACs.

Choose the 'best value' five-a-day

DAY 1		DAY 2	
Fruit/vegetable portion	ORAC	Fruit/vegetable portion	ORAC
⅛ large cantaloupe melon	315	½ pear	2,617
1 kiwi fruit	802	75g (2¾oz) strawberries	2,683
1 medium carrot, raw	406	½ avocado	2,899
55g (2oz) peas, frozen	432	100g (3½oz) broccoli, raw	1,226
30g (1oz) spinach, raw	455	4 asparagus spears, steamed	986
Total score	2,410	Total score	10,411

Reduce your oxidant exposure

The flip side of the antioxidant equation is to reduce your exposure to oxidants – that is, the 'burned' oxygen. Cigarette smoking is an example, but so too is deep-frying or putting cheese on top of a dish and baking or grilling it to go crispy, or grilling, roasting or barbecuing meats until they are brown and crispy. Caramelising, which is burning sugar, is also bad news. Ways of reducing oxidant exposure include poaching, steam-frying (cooking in a covered pan with a little oil or butter and some stock or water) and preparing dishes raw, or only heating them through to serve.

The kind of oil you cook with also makes a big difference. In the next chapter we'll discuss how to optimise your intake of essential fats, found principally in fish, nuts and seeds. Such essential fats are easily oxidised when heated, however, especially at high temperatures. So, when you sauté a food, it is much better to use a source of fat or oil that is saturated, which means it would be solid, or almost solid, at room temperature. Butter, for example, and coconut butter are saturated fats. Olive oil, containing the monounsaturated fat called oleic acid, is close to saturated. Heating these oils creates much fewer oxidants. When a heated fat reaches its 'smoking point' then you are really generating a lot of oxidants.

The best antioxidant supplements

As well as eating a high-ORAC diet, it is worth supplementing these nutrients to ensure your cells have an optimal supply every day. This is especially important if you are over 50 years old, or if you look old for your age, or if taking antioxidant supplements has been recommended in a Good Medicine solution relative to your health issue. I recommend supplementing a combination of all of the antioxidants shown below, rather than putting all your eggs in one basket by just taking in one or two, such as vitamins C and E. This is because they act as 'team players', disarming harmful oxidants, as shown below.

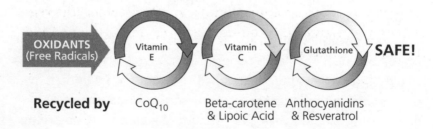

Antioxidants are team players

These are the key players, and an ideal daily intake to supplement on top of a healthy diet and a decent multivitamin, especially when recommended in Part 1 of this book:

Beta-carotene (pre-vitamin A)	7mg
Vitamin E (d-alpha tocopherol acetate)	100mg (126iu)
Vitamin C	1,000–1,500mg
Co-enzyme Q_{10} (CoQ_{10})	10mg (you'll need 90mg if you're on statins)
Alpha lipoic acid	10mg
Selenium	50mcg
L-glutathione (reduced form) or	
N-acetyl-cysteine (NAC)	50mg
Resveratrol	20mg

You can find all-round antioxidant supplements that contain most of these, except vitamin C (see Resources). The amount of vitamin C needed means supplementing this separately, as recommended in Part 1. Some vitamin C tablets also supply berry extracts, high in anthocyanidins, another key antioxidant. (The more purple the tablet, the more it contains.) Other key nutrients, such as B vitamins, zinc and magnesium, as well as extra vitamins A, C and E and selenium, should be provided in good, high-strength multivitamin–minerals. Make sure you supplement, on a daily basis, a total of vitamin A (3,000mcg) provided from both retinol (the animal form) and beta-carotene (the vegetable form), vitamin C (1,500–2,000mg), vitamin E (100mg) and selenium (30–100mcg).

SUMMARY

The key points for increasing your intake of anti-ageing antioxidants and decreasing your intake of oxidants are:

- Eat multicoloured foods every day, aiming to eat foods from each of the different colour groups, from yellow and orange to red, green and purple.

- Eat lots of herbs and spices.

- Aim for seven servings of fruit and vegetables per day.

- Choose daily menus that give you 6,000 ORACs.

- Keep frying to a minimum, choosing steam-frying, light stir-frying or poaching instead.

- Use butter, coconut butter, olive oil or rapeseed oil for cooking.

- Also consider supplementing an extra antioxidant formula, in addition to a high-potency multivitamin, if you are aged 50 or more, if you do a lot of exercise, or if you have any of the conditions listed in Part 1 for which extra antioxidants are recommended.

CHAPTER 3

Increase Your Intake of Essential Fats

There are certain fats that your body needs in plenty and these are called 'essential fats', because they are necessary for each cell to function properly. As you may know, your body is made largely of water, which is contained within cells that have a membrane made of essential fats. The membrane 'perceives' changes in the environment outside the cell and then reacts accordingly. In this way, fats are part of the way our cells 'perceive' and adapt. For many years, fat was believed to be something we must avoid eating for good health, but we now know that essential fats are vital for many processes in the body.

Essential fats are vital for . . .

- A good mood and motivation
- A sharp memory
- A strong immune system
- Hormonal balance
- Reducing the risk of heart disease, strokes, diabetes and cancer
- Keeping your skin velvety smooth and youthful
- Reducing pain and inflammation

Omega-3 and -6 fats

Although larger supplemental amounts are needed to reverse disease processes – for example, if you have heart disease, arthritis or clinical depression – we all need a daily supply of essential fats. As you can see in the diagram below there are two main families of essential fats that we need: omega-3 and omega-6.

Omega-6 fats are made and stored in the seeds and nuts of hot-climate plants, such as sunflower and sesame.

Omega-3 fats are found in colder-climate nut or seed oils, such as chia and flax, as well as walnuts. Pumpkin seeds contain a bit of both. Omega-3s are also richly present in cold-water plankton – the food of little fishes, and especially in oily fish.

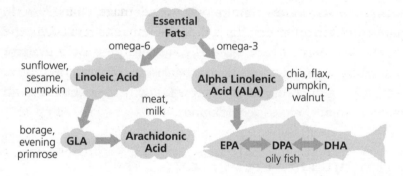

The two essential fat families

Essential fats store sunlight

Sunlight is stored in plankton, which is then passed up the food chain, eaten by little fish which are then eaten by carnivorous oily fish. In the case of seals, they eat the oily fish, and the oils are then stored in their fat and used as an energy source during the winter months – essential because they live in regions of the world that are devoid of sunlight throughout these months. The Inuit survived, and stayed healthy (until they started to eat a more Western diet), in spite of the lack of sunlight, due to their high intake of nutrients in the seal meat they ate. Humans are, in effect, solar-powered. The plants we eat also store the sun's energy in carbohydrate, the body's primary fuel. Both vitamin D and essential fats are dependent on sunlight.

The decline in our oily fish consumption, largely because of a phobia of eating fat, has fuelled an epidemic in deficiencies of both omega-3 and vitamin D. This is doubly bad if you live far away from the equator – for example in the UK – with little strong sunlight and not much desire to expose yourself to the sun's rays during the cold months of winter.

Getting the omega balance right

The further down the essential-fat chain you go, the more 'poly-unsaturated' the fat becomes, which makes it more biologically active, but also more prone to oxidative damage, which is what happens when an oil goes rancid. Alpha linolenic acid (ALA), the vegetarian source of omega-3, is more prone to such damage than linoleic acid (omega-6). In the interests of making foods with a long shelf life, most processed foods have the essential fats removed. Coupled with our fat phobia, we've ended up with a diet that is extremely deficient in omega-3s.

To be healthy you need to focus on getting a source of omega-3 every day.

The best fish

Although it may not be environmentally friendly, with declining levels of fish in the sea and an increasing population, the optimal intake of oily/carnivorous fish we should aim for is three to five servings a week. The National Institute for Clinical Excellence (NICE), which guides NHS policy, recommends all heart-attack patients eat two to four portions of oily fish (herring, sardines, mackerel, salmon, tuna and trout) a week.

In the Holford 100% Health Survey (over 100,000 people have completed the 100% Health Check questionnaire), it was found that a person's chances of being in optimal health goes up by a third for those consuming three or more servings of oily fish a week, compared to two a week. A portion is defined as 140g (5oz), which is a small can of fish or a small fillet of fresh fish, from which one should derive at least 7g of omega-3 essential fats over a week.

If you look at the chart below, you will see that the level of omega-3s is a fraction in canned tuna compared to fresh. This is probably because the oil may be squeezed out, and may be sold to the supplement industry, leaving a drier meat that is disguised by then adding an inferior oil. In the US you can buy tuna in its own oil. It tastes completely different and much better, so don't rely on canned tuna to provide your omega-3 quota, always try to use fresh fish. Another problem with oily fish is the potential for mercury contamination, particularly in very large fish such as tuna. This is particularly relevant for pregnant women, because mercury is a neurotoxin and can induce birth defects. I would recommend tuna once a fortnight during pregnancy and once a week or a fortnight otherwise. The same advice applies to marlin or swordfish. The best all-rounders are probably wild salmon and mackerel. The level of omega-3s in farmed salmon depends on what the fish are fed.

The omega-3 and mercury content of fish

Fish	Omega-3 g/100g	Mercury mg/kg	Omega-3/ mercury ratio
Canned tuna	0.37	0.19	1.95
Trout	1.15	0.06	19.17
Herring	1.31	0.04	32.75
Fresh tuna	1.50	0.40	3.75
Canned/smoked salmon	1.54	0.04	38.50
Canned sardines	1.57	0.04	39.25
Fresh mackerel	1.93	0.05	38.60
Fresh salmon	2.70	0.05	54.00

Source: FSA 2004

Supplements and vegetarian sources

Oily fish has health benefits unrelated to its omega-3 levels, being very high in protein, vitamin E, selenium and choline, from which we make tri-methyl-glycine (TMG), a vital homocysteine-lowering nutrient (as explained on page 420). As well as eating three portions a week I also suggest supplementing, especially on those days that you don't eat fish.

The best vegetarian sources of omega-3 are chia seeds and flax seeds, followed by hemp seeds, pumpkin seeds and walnuts. Regarding pumpkin seeds, the colder the climate they grow in, the more omega-3s they will contain. You also get a small amount of omega-3s in meat, especially if the animals are grass fed and in a colder climate, dairy products, eggs from chickens fed on flax seeds, and cold-climate vegetables, such as kale, cabbage, broccoli, cauliflower and Brussels sprouts. Although this kind of omega-3 (ALA) is not as potent as the kind found in oily fish (EPA, DPA and DHA), a small amount of it will be converted into these more potent forms.

It is best to also take a combined omega-3 and -6 supplement providing the omega-3 fats eicosapentaenoic acid (EPA), docosapentaenoic acid (DPA) and docosahexaenoic acid (DHA) as well as the most potent form of omega-6 fat gamma-linolenic acid (GLA), which is derived from evening primrose oil or borage oil.

The fish-derived omega-3 fats, especially EPA, are the most potent anti-inflammatories, and so for some diseases I recommend that you take high-potency EPA-rich omega-3 fish oil capsules to achieve at least 500mg, if not 1,000mg, of EPA per day.

I like to eat a vegetarian source of omega-3s most days, as well, my favourite being chia seeds. These taste delicious and are high in protein, essential fats and antioxidants, and are also a rich source of soluble fibres. Chia seeds were once a staple food in Central America, but the invading Spanish conquistadores, over 500 years ago, disliked the locals worshipping the seeds and so banned their cultivation. Only now are chia seeds making a comeback. They are available in health-food stores and online (see Resources) and look like dark sesame seeds. They are small in size, and are therefore best ground or soaked to maximise the absorption of their nutrients. Next best for omega-3 are flax seeds.

Most people are deficient in active omega-6 fats (which are different from most of the omega-6 we get in our foods today, which is damaged and oxidised) but they are more deficient in omega-3. As for the 'basic' supplements recommended for everyone, it is better to have a supplement that provides both types of omega fats. I have, however, tried to limit the total number of supplements recommended in Part 1, so if a condition needs primarily omega-3 fats I will sometimes have recommended taking just these and not the combined omegas.

Vital vitamin D

There is another essential fat that many of us are deficient in, especially during the winter: vitamin D. Although you may know that it is essential for keeping your bones strong, this fat-based hormone does so much more. It may prove to be one of the most important cancer preventers, as well as being vital for a healthy nervous system – and hence brain function – and a good all-round immune-booster. Low levels of vitamin D in the winter months may be one of the reasons why we become more susceptible to colds.

The importance of vitamin D, beyond its role in bone health, was noticed when researchers investigated possible reasons why the prevalence of a number of diseases, including many forms of cancer, MS and schizophrenia, increased in relation to the distance people live from the equator.

The minimum level of vitamin D we need for optimal health is around 30mcg a day, although some experts say this is too low. If you expose yourself to moderate sunlight for 30 minutes a day and eat eggs and oily fish, you might achieve 15mcg. From November to February, however, it is unlikely you'll get enough high-intensity sun exposure to make even this if you live in more northerly areas. Hence, it is wise to supplement 15mcg, especially if you live in the UK or another country that is an equivalent distance from the equator, or even further away. You'll find this quantity in a good, high-strength multivitamin–mineral.

The best dietary sources for vitamin D by a long way are oily fish, followed by eggs. I make a point of eating at least three servings of oily fish a week, plus at least six eggs – which, by the way, won't increase your risk of heart disease or raise your blood cholesterol level.

SUMMARY

Use the following list to ensure that you are eating sufficient of the essential omega fats:

- Aim to have at least three servings of unfried oily fish (salmon, mackerel, herring including kippers, sardines) a week, and four or more servings of other fish a week.

- Eat some omega-3-rich raw seeds or nuts every day – a tablespoon of chia or flax seeds, or a small handful of walnuts or pumpkin seeds. If you are a strict vegetarian or vegan you'll need double this amount.

- Have at least six free-range or organic eggs a week, preferably from chickens fed with omega-3s (such as flax seeds).

- Expose yourself to at least 30 minutes of sunlight every day, when possible.

- Supplement essential omegas providing omega-3 (EPA, DPA, DHA) and omega-6 (GLA) oils.

- Supplement a high-potency multivitamin that provides at least 15mcg of vitamin D, and possibly an extra vitamin D supplement to achieve two or three times this amount during winter months.

CHAPTER 4

Improve Methylation and Lower Your Homocysteine

Homocysteine is a naturally occurring amino acid found in the blood, high levels of which are toxic. If your level is too high, this means that your body is not efficient at a process called 'methylation', which is critical for keeping the body's and brain's biochemistry in balance. The net result of high homocysteine is worsening health – including declining memory, energy and bone density, as well as arterial damage, increasing your risk of a heart attack or stroke. Your homocysteine level is therefore one of the best indicators of your overall health.

Keeping homocysteine low depends on having a host of 'methyl' nutrients available for your body to use. Therefore, if your homocysteine score is high, it is an indicator that you are not getting enough of the necessary vitamins for your body to work optimally. In this situation there are some very specific diet and lifestyle changes, plus particular nutrients (which include the B vitamins), that will help to keep your homocysteine score ideal. The first step is to know what your homocysteine score is.

How to measure your homocysteine level

It's unlikely that your doctor will arrange for a homocysteine test for you, unless you have a specific homocysteine-related disease, such as age-related memory loss, cardiovascular disease or osteoporosis, and you also have a switched-on doctor, but you can easily do one at home using a test kit that only involves taking a pin-prick sample of blood (see Resources). Homocysteine is measured in micromoles per litre, written as mmol/l. It used to be thought that a 'high' level was above 15 units (mmol/l). This is what increases your risk of a heart attack and doubles your Alzheimer's risk. Now, however, levels as low as 7 units are being linked to increased disease risk. Basically, there's no official safe level and no guarantee that your diet and the supplements you are currently taking are keeping homocysteine at bay.

Up to 30 per cent of people with a history of heart disease have a homocysteine level above 14 units. A level above 9.5 units is associated with accelerated brain shrinkage. The average level in Britain is 10.5; however, experts believe that a level below 6 units is ideal. If you have any of the associated risk factors listed in the checklist below, it's especially important to get tested. Since homocysteine does go up with age, if you are pursuing optimal health and aiming to minimise your risk of developing any disease, including Alzheimer's, my rule of thumb is to keep your homocysteine score below your age, divided by ten. If you are 80, keep your level below 8. Below 6 or 7 is ideal for most people younger than 80, however.

Signs and symptoms – check yourself out

If you have five or more of the following symptoms, it's almost a certainty that your homocysteine level is moderate to very high (9–15, if not higher):

1 Are you tired a lot of the time?

2 Is your stamina, or ability to keep going, noticeably decreasing?

3 Are you having a hard time keeping your weight stable?

4 Do you often experience physical pain, be it arthritis, muscle aches or migraines?

5   Do you get frequent colds?

6   Is your eyesight deteriorating?

7   Is your mental clarity or concentration decreasing?

8   Are you experiencing more sleeping problems?

9   Is your memory on the decline?

10   Are you often depressed?

11   Do you average two or more alcoholic beverages daily?

12   Do you drink more than three cups of coffee daily?

13   Do you smoke cigarettes?

14   Are you a strict vegetarian?

15   Do you eat red meat at least once a day?

16   Have any members of your first-degree family (mother, father, brothers or sisters) suffered from any of the following:

- Heart disease, especially before 50 years of age
- Stroke
- Alzheimer's disease
- Abnormal blood clots
- Osteoporosis
- Cancer
- Severe depression (especially in women)
- Elevated homocysteine levels

How to reduce a high level of homocysteine

The current vogue in medicine is to recommend taking folic acid to lower homocysteine. Described in the *British Medical Journal* as 'the leading contender for panacea of the 21st century', folic acid alone is, however, far less effective than the correct nutrients in combination. The amount you need also depends on your current homocysteine level. One study found that homocysteine scores were reduced by 17 per cent on high-dose folic acid alone, 19 per cent on vitamin B_{12} alone, 57 per cent on folic acid plus B_{12}, and 60 per cent on folic acid, B_{12} and B_6[1] All this was achieved in just three weeks!

Even better results would have been achieved by including tri-methyl-glycine (TMG). In one New Zealand study, the homocysteine scores of patients with chronic kidney failure and very high homocysteine levels were reduced by a further 18 per cent when 4g of TMG was given along with 50mg of vitamin B_6 and 5,000mcg of folate, compared to patients taking just B_6 and folate. At the Brain Bio Centre my associates and I achieve, on average, reductions in high homocysteine scores of greater than 50 per cent in 8–12 weeks with the combination of these nutrients, plus diet!

Some companies produce combinations of the above nutrients. These are the most cost-effective supplements for restoring a healthy homocysteine level. The inclusion of N-acetyl-cysteine (NAC) is particularly helpful for older people when memory protection is the aim. This is because this vital antioxidant helps the methylation B vitamins to protect brain function.

Nutrients and levels to supplement, depending on your homocysteine score

Nutrient	No risk Below 7	Low risk 7–9	High risk 10–15	Very high risk above 15
Folate	200mcg	400mcg	800mcg	800mcg
B_{12}	10mcg	250mcg	500mcg	750mcg
B_2	5 mcg	10mg	15mg	25mcg
B_6	10 mcg	20mg	25mg	50mg
Zinc	5mg	10mg	15mg	20mg
TMG	–	500mg	750mg	1500g
NAC	–	250mg	500mg	750mg

Follow my H-factor diet

A few years ago, I devised the H-factor diet: eight easy dietary changes that will help to lower your homocysteine level. Here they are:

1 Eat less fatty meat, but more fish and vegetable protein

Eat no more than four servings of lean meat a week; fish (not fried) at least three times a week; and if you're not allergic or intolerant, a serving of a soya-based food, such as tofu, tempeh or soya sausages, plus beans, such as kidney beans, chickpea hummus or baked beans, at least five times a week.

2 Eat your greens

Have at least five servings of fruit or vegetables a day. This means eating at least two pieces of fruit every single day, and three servings of vegetables. Vary your selections from day to day. Make sure half of what's on your plate for each main meal is vegetables.

3 Eat a garlic clove a day

Either eat a garlic clove a day or take a garlic supplement every day. You can take garlic-oil capsules or powdered garlic supplements.

4 Cut back on coffee

Don't drink more than one cup of caffeinated or decaffeinated coffee in a day. Instead, choose from the wide variety of herbal teas and grain coffees available. Drinking two cups of tea or three cups of green tea has not been shown to raise homocysteine.

5 Limit your alcohol

Limit your alcohol intake to no more than 300ml (10fl oz/½ pint) of beer, or one small glass (125ml/4fl oz) of red wine, in a day. Ideally, limit your intake to 1.2 litres (2 pints) of beer or four small glasses (500ml/18fl oz) of wine a week.

6 Reduce your stress

If you are under a lot of stress, or if you find yourself reacting stressfully much of the time, make a decision to reduce your stress load (read Chapter 6).

7 Stop smoking

If you smoke, make a decision to stop, and seek help to do it. There is simply no safe level of smoking as far as homocysteine and your health are concerned. Smoking is nothing less than slow suicide. The sooner you stop, the longer you'll live. Refer to page 280 for guidance on how to do it.

8 Supplement a high-strength multivitamin–mineral every day

Excellent-quality multis are available in every health-food store and online (see Resources). To keep your homocysteine levels in check, you'll need one that gives at least 20mg of vitamin B_6, 200mcg of folic acid and 10mcg of B_{12}.

This diet, lifestyle and supplement plan has the potential to halve your homocysteine score in weeks. If your score is very high, you may need to supplement additional nutrients, as outlined in the table on page 420. The goal is to bring your score to below 6.

Your homocysteine score is probably the best objective measure of whether you are achieving optimum nutrition.

The H-factor diet works seamlessly with my low-GL diet, explained in Chapter 1.

SUMMARY

A low homocysteine score is essential for overall good health. Reducing high levels is easily done with dietary changes and supplementing:

- Test your homocysteine level.

- If it's above 6, supplement the levels of homocysteine-lowering nutrients given in the table on page 420.

- Also, take a high-strength multivitamin–mineral giving at least 20mg of B_6, 200mcg of folic acid and 10mcg of B_{12}, even if your homocysteine score isn't above 6.

- Follow the H-factor diet plan as shown above.

- Re-test yourself every three months until your homocysteine is below 6. Then test yourself once a year (see Resources).

Dig deeper by reading *The Homocysteine Solution* (Patrick Holford and Dr James Braly). *Ten Secrets of 100% Healthy People* (Patrick Holford) also has a whole chapter on homocysteine and methylation.

CHAPTER 5

Personalise Your Supplement Programme

The biggest breakthrough in medicine in the last 100 years was the discovery that large amounts of, and combinations of, naturally occurring nutrients can help restore biochemical balance and reverse disease processes. This approach was first called 'orthomolecular medicine', but I have simplified this to 'optimum nutrition' and it is also often presented as 'functional medicine'. It involves treating diseases by understanding the true underlying causes, then creating an appropriate diet, lifestyle and supplement programme to restore health.

The greatest myth in nutrition is that 'you can get all the nutrients you need from a well-balanced diet'. This fundamental lie is even written into law; for example, no advertisement can claim otherwise. Yet it is wrong. There are many nutrients and many situations in which no amount of food can give you optimal amounts, or even very basic amounts, of nutrients essential to life.

One example is vitamin D. As we have seen in Chapter 3, the further north you live, the greater your risk of heart disease, many cancers, osteoporosis, respiratory infections, multiple sclerosis and other quite common diseases. Why? Because we just don't get enough sun exposure, which makes vitamin D in the skin, and all the above diseases are linked to low levels of vitamin D. You'd have to be eating at least a serving of oily fish a day to get close to the optimum levels of vitamin D.

Another example is vitamin B_{12}. Over half of all people aged over 65 have insufficient vitamin B_{12} in their blood. This lack of B_{12} is linked to brain shrinkage – leading to Alzheimer's disease – as well as bone shrinkage, depression and an increased risk of stroke. This deficiency is due to poor absorption, and therefore no amount of meat, fish, eggs or milk in the diet will provide enough B_{12} for these people.

When you are sick, you need more of specific nutrients; for example, when you have a cold, you need about 1,000mg of vitamin C an hour to get well; when you are well, by comparison, you'll benefit from 1,000mg twice a day. That is consistent with our evolution, during which we obtained high levels of nutrients from the food we ate, but it is unachievable with today's food (1,000mg of vitamin C, for example, equals 20 oranges).

For each disease in Part 1 I've calculated the ideal supplement programme based on 30 years of clinical experience. If you were to consult a nutritional therapist (see Resources) they would work out something similar based on your personal needs and circumstances. These supplements are in addition to the basic supplements that I recommend everyone takes – as I do – every day.

In case you are new to health supplements, here are the basic building blocks of a good nutritional supplement programme, based on my research at the Institute for Optimum Nutrition to establish optimum daily allowances.

Theoretically, at one extreme you could take a mega-mega-multivitamin–mineral that contains everything you could possibly need. The trouble with this is that it would be enormous, impossible to swallow and no doubt give you a lot more than you need of some nutrients. The other extreme is to take one supplement for each nutrient, exactly matching your requirements – but you'd end up with handfuls of pills.

Nutritional therapists use formulas – combinations of vitamins and minerals – that, when combined appropriately, more or less suit your needs. In a typical health-supplement programme you may have four supplements to take. These formulas are like building blocks.

The essential building blocks are shown in the supplement jigsaw below.

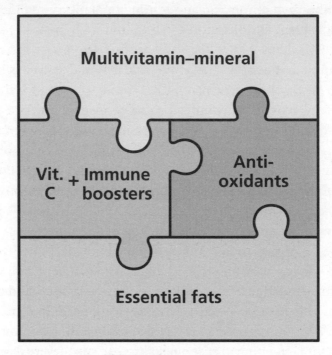

The supplement jigsaw

1 Start with a high-potency multivitamin–mineral

The starting point of any supplement programme is a high-potency multivitamin–mineral. This should provide the following nutrients:

Multivitamins A good multivitamin should contain at least 2,000mcg (6,000iu) of vitamin A*, 10mcg (400iu) of D, 100iu of E, 250mg of C, roughly 25mg each of B_1, B_2, B_3, B_5 and B_6, 10mcg of B_{12}, 200mcg of folic acid and 50mcg of biotin.

* This includes beta-carotene, which converts into vitamin A.

Multiminerals This should provide at least 300mg of calcium, 150mg of magnesium, 10mg of iron, 10mg of zinc, 2.5mg of manganese, 20mcg of chromium and 25mcg of selenium, and ideally some molybdenum, vanadium and boron.

You simply can't fit all of the above vitamins and minerals into one tablet, so good, combined multivitamin–mineral formulas recommend two or more tablets a day to meet these kinds of levels. The bulkiest nutrients are vitamin C, calcium and magnesium. These are often insufficiently supplied in multivitamin–mineral formulas. Vitamin C, in particular, is best taken separately simply because you'll never get 1,000mg into a multi.

2 Add extra vitamin C and other immune-support nutrients

Vitamin C should be supplemented to provide around 1,800mg per day. This means taking a 900–1,000mg vitamin C tablet twice a day. Since vitamin C is water-soluble, and in and out of the body in a few hours, it is much better to take it twice a day than all in one go. Some vitamin C formulas also provide other key immune-boosting nutrients such as bioflavonoids or anthocyanidins in the form of black elderberry, bilberry and zinc. This is especially useful if you are taking large amounts for immune support.

3 Add extra antioxidant nutrients

The evidence is now very persuasive that an optimal intake of antioxidant nutrients slows down the ageing process and prevents a variety of diseases. For this reason it is well worth supplementing extra antioxidant nutrients – on top of those in a good multivitamin – to ensure you are achieving the best possible ageing protection, as discussed in Chapter 2. This is especially important the older you get. The kind of nutrients that are provided in an antioxidant supplement are vitamins

A, C, E and beta-carotene, zinc and selenium, possibly iron, copper and manganese, co-enzyme Q_{10} (CoQ_{10}), the amino acids glutathione and N-acetyl-cysteine (NAC), plus optional phytonutrients such as resveratrol, pycnogenol and grape-seed extract. These plant chemicals, rich in bioflavonoids and anthocyanidins, are also often supplied in more comprehensive vitamin C formulas.

4 Add essential omegas

There are two ways of meeting your essential fat requirements: one is from diet, either by eating a heaped tablespoon of ground seeds such as chia seeds every day, taking a tablespoon of special cold-pressed seed oils and/or eating oily fish (such as salmon, mackerel, sardines, trout, herring or anchovies) at least three times a week; the other is to supplement concentrated oils. For omega-3 this means either flaxseed oil capsules or the much more concentrated and biologically active fish oil capsules providing EPA and DHA. For omega-6 this means supplementing a source of GLA such as evening primrose oil or borage oil. Even better is a combination of all three – giving you EPA, DHA and GLA in one capsule. There is a third potent omega-3 fat called DPA which can convert into either DHA, important for brain building, or EPA, a potent anti-inflammatory. Some fish oil supplements provide EPA, DPA and DHA.

I recommend hedging your bets and eating oily fish three times a week and raw seeds or nuts most days, and supplementing the essential omegas.

Even though these are not all recommended for every health issue in Part 1, I recommend them as the basic building blocks of a good supplement programme, and I take them every day. Then, there are optional extras – to be taken until your health issue resolves – to support the systems of your body that are out of balance.

SUMMARY

Always take a high-potency multivitamin–mineral, extra vitamin C and essential fats (both omega-3 and -6), ideally twice a day. Take supplements every day – there is no logic in 'taking a break'. During the winter, if you live far in the north or south, you may wish to add extra vitamin D. The older you are, the more antioxidants you need, so taking an antioxidant complex is an optional extra. Also, the older you are, the more B_6, B_{12}, folic acid and phospholipids (phosphatidylcholine and serine) you need, so taking a 'brain food formula' is another optional extra.

CHAPTER 6

Reduce Your Stress Level

Most people today have jobs or other aspects of their lives that are stressful, or they feel that they need to work exceptionally hard for fear of losing their employment and endangering the security of their family. The way we deal with the stress in our lives makes the difference between coping and feeling well and floundering under the weight of it and making ourselves ill.

It's important to avoid piling on the stressful situations, but we also need to know how to cope with the unavoidable ones. Freedom from stress comes from knowing you are on track in life. Being positively engaged, and successful, in activities that you believe in makes all the difference. Inevitably, things happen that don't fit in, and it is easy to react stressfully. Some people get aggressive, others become depressed, and others hit the booze or binge on chocolate.

Whatever your reaction, it's possible to reverse negative patterns and manage stress without necessarily changing what's stressing you by following a few simple measures.

Test your stress

Here are some of the classic signs of stress. How many relate to you?

1 Do you have difficulty relaxing?

2 Do you find yourself feeling irritable?

3 Do you worry about little events of the day and are unable to shut your mind off?

4 Do you smoke or drink excessively (especially by others' standards)?

5 Are you competitive and aggressive in the things you do?

6 Do you find it hard to relate to people?

7 Do you find you are impatient with others?

8 Do you eat quickly?

9 Do you take on too much?

10 Do you have difficulty delegating?

11 Do you have aching limbs or recurrent headaches?

12 Do you have digestive problems?

13 Do you have allergies and sinus problems?

14 Do you have a dry mouth and sweaty palms?

15 Do you have a lack of interest in sex?

16 Are your muscles tense?

17 Do you have problems sleeping?

Score:
Below 5: you're in fine shape, able to take life in your stride.

5–10: you are quite stressed, so pay attention to these warning signs. This is the only body you have – treat it well.

More than 10: you are very stressed. It's time to make some positive changes before your stress has serious consequences.

As well as eating a healthy diet to help combat stress, there are a number of strategies that you can use to help lower the toll that stress can have on your health.

Recognise when stress is building up

Stress is often the result of having unfinished business: too many incomplete demands and obligations. Make a list of all the issues that are bothering you, including relationship issues, that you would like to resolve. Particularly stressful are situations where you have a lot of responsibility, but no control; for example, if you have a sick relative in a home, but no control over their care, or you have responsibilities at work, but your boss won't let you make what you feel is the right move. A debt or a mortgage, or a fear of losing your job, is in the same category – you have something to fulfil but you can't easily see the means of fulfilling it.

Other stresses on your life can result from feeling that you are betraying yourself – not living your life in alignment with who you really are. This could arise from feeling stuck in the wrong career or relationship that doesn't fully use your inborn talents or allow you to do what is fulfilling. It is good to be aware of your own needs and work towards designing your life in a way that works for you. Some people have life coaches to help them get there.

At the point where you are stressed or you finally snap, no amount of logical thought is likely to deal with the stress of that moment, but there are some simple techniques that do work.

Transform stress into resilience

A large part of stress is self-induced by perceiving a change of circumstances in a negative way. When we do this we resist the opportunities that life presents us with, rather than embracing them.

One of the leading organisations exploring how stress affects us, and how to turn off stress reactions, is the HeartMath Institute in California. Using a device called an EmWave (more on this on page 434) they monitor a person's heart-rate variability, which is a direct measure of a stressful state, to find out what kind of activities and exercises enable us to get into a 'coherent' state, where you are not overly stressed but are able to fully participate in life, and you are present and open to new experiences. This state – 'coherence' – fits very well with the psychological attributes of those people who live the longest. The word is well chosen, because you can actually measure very coherent or integrated brain-wave patterns, heart-rate patterns and other biological rhythms, and they become in tune, rather like a well-conducted orchestra.

The researchers found that activities, feelings or exercises that were more heart-centred were the most effective at turning off the harmful stress hormones.

The HeartMath Institute runs workshops around the world to help people learn how to transform stressful reactions into resilience (see Resources). You can also consult a practitioner on a one-to-one basis (see Resources). Here are three simple 'quick coherence' techniques from HeartMath that you can learn and then apply whenever you are feeling stressed:

Exercise: heart focus, breathing and feeling

1 Heart focus
   Focus your attention on your heart area   the space behind your breastbone in the centre of your chest between your nipples (your heart is more in the centre than on the left).

2 Heart breathing
   Now imagine your breath flowing in and out of your heart area. This helps your respiration and heart rhythm to synchronise. Focus on this area and aim to breathe evenly; for example, inhale for five or six seconds and exhale for five or six seconds (choose a timescale that feels comfortable and flows easily).

   Take a few minutes to get the hang of the heart focus and heart breathing stages, then introduce step three.

→

3 Heart feeling
As you breathe in and out of your heart area, recall a
positive emotion and try to re-experience it. This could
be remembering a time spent with someone you love,
walking in your favourite spot, stroking a pet, picturing
a tree or scenic location you admire or even just feeling
appreciation that you ate today or have shoes on your
feet. If your mind wanders, just bring it gently back to the
positive experience.

These three steps, when practised daily for five minutes, can
help you to de-stress, feel calmer and more content. Your heart
rhythms will become coherent and your heart–brain communication will optimise to help you think more clearly. For your daily
HeartMath practice, it's a good idea to find a regular time when
you can sit down quietly and undisturbed (such as first thing in
the morning, during your lunch break or when you get home
from work). This way it's more likely to become a habit and you
can give the exercise your full attention.

Once you've got the hang of HeartMath, you can then use
it any time you encounter a stressful event; for example, if you
start to feel tense in heavy traffic, or you become overloaded at
work, or sense you are about to face a difficult emotional situation. Just a few HeartMath breaths can help you to stay calm
and coherent instead of becoming stressed. And you can do it
with your eyes open, as you walk or talk – so you have a tool to
control stress at the direct point you encounter a situation likely
to trigger a negative reaction.

Monitor your state with an EmWave

The HeartMath exercises sound very simple, or basic, but they
can have a deep effect, especially if you use a device called
an EmWave Personal Stress Reliever (PSR), which gives you

instant feedback to enable you to learn how to go into a state of coherence.

The EmWave PSR has an ear clip that attaches to your ear lobe to pick up what is known as your heart-rate variability (HRV), through the pulse in your ear lobes, and then feeds this data through to a hand-held device that tells you how coherent you are. The device easily fits into your pocket.

There are three zones – 'red' or incoherent (the state most of us are in), 'blue' for more coherent, and 'green' for fully coherent. There is a also a 'breath pacer' to help you regulate your breathing, and different levels and modes so that you can adapt your practice as you get the hang of it.

Using the EmWave PSR gives you an objective measure of what works, and even the very act of knowing, through this 'biofeedback', can help you calm down. You can also plug it into the USB port of your computer and track your state. In this way you can try out different techniques for changing your state. One woman found that stroking her cat immediately brought her into a state of coherence. If you own a cat, this might be a useful way of bringing yourself back into a positive state. If not, try one of the exercises above.

Get into the stress-free zone

We are all different, and the trick is to find what really gets you into the zone where you leave your stresses behind. It might be through exercising, listening to music, gardening and growing your own vegetables, walking the dog, being in beautiful natural environments, learning pottery, painting, playing a musical instrument, practising yoga and t'ai chi, helping others or studying a particular subject. (The EmWave can also help with this because it can find out what really does it for you. I recommend it as an anti-ageing device. It is also excellent to use as you go to sleep, as it trains you to let go of your stresses.)

Practise meditation

Another way to find a more coherent, less stressful state is through meditation. In meditation, you become aware of your thoughts, emotions and physical sensations and, in the process, become detached. The purpose in meditation is to become aware of everything that occurs – be it a thought, a feeling, a sound or a physical sensation – anything that happens in the space of your awareness. In the same way that the space in a room is not affected by different people coming and going, in meditation the purpose is to rest in that 'space' or awareness, and let each thought, or perception, arise and subside without attachment.

There are many ways to approach meditation, and detach from thoughts, feelings, perceptions and sensations. In some meditative techniques you focus on the breath, in some the heart, and in others on the vital-energy centre of the body, known as the *tan tien* in t'ai chi and also called the Kath™ point by the philosopher Oscar Ichazo. (Ichazo has thoroughly researched methods of generating vital energy, known as 'chi', and of attaining higher states of consciousness.) Some people also repeat a word or a mantra silently. In any event it is good to get instruction (see Resources).

Diakath Breathing™

An example of a technique to induce a more coherent and meditative state is Oscar Ichazo's Diakath Breathing, based on focusing on one part of the body, known as the Kath point. Although not an anatomical point as such, the Kath point is the body's centre of gravity, and by placing one's awareness at this point, rather than in the head as we most often do, it is possible to become aware of the whole body. All the martial arts, in their pure form, are practised with this awareness, which gives a more complete and grounded experience of oneself. You can experience this for yourself by practising the simple breathing exercise shown on page 437.

Exercise: Diakath Breathing

This breathing exercise (reproduced with the kind permission of Oscar Ichazo) connects the Kath point – the body's centre of equilibrium – with the diaphragm muscle, so that deep breathing becomes natural and effortless. You can practise this exercise at any time, while sitting, standing or lying down, and for as long as you like. You can also practise it unobtrusively during moments of stress. It is an excellent, natural relaxant and energy booster, helping you to feel more connected and in tune.

The diaphragm is a dome-shaped muscle attached to the bottom of the rib cage. The Kath point is located three finger-widths below the belly and 2.5cm (1in) in. If you place your index finger in your belly button your little finger will be in the Kath point. When you put your awareness in this point, it becomes easy to be aware of your entire body.

Ideally, find somewhere quiet first thing in the morning. When breathing, inhale and exhale through your nose. As you inhale, you will expand your lower belly from the Kath point and your diaphragm muscle. This allows the lungs to fill with air from the bottom to the top. As you exhale, the belly and the diaphragm muscle relax, allowing the lungs to empty from top to bottom.

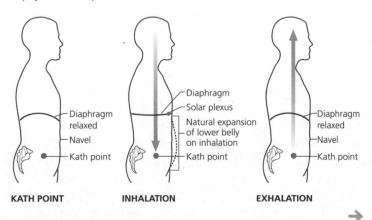

Diaphragm
relaxed
Navel
Kath point

KATH POINT

Diaphragm
Solar plexus
Natural expansion
of lower belly
on inhalation
Kath point

INHALATION

Diaphragm
relaxed
Navel
Kath point

EXHALATION

→

1 Sit comfortably, in a quiet place with your spine straight.
2 Focus your attention on your Kath point.
3 Let your belly expand from the Kath point as you inhale slowly, deeply and effortlessly. Feel your diaphragm being pulled down towards the Kath point as your lungs fill with air from the bottom to the top. On the exhale, relax both your belly and your diaphragm, emptying your lungs from top to bottom.
4 Repeat at your own pace.
- Every morning, sit down in a quiet place before breakfast and practise Diakath Breathing for a few minutes.
- Whenever you are stressed throughout the day check your breathing. Practise Diakath Breathing for nine breaths. This is great to do before an important meeting or when something has upset you.

Diakath Breathing is part of a series of exercises and techniques, developed by Oscar Ichazo, that help to generate vital Kath energy. There is a one-day training session called 'Kath State – The Energy of Inner Fire™' which teaches these exercises, and a complete exercise system that takes about 15 minutes to do, called Psycho-calisthenics®. It can be learned either in a training session or from a DVD. To find out more about these excellent de-stressing and energising exercises, see Resources under Psychocalisthenics®.

(© 1972, 2002, 2013 Oscar Ichazo. Psychocalisthenics is a registered trademark; and Diakath Breathing, the Diakath Breathing illustration, Kath, and Kath State – The Energy of Inner Fire are trademarks of Oscar Ichazo. Used by permission.)

The purpose of such practices is to centre yourself, become more energised and aware, giving you perspective on stressful and fearful thoughts. There are, of course, many different ways of doing this, as discussed above. Finding what works for you is essential to put the stresses of life into perspective.

Exercise beats stress

As well as keeping your body in shape, building regular exercise into your life will help you to keep control of stress. Although there are lots of ways to exercise alone, joining a group or class can add a social aspect to your exercise. Here are a few to try:

Pilates usually involves tuition in a small group. It helps develop 'core' strength.

Yoga is excellent for stretching and maintaining suppleness. Some forms of yoga, such as hatha, include meditation and visualisation. It is best to join a class rather than trying at home from a book or DVD.

Aerobics and dance fitness These classes are taught in gyms and on DVDs, and are obviously designed to keep you fit, with stamina and a degree of strength, depending on the muscles being used.

Jogging and walking The trick with jogging and walking is to build up your speed and distance to achieve a good level of fitness. Hill walking is especially good for enhancing cardiovascular health.

Toning exercises are specific exercises designed to tighten, for example, bum, tum and thigh muscles and also improve your muscle mass and strength. The more muscle mass you have, the more fat you will burn.

Swimming is an excellent all-round exercise, developing strength, stamina and suppleness.

Cycling is good for improving cardiovascular health, although make sure you don't spend too long on busy roads breathing in exhaust fumes (oxidants).

I used to have ...

Robert, aged 66, took up t'ai chi when he retired. Here's how he describes the benefits:

'I've never been an athletic person or good at anything physical. T'ai chi, however, I enjoy immensely. I like the feeling of being "in control" of my body. It gives me an aesthetic pleasure. I do it almost every day for 20 minutes. It increases my energy and clears my mind. It gives me a kind of equilibrium that has many benefits, such as helping me to play my violin better and helping me to stay detached when things are bad. I find it very calming when I'm stressed or feeling fraught.'

Take positive action on your current stresses

Although these exercises and techniques can all help to reduce stress, it is important to recognise that sometimes you need to do something about the circumstances in your life that are causing it.

Make a list of the people and situations that cause you to react stressfully. Are there some that you can change by changing your circumstances, or by changing your attitude towards them, or by taking a positive action? Often we hold people or circumstances in a negative mind-frame, blaming them for our discomfort. Can you think of a more positive interpretation of something that you consider stressful? If you are in an 'impasse' where no obvious solution presents itself, be aware that nothing stays the same for ever, and perhaps hold the circumstance in your mind during meditation and see if an alternative solution arises. The prayer of St Francis is quite apt in these circumstances: 'Lord, give me the courage to change the things I can, the patience to accept the things I cannot change, and the wisdom to know the difference.'

SUMMARY

Become aware of when you are stressed. Find a practice that helps you to de-stress; for example, meditation, Diakath Breathing, the HeartMath techniques, yoga, t'ai chi or Psychocalisthenics, or go out and take some exercise that will get you puffed out and warm. Practise these regularly, ideally daily. Identify what is causing you stress and do something about it if you can.

References

Part 1

Acne

1. E. Spencer, et al., *International Journal of Dermatology*, Apr. 2009;48(4):339–47

ADHD

1. A. Richardson and B. Puri, 'A randomized double-blind, placebo-controlled study of the effects of supplementation with highly unsaturated fatty acids on ADHD-related symptoms in children with specific learning difficulties', *Progress in Neuro-psychopharmacology & Biological Psychiatry*, 2002;26(2):233–9
2. N.I. Ward, 'Assessment of clinical factors in relation to child hyperactivity', *Journal of Nutritional & Environmental Medicine*, 1997;7:333–42

Alcohol Dependence/Cravings

1. V. Coiro, et al., 'Alcoholism abolishes the growth hormone response to sumatriptan administration in man', Center for Alcohology, University of Parma, Italy, Metabolism Clinical and Experimental, 1995; A. Heinz, et al., 'Blunted growth hormone response is associated with early relapse in alcohol-dependent patients', *Alcoholism, Clinical and Experimental Research*, 1995;19(1):62–5

Allergies

1. Y.B. Shaik, et al., 'Role of quercetin (a natural herbal compound) in allergy and inflammation', *Journal of Biological Regulators & Homeostatic Agents*, Jul.–Dec. 2006;20(3–4):47–52

Angina

1. R.N. Iyer, A.A. Khan, et al., 'L-carnitine moderately improves the exercise tolerance in chronic stable angina', *Journal of the Association of Physicians of India*, Nov. 2000;48(11):1050–2
2. A. Mager, et al., 'Impact of homocysteine-lowering vitamin therapy on long-term outcome of patients with coronary artery disease', *American Journal of Cardiology*, 2009;104:745–9

Colds and Flu

1. H.C. Gorton, and K. Jarvis, 'The effectiveness of vitamin C in preventing and relieving the symptoms of virus-induced respiratory infections', *Journal of Manipulative and Physiological Therapeutics*, Oct. 1999;22(8):530–3

2. D. Hulisz, 'Efficacy of zinc against common cold viruses: An overview', *Journal of the American Pharmaceutical Association*, Sep.–Oct. 2004;44(5):594–603

3. Z. Zakay-Rones, et al., 'Randomized study of the efficacy and safety of oral elderberry extract in the treatment of influenza A and B virus infections', *Journal of International Medical Research*, Mar.–Apr. 2004;32(2):132–40

4 A. Ginde, et al., 'Association between serum 25-hydroxyvitamin D level and upper respiratory tract infection in the Third National Health and Nutrition Examination Survey', *Archives of Internal Medicine*, 23 Feb. 2009;169(4):384–90

Eating Disorders

1. C.L. Birmingham and S. Gritzner, 'How does zinc supplementation benefit anorexia nervosa?', *Eating and Weight Disorders*, Dec. 2006;11(4):e109–11

Eczema

1. G. Hardman and G. Hart, 'Dietary advice based on food-specific IgG results', *Nutrition & Food Science*, 2007;37(1):16–23

2. A. Soutar, 'Bronchial reactivity and dietary antioxidants', *Thorax*, 1997;52:166–70

3. I. Kunitsugu, et al., 'Self-reported seafood intake and atopy in Japanese school-aged children.' *Pediatrics International*, Apr. 2012;54(2):233–7

4. D.J. Palmer, et al., 'Effect of n-3 long chain polyunsaturated fatty acid supplementation in pregnancy on infants' allergies in first year of life: Randomised controlled trial', *British Medical Journal*, 30 Jan. 2012;344:e184

5. E. Grandjean, et al., 'Efficacy of oral long-term N-acetylcysteine in chronic bronchopulmonary disease: A meta-analysis of published double-blind placebo-controlled clinical trials, *Clinical Therapeutics*, 2000:22(2):209–21

6. E. Middleton and G. Drzewiecki, 'Flavonoid inhibition of human basophil histamine release stimulated by various agents', *Biochemical Pharmacology*, 1984;33(21):3333–8

7. B.B. Aggarwal and S. Shishodia, 'Suppression of the nuclear factor-kappaB activation pathway by spice-derived phytochemicals: Reasoning for seasoning', *Annals of the New York Academy of Sciences*, 2004;1030:434–41, Review

Eyesight Deterioration

1. M. Larkin, 'Vitamins reduce risk of vision loss from macular degeneration', *Lancet*, 2001;358(9290):1347; 'National Eye Institute of America, Age-Related Eye Disease Study (AREDS)', *Archives of Ophthalmology*, 2001;119:1417–36

2. K.M. Cornish, et al., 'Quercetin metabolism in the lens: Role in inhibition of hydrogen peroxide', *Free Radical Biology and Medicine*, 2002;33(1):63–70

3. A. Jacadzadeh, et al., 'Preventive effect of onion juice on selenite-induced experimental cataract', *Indian Journal of Ophthalmology*, 2009;57(3):185–9

4. J. M. Seddon, et al., 'Dietary fat and risk of advanced age-related macular degeneration', *Archives of Ophthalmology*, 2001;119:1191–9

Fibromyalgia

1. K.G. Henriksson and A. Bengtsson, 'Fibromyalgia: A clinical entity?' *Canadian Journal of Physiology and Pharmacology*, 1991;69(5):672–7

2. A. Bengtsson and K.G. Henriksson, 'The muscle in fibromyalgia: A review of Swedish studies', *Journal of Rheumatology*, 1989;19(suppl.):144–9

3. W.B. Weglicki, et al., 'Immunoregulation by neuropeptides in magnesium deficiency: Ex vivo effect of enhanced substance P production on circulating T lymphocytes from magnesium-deficient mice', *Magnesium Research*, 1996;9(1):3–11

4. M.S. Seelig, 'Consequences of magnesium deficiency on the enhancement of stress reactions: Preventive and therapeutic implications (a review)', *Journal of the American College of Nutrition*, 1994;13(5):429–46

5. G.E. Abraham and J. Flechas, 'Management of fibromyalgia: Rationale for the use of magnesium and malic acid', *Journal of Nutritional Medicine*, 1992;3:49–59; V. Bobyleva-Guarriero and H.A. Lardy, 'The role of malate in exercise-induced enhancement of mitochondrial respiration', *Archives of Biochemistry and Biophysics*, 1986;245(2):470–6

6. J. Eisinger, et al., 'Glycolysis abnormalities in fibromyalgia', *Journal of the American College of Nutrition*, 1994;13(2):144–8

7. M. Nicolodi and F. Sicuteri, 'Fibromyalgia and migraine. Two faces of the same mechanism: Serotonin as the common clue for pathogenesis and therapy', *Advances in Experimental Medicine and Biology*, 1996;398:373–9; P. Sarzi Puttini and I. Caruso, 'Primary fibromyalgia syndrome and 5-hydroxytryptophan: A 90-day open study', *Journal of International Medical Research*, 1992;20(2):182–9; K. Lawson, 'Tricyclic antidepressants and fibromyalgia: What is the mechanism of action?', *Expert Opinion on Investigational Drugs*, 2002;11(10):1437–45; I. Caruso, et al., 'Double-blind study of 5-hydroxytryptophan versus placebo in the treatment of primary fibromyalgia syndrome', *Journal of International Medical Research*, 1990;18(3):201–9

8. M. Nicolodi and F. Sicuteri, 'Eosinophilia myalgia syndrome: The role of contaminants, the role of serotonergic set up', *Advances in Experimental Biology and Medicine*, 1996;398:351–7

9. B. Regland, et al., 'Increased concentrations of homocysteine in the cerebrospinal fluid in patients with fibromyalgia and chronic fatigue syndrome', *Scandinavian Journal of Rheumatology*, 1997;26(4):301–7

Gastroenteritis (Stomach Bugs)

1. P. Kyme, et al., 'C/EBPε mediates nicotinamide-enhanced clearance of *Staphylococcus aureus* in mice', *Journal of Clinical Investigation*, 4 Sep. 2012;122(9):3316–29 [http://www.ncbi.nlm.nih.gov/pubmed/22922257]

Gout

1. H.K. Choi, S. Liu and G. Curhan, 'Intake of purine-rich foods, protein, and dairy products and relationship to serum levels of uric acid: The

Third National Health and Nutrition Examination Survey', *Arthritis & Rheumatism*, 2005;52(1): 283–9

2. http://www.acumedico.com/purine.htm
3. http://www.acumedico.com/purine.htm
4. R.A. Jacob, et al., 'Consumption of cherries lowers plasma urate in healthy women', *Journal of Nutrition*, 2003;133(6):1826–9
5. H.K. Choi, et al., 'Alcohol intake and risk of incident gout in men: A prospective study', *Lancet*, 2004;363(9417):1277–81

High Blood Pressure

1. B. Altura and B. Altura, 'Magnesium in cardiovascular biology', *Scientific American*, May/June 1995:28–36
2. D. Almoznino-Sarafian, S. Berman, et al., 'Magnesium and C-reactive protein in heart failure: An anti-inflammatory effect of magnesium administration?', *European Journal of Nutrition*, Jun. 2007;46(4):230–7
3. L. Hooper, et al., 'Advice to reduce dietary salt for prevention of cardiovascular disease', Cochrane Database of Systematic Reviews, CD003656 (2004)
4. http://news.bbc.co.uk/1/hi/health/6570933.stm
5. S.P. Juraschek, 'Effects of vitamin C supplementation on blood pressure: A meta-analysis of randomized controlled trials', *American Journal of Clinical Nutrition*, May 2012;95(5):1079–88
6. D.A. Hobbs, et al., 'Blood pressure-lowering effects of beetroot juice and novel beetroot-enriched bread products in normotensive male subjects', *British Journal of Nutrition*, 14 Dec. 2012;108(11):2066–74
7. A.J. Webb, et al., 'Acute blood pressure lowering, vasoprotective, and antiplatelet properties of dietary nitrate via bioconversion to nitrite', *Hypertension*, Mar. 2008;51(3):784–90
8. R. McCraty, et al., 'The impact of a new emotional self-management program on stress, emotions, heart-rate variability, dhea and cortisol, integrative', *Physiological and Behavioural Science*, 1998;33(2):151–70
9. R. McCraty, et al., 'Impact of workplace stress reduction program on blood pressure and emotional health in hypertensive employees', *Journal of Alternative and Complementary Medicine*, 2003;9(3):355–69
10. R.H. Schneider, et al., 'Stress reduction in the secondary prevention of cardiovascular disease', *Archives of Internal Medicine*, 2011. doi: 10.1001/archinternmed.2011.310

High Cholesterol

1. A. Lewis, et al., 'Treatment of hypertriglyceridemia with omega-3 fatty acids: A systemic review', *Journal of the American Academy of Nurse Practitioners*, Sep. 2004;16(9):384–5
2. M.D. Ashen and R.S. Blumenthal, 'Low HDL cholesterol levels', *New England Journal of Medicine*, Sep. 2005;353:1252–60
3. I. Singh, et al., 'High-density lipoprotein as a therapeutic target: A systematic review', *Journal of the American Medical Association*, Aug. 2007;298:7

4. G. Yang, et al., 'Longitudinal study of soy food intake and blood pressure among middle-aged and elderly Chinese women', *American Journal of Clinical Nutrition*, 2005;81(5):1012–1017

Infections
1. P. Kyme, et al., 'C/EBPε mediates nicotinamide-enhanced clearance of *Staphylococcus aureus* in mice', *Journal of Clinical Investigation*, 4 Sep. 2012;122(9):3316–29 [http://www.ncbi.nlm.nih.gov/pubmed/22922257]

Infertility
1. T. Jensen, et al., 'Does moderate alcohol consumption affect fertility? Follow-up study among couples planning first pregnancy', *British Medical Journal*, 1998;317:505–10
2. A. Wilcox et al., 'Caffeinated beverages and decreased fertility', *Lancet*, 1988; 2(8626–27):1453–5
3. D. Hamilton-Fairley, et al., 'Association of moderate obesity with a poor pregnancy outcome in women with polycystic ovary syndrome treated with low dose gonadotrophin', *British Journal of Obstetric Gynaecology*, 1992;99:128–31
4. B.V. Sastry and V.E. Janson, 'Depression of human sperm motility by inhibition of enzymatic methylation', *Biochemical Pharmacology*, 1983;32:1423–32

Irritable Bowel Syndrome (IBS)
1. S.A. Gaylord, et al., 'Mindfulness training reduces the severity of irritable bowel syndrome in women: Results of a randomized controlled trial', *American Journal of Gastroenterology*, Sep. 2011,106(9):1678–88

Osteoporosis
1. J. Prior, 'Progesterone as bone-trophic hormone', *Endocrine Reviews*, 1990;11(2):386–98

Prostate Cancer
1. http://www.nejm.org/doi/full/10.1056/NEJMoa0810696
2. http://www.ncbi.nlm.nih.gov/pubmed/19297566
3. J.L. Stanford, et al., 'Prostate cancer trends 1973–1995', SEER Program, National Cancer Institute, NIH Pub. No. 99–4543. Bethesda, MD, 1999

Prostate Enlargement and Hyperplasia
1. P. Terry, et al., 'Fatty fish consumption and risk of prostate cancer', *Lancet*, 2001;357(9270):1764–6
2. F. Meyer, et al., 'Antioxidant vitamin and mineral supplementation and prostate cancer prevention in the SU.VI.MAX trial', *International Journal of Cancer*, 2005;116(2):182–6

3. W. H. Goldmann, et al., 'Saw palmetto berry extract inhibits cell growth and Cox-2 expression in prostatic cancer cells', *Cell Biology International*, 2001;25(11):1117–24

4. T.L. Wadsworth, et al., 'Saw palmetto extract suppresses insulin-like growth factor-I signaling and induces stress-activated protein kinase/c-Jun N-terminal kinase phosphorylation in human prostate epithelial cells', *Endocrinology*, 2004;145(7):3205–14

5. F. Yablonsky, et al., 'Antiproliferative effect of *Pygeum africanum* extract on rat prostatic fibroblasts', *Journal of Urology*, 1997;157(6):2381–7

Sinus Problems

1. H. Sharp, et al., 'Treatment of acute and chronic rhinosinusitis in the United States, 1999–2002', *Archives of Otolaryngology – Head and Neck Surgery*, 2007;133:260–5

2. T.M. Nsouli, et al., 'Role of food allergy in serous otitis media', *Annals of Allergy*, 1994;73:215–19

3. A. Yerushalmi, S. Karman and A. Lwoff , 'Treatment of perennial allergic rhinitis by local hyperthermia', *Proceedings of the National Academy of Sciences*, 1982;79:4766–9

Stomach Ulcers and *Helicobacter pylori* Infection

1. K.Y. Wang, et al., 'Effects of ingesting Lactobacillus- and Bifidobacterium-containing yogurt in subjects with colonised *Helicobacter pylori*', *American Journal of Clinical Nutrition*, Sept. 2004;80(3):737–41

2. S. Parascho, et al., 'In vitro and in vivo activities of chios mastic gum extracts and constituents against *Helicobacter pylori*', *Antimicrobial Agents and Chemotherapy*, 2007;51(2):551–9

3. J. Xing, et al., 'Effects of sea buckthorn (*Hippophaë rhamnoides L.*) seed and pulp oils on experimental models of gastric ulcer in rats', *Fitoterapia*, Dec. 2002;73(7–8):644–50

Stroke

1. A. Cherubini, et al., 'Antioxidant profile and early outcome in stroke patients', *Stroke*, 2000;31:2295

2. Y. Wang, et al., 'Dietary supplementation with blueberries, spinach, or spirulina reduces ischemic brain damage', *Experimental Neurology*, May 2005; 193(1):75–84

Part 2

Chapter 4: Improve Methylation and Lower Your Homocysteine

1. K. Koyama, et al., 'Efficacy of methylcobalamin on lowering total homocysteine plasma concentrations in haemodialysis patients receiving high-dose folic acid supplementation', *Nephrology, Dialysis, Transplantation*, 2002;17(5):916–22

Resources

Sources of information and advice

Beat
(Beating Eating Disorders) Beat provides a helpline, online support and a network of UK-wide self-help groups to help adults and young people beat their eating disorders. Visit www.b-eat.co.uk

The Brain Bio Centre
The outpatient clinic of the charitable Food for the Brain Foundation in London (see below), the Brain Bio Centre specialises in the nutritional treatment of mental health issues, ranging from depression to insomnia, Parkinson's disease and ADHD. Support is available for people both in the UK and all over the world via Skype. Visit www.brainbiocentre.com or tel.: 020 8332 9600.

Buteyko method
For more information on this method visit www.buteykobreathing.org

***Candida* checklist**
To find out whether you are likely to have *Candida* you can complete an online checklist at www.patrickholford.com/candida

The Food for the Brain Foundation
This is a non-profit educational charity directed by Patrick Holford, which aims to promote awareness of the link between learning, behaviour, mental health and nutrition. The website has a free online Cognitive Function Test that takes 15 minutes to complete. It also has a free online hyperactivity/ADHD check to help you decide whether your child is hyperactive. For more information visit www.foodforthebrain.org

HeartMath

You can attend a 'Transforming Stress' half-day workshop. See the events section of www.patrickholford.com. Also, the EmWave Personal Stress Reliever is available from this website. For further details visit www.heartmath.com

Herbal remedies/medical herbalists

For more detailed advice about herbal remedies, find a medical herbalist in your area – visit the National Institute of Medical Herbalists for details at www.nimh.org.uk

Intravenous vitamin C

For details of doctors in the UK providing this therapy visit www.patrickholford.com/IVtherapy

Multiple Sclerosis Resource Centre

To find out more about MS, visit the charity's website at www.msrc.co.uk

Natural progesterone

For more information contact the Natural Progesterone Information Service at www.npis.info

Nutritional therapy and consultations

To find a recommended nutritional therapist near you, visit the advice section at www.patrickholford.com. This service gives details on who to see in the UK as well as internationally. If there is no one available nearby, you can always take an online assessment – see below.

Online 100% Health Programme

Are you 100% healthy? Find out with our health check and comprehensive 100% Health Programme, giving you a personalised action plan, including diet and supplements. Visit www.patrickholford.com

Pernicious Anaemia Society
For more information on the condition and a checklist of
symptoms visit www.pernicious-anaemia-society.org

Psychocalisthenics®
This is an excellent exercise system that takes less than 20 minutes
a day, and develops strength, suppleness and stamina, as well
as generating vital energy. The best way to learn it is to do the
Psychocalisthenics® training. For further information see www.
pcals.com, which lists training sessions and trainers in your area.
You can also teach yourself from the Psychocalisthenics® DVD,
available from www.patrickholford.com (shop). There is also a CD
with music and instructions to follow once you have learned the
exercises, and a book which explains each exercise. In the UK you
can also attend a one-day 'Kath State – The Energy of Inner Fire
Training™' that gives you exercises for awakening, generating and
revitalising oneself with the Kath energy (chi). See www.pcals.com
and select 'Training Information', then 'Integral View'.
(© 1972, 2013 Oscar Ichazo. Psychocalisthenics is a registered
trademark; and Kath and Kath State – The Energy of Inner Fire are
trademarks of Oscar Ichazo. Used by permission.)

Salvestrols
To find a practitioner near you who is knowledgeable in the use of
salvestrols or to obtain both maintenance and higher therapeutic
dosage levels of salvestrols, visit www.1880life.com or
tel.: 0845 0896470.

Testosterone deficiency
There is a good online test for factors that predict testosterone
deficiency at www.centreformenshealth.co.uk

Weight gain and obesity
There are a number of online support services to help keep you on
track, motivated and informed. Visit
www.patrickholford.com/weightloss. Also see Zest4Life (below).

Yoga

To find hatha yoga class (which usually includes meditation), visit the British Wheel of Yoga at www.bwy.org.uk. Or for an Iyengar yoga class (which uses props to help with the postures), visit the Iyengar Yoga Association at www.iyengaryoga.org.uk

Zest4Life

A health and nutrition club, based on low-GL principles, Zest4Life provides advice, coaching and support for losing weight and gaining health. For more information, visit www.zest4life.eu

Products

Cherry Active

This is sold in a highly concentrated juice form. Mix a 30ml serving with 250ml water to make a deliciously healthy, low-GL cherry juice. Each 946ml bottle contains the juice from over 3,000 cherries – that's half a tree's worth – and equates to a month's supply. Cherry Active is also available as a dried cherry snack and in capsules. Other flavours – Beet Active and Blueberry Active – are also now available. For more information and to order, visit www.totallynourish.com

Environ

Developed by the cosmetic surgeon Dr Des Fernandes, Environ products help prevent skin cancer and address the damaging effects of the environment on our skin. Formulated with scientifically proven active ingredients, including vitamin A and the antioxidant vitamins C and E and beta-carotene, which are used in progressively higher concentrations, Environ will help maintain a normal healthy skin, especially where there are signs of ageing, pigmentation, problem skin and scarring. Some Environ products are available from www.totallynourish.com or direct from an Environ skincare therapist. See www.iiaa.eu or tel.: 020 8450 2020 to find one near you in the UK and Ireland. In South Africa tel.: 0800 220 402. For international enquiries tel.: +27 11 2685711 or email tollfree@environ.co.za or visit www.environ.co.za

Eye health

A micro-current stimulator (MCS) can help provide protection against age-related macular degeneration. Electrical stimulation, which encourages cellular regeneration, is applied to acupressure points around the eyes using the MCS. Visit www.dovehealth.com.

Pinhole glasses can help with most focusing problems, even if you already use spectacles or lenses. Visit www.trayner.co.uk

Glucomannan

Glucomannan fibre is found in Patrick Holford's Carboslow – available in powder or capsule form. For further information and to order online visit www.totallynourish.com. In North America PGX, based on glucomannan, is widely available. See www.pgx.com

Probiotics/digestive enzymes/gut repair

Probiotics are supplements of beneficial bacteria, the two main strains being *Lactobacillus acidophilus* and *Bifidobacterium bifidus*. There are various strains within these two – some more important in children, others in adults. There is quite some variability in amounts of bacteria (some labels say, for example, 'a billion viable organisms per capsule') and quality. For a good-quality product try Patrick Holford's Digestpro, which also contains digestive enzymes and glutamine – available from www.totallynourish.com. BioCare (see details below) also has a range of probiotic supplements, including Bio-Acidophilus.

Silence of Peace **CD**

Based on centuries-old use of specific musical scales and arrangements, the music of John Levine helps you enter a more relaxed and peaceful state of mind – excellent as an aid to a good night's sleep. To find out more and purchase, visit www.patrickholford.com (shop)

Tests

Celiac test
A home test kit, the BioCard Celiac Test, is available from www.totallynourish.com

Food intolerance test
YorkTest Laboratories sells FoodScan, a convenient finger-prick mail-order service. This is the only food intolerance test endorsed by Allergy UK. The First Step FoodScan will generate a positive or negative result. If positive, your sample is then upgraded to the Second Step FoodScan 113 Test, which identifies the actual foods causing the intolerance and the level of intolerance. In addition, the service includes nutritionist consultations and comprehensive support and advice. To order, call YorkTest Laboratories on 0800 130 0580 or visit www.yorktest.com

Homocysteine, food and inhalant allergy tests
YorkTest also sells home testing kits for homocysteine, food and inhalant allergies (AllergyCheck). To order, call YorkTest Laboratories on 0800 130 0580 or visit www.yorktest.com

Hormone tests
Based on saliva, hormone tests are available from Genova Diagnostics, ranging from a 12-sample test over a monthly cycle (Rhythm test) to single hormone tests and thyroid function tests. Visit www.gdx.net/uk/. A nutritional therapist can both arrange and interpret the results of these tests.

Vitamin D
This can be tested for £20 via www.vitamindtest.org.uk and is available through your doctor.

Supplement suppliers

The following companies produce good-quality supplements that are widely available in the UK.

BioCare
Offering an extensive range of nutritional and herbal supplements, as well as probiotics, BioCare's products are stocked by most good health-food stores. They are also available by mail order from Totally Nourish (www.totallynourish.com) – see below.

Higher Nature
Available in most independent health-food stores or visit www.highernature.co.uk; tel.: 0800 458 4747 (freephone within the UK).

Patrick Holford
This range of daily 'packs' includes the convenient Optimum Nutrition Pack and the 100% Health Pack, containing a strip of the basic supplements – high-potency multivitamin–mineral, vitamin C and essential fats. The range includes many combination formulas such as Allex, Digestpro, Glucosamine Support, Bone Support, Mood Food, Brain Food, Chill Food, Awake Food (with tyrosine for thyroid support) and Connect, containing homocysteine-related nutrients. They are stocked by most good health-food stores. They are also available by mail order from Totally Nourish (www.totallynourish.com) – see below. See www.patrickholford.com/supplementsandtests for suppliers.

Solgar
Available in most independent health-food stores or visit www.solgar-vitamins.co.uk; tel.: 01442 890355.

Totally Nourish
This is an e-health shop that stocks many high-quality health products, including home test kits and supplements. Visit www.totallynourish.com; tel.: 0800 085 7749 (freephone within the UK).

Viridian
For stockists visit www.viridian-nutrition.com; tel.: 01327 878050.

And in other regions

South Africa
The original Patrick Holford vitamin and supplement brand from the UK is now available in South Africa through leading health-food stores, Dis-Chem and Clicks retail pharmacies. They are also available online from www.holforddirect.co.za; tel.: 011 2654 554 and are delivered by post or courier direct to your door.

Australia
Solgar supplements are available in Australia. Visit www.solgar.com.au; tel.: 1800 029 871 (free call within Australia) for your nearest supplier. Another good brand is Blackmores.

New Zealand
BioCare and Patrick Holford products are available in New Zealand through Pacific Health, PO Box 56248, Dominion Road, Auckland 1446. Visit www.pachealth.co.nz; tel.: 9815 0707.

Singapore
BioCare, Patrick Holford and Solgar products are available in Singapore through Essential Living.
Visit www.essliv.com; tel.: 6276 1380.

UAE
BioCare and Patrick Holford supplements are available in Dubai and the UAE from Organic Foods & Café, PO Box 117629, Dubai, United Arab Emirates. Visit www.organicfoodsandcafe.com; tel.: +971 44340577.

Kenya
Patrick Holford supplements are available in all Healthy U stores. Visit www.healthy-U2000.com

Index